George III's Illnesses
and His Doctors

George III's Illnesses and His Doctors

A Study in Early Psychiatry

Michael Ramscar

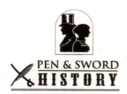

PEN & SWORD
HISTORY

First published in Great Britain in 2023 by
Pen & Sword History
An imprint of
Pen & Sword Books Ltd
Yorkshire – Philadelphia

Copyright © Michael Ramscar 2023

ISBN 978 1 39906 027 1

Typeset by Mac Style
Printed in the UK by CPI Group (UK) Ltd, Croydon, CR0 4YY.

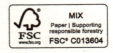

Pen & Sword Books Limited incorporates the imprints of Atlas,
Archaeology, Aviation, Discovery, Family History, Fiction, History,
Maritime, Military, Military Classics, Politics, Select, Transport,
True Crime, Air World, Frontline Publishing, Leo Cooper, Remember
When, Seaforth Publishing, The Praetorian Press, Wharncliffe
Local History, Wharncliffe Transport, Wharncliffe True Crime
and White Owl.

For a complete list of Pen & Sword titles please contact

PEN & SWORD BOOKS LIMITED
47 Church Street, Barnsley, South Yorkshire, S70 2AS, England
E-mail: enquiries@pen-and-sword.co.uk
Website: www.pen-and-sword.co.uk

Or

PEN AND SWORD BOOKS
1950 Lawrence Rd, Havertown, PA 19083, USA
E-mail: Uspen-and-sword@casematepublishers.com
Website: www.penandswordbooks.com

For Jan

Contents

Introduction

'Something disgraceful, nay, almost amounting to criminality, becomes attached to the person, and even to the family of an unhappy lunatic.'[1] Sir Alexander Halliday. *A General View of the Present State of Lunatics and Lunatic Asylums in GB and Ireland.* London 1827.

King George III has been defined by his insanity and comes to us as a caricature courtesy of Rowlandson, Gillray and others. He is the 'mad' king who lost Britain's American colonies and as 'tyrant' is integral to the founding myth of the United States. We forget his less than tyrannical comment from 1788 however, '(Lord North) poor fellow, has lost his sight, and I have lost my mind. Yet we meant well by the Americans; just to punish them with a few bloody noses, and then make bows for the mutual happiness of the two countries.'[2] We also forget that this 'mad' king would walk beside the Thames discussing the latest scientific developments with Sir Joseph Banks the President of the Royal Society. The latter may have had to become more involved with the breeding of merino sheep than he might have wished, but King George's genuine interest in improvements in agriculture and many other scientific subjects is not in doubt.[3]

This book is not intended as an analysis of the political implications – real and imagined – of George III's insanity. Nor is it intended as an analysis of the subsequent attempts to arrive at a clear historical diagnosis of the king's illness; although this will be covered in an Afterword. Its aim is to examine how the diagnosis and treatment of this most famous, and almost certainly best documented, case of 'insanity' in history had such a profound impact on popular and professional perceptions of insanity and on how it should be managed. For George III was too visible and too important simply to be confined and hidden in some private asylum, workhouse or even prison as so often happened to his less exalted contemporaries. Constitutionally the king was required to fulfil his role and the government and the royal family were expected to do all they could to ensure that happened. The problem could not be ignored and the way it was dealt with would be all too public.

In 1789 Dr Francis Willis had declared, following George III's recovery from his first crisis, that insanity was a disease and that like any other disease it could be treated and patients cured. Willis even claimed an impressive rate of 'cure' for the patients at his asylum in Lincolnshire. With the king recovered, apparently as a direct response to the ministrations of Willis and his team of orderlies, his assertions seemed to carry the weight of authority.

It was a long way from the seventeenth and earlier eighteenth century explanations of insanity as the reflection of demonic possession or an indication of divine punishment; from moral judgements of the sufferers rather than an assessment of pathology. Yet as Sir Alexander Halliday, an eminent specialist in the treatment of the insane, considered more than a generation after George III's first mental crisis in 1788 in the quotation at the opening of this introduction, the popular view was one which still involved moral rather than purely medical perceptions of the disease.

Even for those who saw insanity as an illness it had been generally assumed to be incurable. The fact that the king, in 1788/9 had been diagnosed as insane, treated and had apparently recovered changed understanding of the illness fundamentally. It was no longer a hopeless case and expectations were raised about the treatment of the insane. George Mann Burrows, probably the preeminent 'mad-doctor' of the late 1810s and 1820s set out in the clearest terms just how important George III's illness had been in changing perceptions. 'This one case exemplified like no other that anyone and everyone was vulnerable to mental illness irrespective of their rank in society or their moral status.'[4] His case had brought insanity into the open. Burrows argued that George III's illness was a case of good coming out of evil. 'The attention of the learned was directed to a malady but little understood.'[5] Burrows identified a heightened awareness of the problem after George's first crisis in 1788–9 and a marked increase in the number of patients recorded with a diagnosis of insanity. The fact that it was the king who had suffered insanity had contributed to a greater willingness to acknowledge that lesser mortals suffered too.

Burrows' perspective of assumed progress in the treatment of the insane was not, however, a perception universally or uncritically accepted at the time. Francis Willis' claim in 1789 that insanity could be treated and cured had raised expectations which were not fulfilled during the succeeding quarter century. The method of treatment which he had used did not prove to be generally successful, despite becoming the standard approach and one which was used on George III when he suffered brief relapses in 1801 and 1804. Indeed many people, including some members of the medical profession, questioned whether it was directly effective in curing insanity at all. Others, including members of the royal family, came to see the intimidation and fear used to condition patients into recovery and the reliance on physical restraint to manage manic episodes as morally unacceptable as well as ineffective. Restraint and intimidation seemed to conflate therapy with punishment.

In 1789 there was simply relief at the king's recovery. The methods by which it had been achieved were not questioned. By 1810, when George had his final relapse, attitudes had changed and there was great reluctance in his family and amongst officials to allow the king to undergo the systematic treatment of the specialist 'mad-doctors'. Indeed the king's case and the way he was treated added to the low standing in which practitioners of the nascent speciality which became psychiatry were held in the early nineteenth century.

George III's final crisis and illness came at a time of transition in attitudes towards the inheritance of the ancient Greeks or the nostrums of medieval medicine. While the king was purged, bled and cupped during the early stages of illness in 1810 and 1811, it was done with less conviction than twenty years before. Empirical evidence was gradually seen to be of value; even if it did contradict the wisdom of Galen. It was a time of experimentation and insanity was the subject of new treatments intended to manage or even cure this elusive illness. Insanity came to be seen as not simply a single illness but a series of distinct complaints, although a range of behaviours were still included in the diagnosis of 'insanity' which had no business to be there.

The fallibility of much medical practice in the early nineteenth century did not reflect incompetence on the part of the practitioners. Much of the 'cruelty' imposed on the king reflected the fundamental difficulties of dealing with patients; particularly in a manic state. The limited options then available meant that the onset of mania made physical restraint of the patient an almost inevitable consequence. Certainly this is what happened to George. Water based treatments and electric shock treatment had been experimented with in the hope that they would prove beneficial in the control of mania, even if they did not represent an outright cure for insanity. The thrust of much of the experimentation in treatment of insanity focused on shock or surprise as a basis for changing or breaking cycles of aberrant behaviour. The fact that George III's case was so well documented and publicised provided a focus for and an encapsulation of the arguments on how to treat the insane.

The opening chapters of this book cover the onset of George III's final illness in October 1810 and the early confidence that the king would recover. But as the illness continued and concern mounted the focus of the king's care gradually shifted from recovery to an increasingly desperate battle to manage the intensifying symptoms of his deteriorating condition. Indeed at the height of the crisis it was considered that the king could die at any moment. There were dissenting voices, even within the team of royal doctors, over what the appropriate treatment of the king should involve. The decision in mid-1811 that specialist 'mad doctors' should take charge of the king's case was an act of desperation on the part of the authorities responsible for the king's care. As it turned out the specialists had nothing helpful to contribute.

In this charged atmosphere the Duke of Kent, father of the future Queen Victoria, and his brother the Duke of Sussex began to look for alternative treatments and practitioners. The action of these two sons of George III amounted to a rejection of the orthodox methods for treating the insane and an endorsement of the need for a more effective and more humane treatment for such patients. In the pursuit of alternatives they engaged with a practitioner, James Lucett, who was from outside the ranks of regular medicine but who offered a 'cure' for insanity for possible use on the king. The relationship began discreetly, but the king's sons were soon joined by a group of eminent men who together underwrote a controlled, scientific trial to test whether the treatment Lucett offered really would cure insanity. The account of this experiment is drawn from the surviving archival record.

The experiment has been referred to as 'psychiatry's first therapeutic trial'.[6] Its ambitious aim was to determine whether the treatment offered by Lucett represented a cure for insanity which might be made available to the whole of mankind. What was not stated but was clearly understood to be the immediate aim of the whole enterprise was to determine whether the treatment was suitable for use on George III. It is also possible that the trial reflected concern from within the royal family that the king's illness might affect others in the Hanoverian dynasty including the king's children.

The story of Lucett and the therapeutic trial has never been fully told, despite the trial being carried out publicly. In the establishment and management of the trial and the assessment of Lucett's curative process, the experiment anticipated many later developments in scientific methods. Although the trial promoted by the Duke of Kent and his brother was not successful in its immediate objective and Lucett never treated the king as his patient, the trial contributed directly to the movement away from the automatic use of mechanical restraint to manage patients. It also launched the career of the irregular or 'quack' practitioner, James Lucett, who had attracted the attention and support of members of the royal family.

Lucett was representative of a number of people from different backgrounds who were involved in efforts to improve conditions or treatment for the insane and to dispense with physical restraint. The early nineteenth century was a moment of opportunity when the lay practitioner could and did drive innovation forward. Some of the initiatives have become celebrated, such as the foundation of an asylum, The Retreat, in York by local Quakers where the humane regime rapidly became mainstream in the management of insanity.

Lucett, for all his far-sightedness, was no starry-eyed idealist. While he went on to highlight and confront the most egregious ills in the treatment of the insane, he was also trying to make a living, promoting his own claims as a lay practitioner in outright defiance of the medical establishment. As time went by, he became increasingly involved in unscrupulous and probably criminal activity, although this did not apparently directly involve his treatment of his patients. He was in many ways an astonishing figure to have come close to treating the king. He was not 'qualified', but arguably nobody was qualified to treat insanity at the time.

For all his faults, however, Lucett was an early exponent of what was to become the defining characteristic of psychiatry in the United Kingdom, namely the absence of physical restraint. This book places Lucett and the experiment with his 'curative process' in the context of the wider efforts to ameliorate the condition of the insane and more particularly in the context of George III's final illness and the impact which conventional treatment was having on him. It will seek to demonstrate that Lucett should be better known now for he was practising care for the insane without mechanical control long before the practitioners who were lauded in the mid-nineteenth century for being in the vanguard of reform.

Chapter One

Assuming His Inheritance

'George III was twenty-two years old when he succeeded his grandfather but mentally and emotionally he was little more than a boy. His tutors had found him a difficult pupil, not exactly unwilling, but lethargic and incapable of concentration. He was eleven before he could read fluently and at twenty he wrote like a child. He possessed, however, a strange emotional nature. He was deeply attached to his brother, Edward, and could not be parted from him.'[1]

The First Four Georges. J.H. Plumb. 1956.

The sudden death of Frederick Prince of Wales in 1751 changed everything for the future George III. That unexpected death propelled George at the age of thirteen to the position of heir to the throne and given that his grandfather George II was sixty-eight, elevation to the throne could have come at any time. As Prince of Wales George felt the enormity of what would be expected of him. As a boy he had been shy and retiring and the death of his father and the sense of his impending responsibilities added to the rather withdrawn nature which he instinctively displayed as he grew up. The fact that his grandfather left him in the household of his mother added to his isolation from outside contacts and influences. George's mother, Princess Augusta, had supported her husband Frederick in his political machinations and had accepted the total hostility between him and George II. Whether it was a hang-over of this antipathy or just a lack of care on his part, George II took little interest in his heir and did little to ensure that he was prepared for his future responsibilities. The one initiative which George II did take was in 1756 when he offered his heir an independent establishment at St James' Palace, the ceremonial centre of the monarchy, from which he might gradually have taken up a role in society. The offer was rejected and George II may have considered he had done his duty as there were no further initiatives. So the future George III was left with his mother and her other children in the isolation which she had embraced.

The education which the future king received was for the most part what a gentleman of the age might have received. Today it would be seen as 'cramming' and George did complain that there was a greater emphasis on the translation of the works of Julius Caesar than he would have wanted. He did, however, cover science and mathematics in a way that none of his predecessors had done and his architectural drawings which survive in the Royal Collection reflect an interest which remained with him for the rest of his life. His education was not joyless as he and his siblings were taught to draw and paint and all sang and played musical instruments. The perception that George lacked enthusiasm for his tutoring was probably accurate. He seems to have been uncomfortable with highly structured and formal learning and it is possible that the combination of enforced rigour and the deference with which he was treated by his tutors as well as the isolation in which it all took place made it difficult for him to engage. The idea that the future king was backward and barely literate when he assumed the throne advanced in the quotation at the beginning of this chapter is unsustainable. The reality was very different. He had mastered both written and spoken English and German before he was ten, while even a glance at the correspondence between him as Prince of Wales and Lord Bute is enough to dispel the idea that he 'wrote like a child' when he was twenty as nonsense.[2]

Bute was a crucial and late influence in the development of the future king. He had been a member of the political circle of George's father but he remained in contact with Princess Augusta who used Bute's extensive botanical knowledge for advice on planting in the gardens at Kew. With encouragement from Augusta, Bute took on an unofficial role as mentor for her eldest son and the relationship developed rapidly. In 1756 Bute's position was endorsed officially, if reluctantly, by George II. The correspondence between the Prince of Wales and Bute demonstrates the dependence of the younger man not simply for political guidance but also for moral certainty. There is no doubt that George considered Bute as his friend, but the intensity of the relationship reveals a strong element of desperation to it which highlights the dreadful isolation in his life which the future George III had felt. The emotional charge to some of the views which George expressed is startling. George felt a sudden strong attraction for Lady Sarah Lennox after meeting her and candidly submitted his feelings to the judgement of Bute, knowing that he would oppose any involvement with the lady. He wrote, 'for if I must lose my friend or my love, I will give up the latter, for I esteem your friendship above earthly joy'.[3] The interest in Sarah Lennox was actually more revealing of George's judgement than some of the prurient commentary has suggested over the years.

Much has been made of the brief infatuation with Lady Sarah Lennox. Certainly his comments on her attractiveness in a letter to Bute, 'She is everything I can form to myself lovely',[4] seem to suggest a young man who had lived an adolescence of almost monastic isolation before suddenly 'discovering' women for the first time. There have been attempts to use the infatuation with Lennox as a counterpoint to George's choice of partner in marriage and to suggest that this had not been a fulfilling relationship. The reality is that George himself recognised the superficiality of his admiration for Sarah Lennox and that he was not going to risk an involvement which would have had domestic political implications. Nor was he going to indulge his sexual appetite as his father, his grandfather and his great grandfather had all done and his sons were to do, by taking a mistress. What George's resolution of the Lennox 'affair' demonstrates is that he was not prepared to indulge appetite at the expense of responsibility. He also placed an absolute block on his grandfather having any part in securing a wife. George was determined that when a decision was made the choice would be his.[5]

George was not allowed to profit from the relationship with Bute without painful controversy. Bute was vilified for supposedly taking the Princess Dowager of Wales as his mistress and for poisoning her son's mind while pursuing his political ambitions. Salacious cartoons appeared ridiculing Bute and Augusta. The idea that Princess Augusta was Bute's mistress was part of an attack by Bute's political opponents, but George and his mother certainly suffered collateral damage. George would have been more reserved in response to the attacks and more hostile towards the Whig opposition and to the political world in general. The idea was a propaganda fantasy as well as a practical improbability. George's strict moral code would not have allowed him to associate with a man who was in an illicit relationship with his mother while how such a relationship between two such conspicuous individuals as Bute and the Princess could have been carried on is not obvious!

Bute was certainly not without serious faults of personality and judgement, and many of these were shown in relief when he became George III's prime minister. It was easy to dismiss Bute as pompous, pretentious and ambitious and unable to cope with the brutal rivalries of politics, yet without him the future George III would have been very much less well prepared to take on the real executive responsibilities of kingship in mid-eighteenth century Britain. It was from Bute that George gained an understanding of statecraft, the constitution and the political role of the crown. Bute was also responsible for bolstering George's natural commitment to moral kingship and leadership which was to stay with him for the whole of his reign. It would be fair to say that George got through his upbringing and survived. He was socially conservative, sexually restrained, dutiful, warm-hearted and decent when he ascended the throne. He was an accomplished amateur musician playing the flute and the harpsichord as well as enjoying singing. His perception of his future role as he saw it was set out in a frequently quoted piece in a letter to Bute. 'The interest of my country ever shall be my first care, my own inclinations shall ever submit to it. I am born for the happiness of a great nation, and consequently must often act contrary to my passions.'[6] This was a fair commitment to being a constitutional monarch.

Once George III became king, in October 1760, marriage was pushed towards the top of his agenda. It was to be an arranged marriage in which he chose from a list of eligible German princesses on whom he commissioned reports of their accomplishments and character. Candidates were rejected for a range of reasons including personality and ironically in one case due to insanity in the family. (See Chapter Ten.) Although she was not on the initial list, George's choice in the end was for Princess Charlotte of Mecklenburg-Strelitz. She was seventeen and brought neither glamour nor prestige to the marriage, but she brought more important qualities which enabled her and the marriage to survive the anticipated strains of marriage to a reigning head of state as well as the unexpected horror of her husband's decline into apparent insanity. Charlotte had not had a serious education and was no court sophisticate. More importantly, however, she was both tough and clever, bookish and conservative. She was also compliant politically, resilient and loyal and she liked Handel! Charlotte had no interest in politics and was happy to comply with her husband's order to keep out of domestic politics – that is until after his first serious illness when he began to discuss politics with her and to value her judgement. What had begun as an arranged marriage turned into a love match of mutual interdependence which only began to fray under the unbearable pressure of the king's illness twenty-seven years after their marriage.

Attempts have been made to implicate Charlotte in her husband's illness and mental decline. These have centred on the idea that the king's insanity was the result of sexual frustration born of his dissatisfaction with his wife and marriage. Perhaps the clearest expression of this idea lay in the comment that the king's insanity was the result of various failings of character and his 'resolute fidelity to a hideous queen'.[7] This was not a perspective which had currency during George's lifetime. Instead Charlotte impressed from her first day in Britain when she journeyed from Chelmsford in Essex to London on the last stage of her journey from Mecklenburg. On arrival at St James' Palace, in the middle of the afternoon of the 8th September 1761, she met her future husband for the first time and was introduced to the immediate members of the royal family with whom she dined. The almost unreal swirl of events continued with the dressing and briefing on the marriage ceremony which followed at nine o'clock in the evening. Supper followed with guests and Charlotte, now the queen, sang and played the harpsichord to the assembly. The king and queen finally retired in the early hours of the following morning. It would be difficult to overstate the resilience, charm and stamina which Charlotte had displayed in what must have been an extraordinary endurance test amongst strangers, including her husband, with every eye watching for some mistake or error. Charlotte had passed this test as observers agreed. 'She is easy, civil and not disconcerted' was Horace Walpole's summing up of his first impressions.[8]

George III had been born two months prematurely and was not expected to live; but he did and thrived and he always gave credit for his survival to his wet nurse. After his unpromising beginning he developed through a healthy childhood to reach adulthood as a robust and active individual who was to outlive his siblings. He was careful about his diet and took regular physical exercise. In general, his health was very good. Four episodes of illness, during which the king lost his reason, were recorded during his sixty-year reign. The first documented episode came in the crisis of 1788 to 1789 when the king was fifty and when he had been on the throne for twenty-seven years. Over all this episode lasted for approximately six months although for the most part during this time George was 'sane' while nevertheless clearly ill. Shorter episodes of illness involving manifestations of 'insanity' came in 1801 and 1804. There have been attempts to argue that the problem started earlier and was more serious in its impact. Some commentators have asserted and others continue to argue that during a period of illness in 1765 George had experienced episodes of mental instability. The absence of any record or even reference to the king suffering any mental aberrations in 1765 is taken as an indication of a cover-up by those wishing to extend the impact of the king's illness. This is despite the fact that during the crisis of 1788 to 1789 there was no hesitation over admitting the mental impact of the king's illness and the shock and surprise this caused at the time. The final episode of illness during which the king lost his reason came in late 1810. George III never recovered from this final illness and the loss of reason which is generally taken as having lasted until his death in January 1820.

The king's illness in 1788, when he first lost his reason, came as a shock and the multiplicity of physical symptoms which he displayed actually caused his principal personal physician, Sir George Baker, to panic. Baker described the onset of illness and the gradually intensifying physical symptoms which accompanied the deterioration towards eventual derangement. In his manuscript entries for 17th October and 21st October 1788, Baker set out a complex and confusing mass of physical symptoms.[9] The king's behaviour was changed with the impact of increasing mania causing a stupendous acceleration in his thought processes and an irresistible need to express his thoughts for days and nights continuously. Perhaps the most disturbing impact of the illness was the apparent change in his personality. The king's language became foul and offensive and an apparently unbridgeable gap opened between the highly sexualised indecency of his utterances and the restrained decorum of his normal conversation. From late November 1788 George had become unrecognisable as a personality to his familiars and it was this which drove the decision to bring in a specialist 'mad-doctor' rather than continue to leave the task to the ministrations of the general physicians.[10]

It was probably at the suggestion of Lady Harcourt [11] that Dr Francis Willis was called in. He had treated Lady Harcourt's mother for a 'nervous complaint' which was a euphemism for insanity. He kept a private asylum in Lincolnshire where he specialised in the treatment of the insane. This was a crucial decision as the involvement of Willis and giving him the management of the king's case was tantamount to making an official statement that the king had been diagnosed as suffering from insanity. There was simply no other possible explanation for the involvement of Dr Francis Willis – especially as it meant side-lining the court doctors who despised Willis and tried to patronise him. It was also an indication of the seriousness of the king's case as it was assessed at the time.

In simple terms the thrust of the Willis approach to the king's case was to substitute the destructive chaos of the patient's mania with the imposition and enforcement of the physician's authority and order. This was absolutely mainstream thinking amongst specialists treating insanity during the last quarter of the eighteenth century. Francis Willis did not set out his thinking on the treatment of insanity either in a record of the king's case or in a text book. Others did, and Dr Joseph Mason Cox' account can be taken as a fair example of the methods and purpose of imposing the authority of the physician. 'Fear is excited by firmness, and menaces producing strong impressions on both mind and body, while confidence and veneration often result from soothing and gentleness.' Cox adds one specific rider which had particular significance in George's case. 'No promise should remain unfulfilled, no threat unexecuted.'[12]

Much was made of the power of enforcing the physician's authority through mental intimidation of 'the Eye'. The often repeated story of Francis Willis' encounter with Edmund Burke in which the 'mad-doctor' cowed the philosopher with a single glance highlights the theatrical nature of some of the aspects of the management of patients at the time. Dr William Pargeter wrote of his achieving ascendancy over a raving lunatic by rushing suddenly into the room where the unfortunate individual was being held and catching his eye with an instant calming impact. Pargeter comes close to setting out the therapeutic aim of the physician's authority over his patient by saying it could be achieved by 'mildness or menaces as circumstances direct'.[13] The imposition of the physician's authority was tantamount to the imposition of sanity on the patient and the reality was that the 'authority' was power assisted. The force of physical restraint was crucial and universal in the management of manic patients by 'mad-doctors' in the period when George III was diagnosed as suffering from insanity. Chains, straight waistcoats, manacles and fixed furniture to which the patient was secured were normal methods of managing patients. Almost all were applied to George III himself. It would be fair to say that a therapeutic effect had been achieved when the mere threat of restraint had a desired effect on the patient's behaviour. Joseph Mason Cox, a contemporary of Francis Willis, set out his thinking on the therapeutic impact of restraint in his comment, 'I have known instances in which furious maniacs in consequence of being liberated from their shackles by my direction [become] so attached and devoted to me as never again to require coercion.'[14]

This was an advance on the treatment which might have been 'administered' to a patient suffering from insanity at the beginning of the eighteenth century. At that time the explanation of insanity as the result of demonic possession was being replaced by insanity as an indicator of moral degeneracy, but in either case the combination of beatings and neglect seem to have emphasised punishment rather than care. Willis did not see insanity in these terms but his treatment of George and other patients depended on the rigorous use of intimidation and physical control to secure order which might at best be seen as creating the conditions in which recovery became possible. Whatever Cox might argue and Francis Willis practice there was no causal relationship between restraint and cure and as time passed the voices raised against restraint became stronger and more numerous.

The determination that the king's illness was insanity was not, however, based simply on the clear displays of mania and the change in his personality. Crucial to the assessment of the king's illness and indeed to his recovery was the delusional element of his thinking when he was ill. George's obsession with Lady Pembroke when he was ill has attracted enormous, almost prurient interest, in part because it was so utterly uncharacteristic. There were other areas of manifestly unreal thinking as will be seen in later chapters, but the delusion centred on the fantasy relationship with Lady Pembroke does deserve to be considered in some detail because it was so hurtful to the queen and so damaging to her relationship with her husband. The obsession developed when George III was at his most delirious during the crisis of 1788–9. The choice of Lady Pembroke as his so called 'preferred partner' could hardly have been more sensitive as she was a friend of the queen and one of her companions as a Lady in Waiting. She had been effectively abandoned by her husband who was a serial womaniser. Perhaps the worst episode in the whole Pembroke saga was an occasion when Francis Willis persuaded Queen Charlotte to visit her husband in late December 1788. The queen was unwilling to meet her husband at that time because he was in a generally excitable state and had already told her that he preferred Lady Pembroke during an earlier encounter. Dr Willis had, however, reassured the queen so she agreed.

The meeting was supposed to be for a quarter of an hour and was intended to be a brief opportunity to maintain the family relationships at a time when the king was being kept separate from his family while he was treated by Willis. The encounter actually lasted an hour and was conducted in German but the king told Willis and others afterwards with unguarded enthusiasm what he had apparently said to his wife. After twenty-seven years of marriage and twelve children and while the queen was pregnant with Octavius, George announced that he didn't like Charlotte, that he preferred another woman, that Charlotte was mad and had been for three years and most bizarrely of all that Charlotte was not to come to his bed again until 1793. It would have been impossible for the queen to look at this last statement with the detachment which would have enabled her to see it as reflecting an unreality brought on by her husband's illness. The problem was that the king seemed to relish expressing these damaging views and Queen Charlotte's humiliation must have been complete when in a separate meeting the king abused his wife in front of three of their daughters and said he preferred Lady Pembroke.[15]

The full impact of this rejection by her husband on Queen Charlotte is difficult to imagine. It was both so public in its execution and so personal in its expression that it can only have undermined the marriage which Charlotte had so conscientiously and completely committed to. Her standing within her family and the court would have been horribly damaged and it would not really have removed the hurt to have rationalised the king's behaviour as the reflection of his illness. In a pre-Freudian era distinctions between conscious and unconscious thoughts and the repression of painful or difficult feelings would not have had the currency they might have now, but Charlotte could only have wondered whether her husband had expressed his real wishes and desires – however unreal they might have been. And they were unreal. Robert

Fulke Greville was the king's equerry and was a confidant. Greville sadly described the king being oblivious to the hurt and embarrassment he was causing while he was ill but was able to describe the uncomfortable sense that the king felt that he had said painful things to his wife and expressed inappropriate comments about Lady Pembroke as his mental condition improved.[16] The separation of the delusion from reality in the case of Lady Pembroke was particularly perplexing for the king as his recovery became complete during the spring of 1789. In the end he could only resolve the matter in his mind by asking the lady herself. Lady Pembroke was able to assure him that in the real world the king had done nothing to compromise his marriage vows and George's understanding of his former delusions was complete.[17]

The relationship between the king and the queen was changed in other ways by the crisis. The queen had been forced to take responsibility for her husband's welfare and some of the problems involving management of the king by Willis and his attendants were particularly difficult. The regular employment of restraint may have seemed justified when the king was in an explosively manic state, but the sense of humiliation which George felt when the crisis had passed nagged at him. He made Charlotte promise to keep him out of the clutches of the mad-doctors if he had a relapse. It was an unrealistic demand which events were later to demonstrate, but the fact that the government of the day would have to consult the queen during any relapse subtly changed her status. George had given Charlotte an instruction when the couple were first married that the queen should keep out of politics. After 1789 George broke his own edict and began to discuss the political issues with his wife. It is possible that her resilience in the face of the awful pressure of his illness prompted George to appreciate her judgement as well as her strength of character.

The crisis of 1788–9 had been a shattering blow to the king, his marriage and his family. There may have been some weakening of the king's constitutional position simply because a regency bill had been examined in detail by parliament. George III forestalled the implementation of the regency by his recovery, but there could have been no confidence that the king would not suffer a relapse. Nevertheless, there was the appearance of an explanation for George's recovery in 1789 and the sense that his illness was manageable was strengthened by the much milder recurrences in 1801 and 1804. The king's advancing age and the fact that he was rapidly losing his sight because of cataracts were taken as positive developments in the conventional medical wisdom of the age. It was thought he would be less susceptible to outside stimulus and stress. There was a sense though that if the worst happened then the appropriate response was known. Close members of George's family and his medical and other attendants were not complacent however. All those around the king watched for and tried to manage threats to his composure. They constantly looked for signs of his metabolism speeding up and of increases in his energy levels. These were sure signs of approaching trouble.

Chapter Two

The Onset of the Crisis

'The King himself told her [Princess Amelia] not long before her death,
that he felt as if his reason would sink beneath the weight of his sorrow.'[1]
Memoires of the Life and Reign of King George the Third.
John Heneage Jesse. 1867.

'O n Wednesday, the 24th of October 1810, the King's excited manner,
and loud rapid utterance, seem to have given the first warning of
a return of the same dreadful malady which had afflicted him on
former deplorable occasions.'[2] This brief record from the diaries of eminent
MP and friend of the king, Sir George Rose, tracks the onset of George III's
final descent into illness. On 26th October the king continued to display the
same symptoms. The pattern of normality was being maintained at Windsor,
but knowledge that something was wrong was beginning to spread. In a letter
to his brother the Marquis of Buckingham on the same day, Lord Grenville
gave the following news, 'I have this day received, as a mark of friendship and
with liberty to communicate it to you alone, the information that the King's
former indisposition is returning upon him. You may guess from whom I
heard it. The person who mentioned it to me ... tells me that he himself met
the King in his ride yesterday talking so loud and fast as to be remarked at a
considerable distance.'[3] While some pretence at least of discretion was being
maintained it could not be long before the return of the king's illness was
generally known.

On the evening of 25th October the queen had organised a family party
at Windsor which George was well enough to attend. There was a savage
irony in that this date and this party marked the celebration of the 50th
anniversary of George III's accession to the throne. Although none of those
involved could have known it, this was to be his last public engagement.
It was to be stage managed, so far as possible, by the queen. When he
entered the drawing room, an eyewitness recorded that it was with the
queen holding his arm. This was normal given that the king had been blind
since about 1805, but the difference in the king's manner was immediately

apparent. 'As he went round the circle as usual it was easy to perceive the dreadful excitement in his countenance. As he could not distinguish persons, it was the custom to speak to him as he approached that he might recognise by the voice whom he was about to address. I forget what it was I said to him, but shall ever remember what he said to me. "You are not uneasy about Amelia, I am sure. You are not to be deceived, but you know that she is in no danger." At the same time he squeezed my hand with such force that I could scarcely help crying out. The Queen however dragged him away. When tea was served, I perceived how much alarmed I had been, for my hand shook so that I could hardly hold the cup. When the King was seated, he called to him each of his sons separately, and said things to them equally sublime and instructive, but very unlike what he would have said before so many people had he been conscious of the circumstance. I never did and never will repeat what I then heard, and sincerely believe that all present felt as I did on that occasion.'[4] Miss Knight, who was a lady in waiting to the queen, would have been very familiar with the king's normal behaviour. Her comment on his 'dreadful excitement' is important as it highlighted the great change which illness immediately brought in the king's behaviour. It also makes it clear that the king's indiscretion in talking to his sons on private matters in the middle of a large gathering was not caused by his blindness making him unaware of his surroundings, but by the impact of the onset of illness.

There was general agreement at the time that the long illness and the inevitable death of Princess Amelia, his youngest child, had been the trigger for the king's relapse. Princess Elizabeth wrote to Lady Harcourt that 'his excess of feeling has been too much to bear'[5] while Lord Wellesley, waiting to call on the king at Windsor on 1st November recorded 'the sight, but still more the *hearing* of him before he went into the room, as most dreadful – a sort of *wailing*, most horrible and heartrending to hear'.[6] Robert Huish in his 1821 biography of George III provides some additional detail which, if it is correct, would add greatly to the already huge emotional charge of the king's predicament. Huish described the king's reaction to Amelia's illness, 'He dwelt upon it with harassing and weakening grief and despair, till at length the powers of his understanding gave way, and he fell a prey to the mental disorder under which he had suffered so much about twenty years ago.'[7] This is a fair replay of what became the accepted account of the events. However, Huish specifically links the critical moment to Amelia's presentation of a ring to her father which she had asked to be engraved with 'Remember Me'.[8] Huish emphasises that the king had not been prepared for the presentation of the ring and that the emotional shock when he realised what he had been given was too much for him. Certainly George had become deranged before Amelia's actual death and Huish's account with its combination of simplicity and pathos, provides an apparently convincing explanation for the king's mental decline.

When George III first became ill during the crisis of 1788 the royal doctors were at a total loss as to how they should deal with their patient. The range of physical symptoms was so great and the intensity of some of the symptoms was so severe that they were unsure how to intervene. The symptoms included abdominal pains, rheumatic pains, weakness and swelling of the legs, disturbed vision, rapid pulse, constipation, extreme agitation and confusion, fever and loss of hearing. With no obvious diagnosis to account for this bewildering range of physical symptoms they feared that any intervention might kill the king while at the same time the crisis was at times so severe that doing nothing seemed equally dangerous for the king's survival. It was the development of the behavioural changes in the king, most importantly the onset of delirium, which seem to have given meaning to the illness and to have enabled the royal doctors to act. In a sense the behavioural changes, particularly the persistence of derangement, gave coherence to the otherwise random series of symptoms and made possible a diagnosis. It also provided a focus for subsequent treatment. The diagnosis was that the king was suffering from insanity.

Less fully documented is the fact that, as with earlier crises, the onset of illness leading to behavioural changes coincided with George having apparently caught a cold or a chill. In 1810 the fact that the king had not changed out of wet stockings was quickly used as a convenient explanation for his having caught a cold. What was going on was the separation of the whole series of physical symptoms from the onset of serious behavioural changes. Just as in 1788, the physical symptoms were put to one side in 1810 and the focus was on what were believed to be the defining characteristics of what had become accepted as a case of insanity.

Although it was some years since George had last been ill with symptoms of derangement, his physicians were constantly on the look-out for anything which might trigger a crisis. Indeed an incident had occurred a little earlier in Princess Amelia's own illness which it was thought had had the potential to seriously disturb the king's mental stability. In early September 1810, Amelia had written to Sir Henry Halford, physician to the royal family, asking for his views on her proposal that she should ask the king for permission to marry, on her deathbed as it turned out, General Charles Fitzroy for whom she felt an obsessive passion. While Amelia's request had ostensibly been for advice in reality she had wanted Halford's active assistance in persuading her father to allow her to marry. The Royal Marriages Act of 1772, which George III had personally underwritten, meant that immediate relatives of the sovereign had to seek permission from the king to marry. This was unlikely to be forthcoming in this instance and Halford knew this. In his response to Amelia he refused to endorse the proposal for raising the matter with the king. Halford advised strongly against it on the basis that, 'I am satisfied that this blow to the King's peace of mind must be so heavy as to endanger the loss not only of His Majesty's happiness but of his health.'[9] In approaching Halford, Princess Amelia was repeating a similar manoeuvre she had made in 1807 when the royal doctor in that instance had been Sir Francis Milman.

Marriage at this time was essentially an issue of duty for the members of the inner circle of the royal family and perhaps unfeelingly Halford opposed passion with duty while at the same time remarking that he would not want to see Princess Amelia 'becoming the object of impertinent conversation and remark at the corner of every street in every town in the island'.[10] Poor Amelia simply wanted to have her way and not be lectured on her duty as her response of 9th September showed. She considered herself to be married to Fitzroy and wanted legal confirmation of that status before she died. She berated Halford in a withering critique of his comments and ended with the comment that she would hold him to secrecy on the issue, but would otherwise never discuss it with him again. This poignant little episode is a marker of the sensitivity which surrounded George with physicians and family almost conspiring to protect the king from unwanted emotional shocks. While people might rationalise the onset of the king's illness by linking it with flu or a chill, the royal family and household were in no doubt in thinking that emotional shocks were dangerous and threatened the king's mental stability. Princess Mary, who had been in on Amelia's initiative, wrote to Halford, probably on 10th September, to thank him for doing *his* duty. The irony of the episode is that the king was to be protected from the knowledge of a relationship which had been known to the rest of the royal family, including the queen, for years.[11]

On Monday, 29th October 1810 the Lord Chancellor, Lord Eldon, and the Prime Minister visited the king at Windsor. On return to Westminster, Spencer Perceval reported to the Speaker, 'that though the King's conversation had been neither 'unconnected nor irrational' yet it had been so hurried and different from his normal manner to convince'[12] the Prime Minister that the king could not handle his constitutional duties. Perceval went on to say that rather than dwell on his own afflictions the king had asked about the Prime Minister's family. Perceval also said that he had been told by the physicians that while the illness of Princess Amelia had been an all-consuming worry for the king, even as illness returned to him, once the mental disturbances appeared he ceased to mention her. When eventually he was led to discuss Amelia he seemed to be under the 'happy delusion' that she was alive in Hanover where she had been endowed with the gifts of perpetual youth and health.[13]

What these accounts record is the gradual and uneven progress in the onset of illness. Initially the king's metabolism seemed simply to go into overdrive but the rationality of his thought processes was apparently not immediately affected. They were simply expressed at a frenetic rate. As the crisis continued, however, the changes in the king's behaviour became more distorted and extreme. George was a decorous, man who was normally calm and controlled and who spoke generally in formal gentlemanly terms. As illness took hold, however, this all changed. He became aggressive and irritable while his language became foul and sexually explicit. All restraint disappeared, but more sinister was that the delusional impact became more obvious. There is a wide difference between the gentle delusion, or perhaps wishful thinking, that Amelia was in 'no danger' and the full-blown 'madness' of her becoming immortal and living in Hanover. In the royal household the initial reaction had been almost relaxed. The doctors who dealt with the routine illnesses of the household remained in sole care of the king. After all, the problem was beginning to become almost routine.[14]

The reaction of the Prime Minister was crucial as he had to assess the potential impact on the king's constitutional role. He was in no doubt that, five days on from the onset of illness, the king was incapable of handling his constitutional duties. This was even though the Prime Minister seems not to have considered the king was actually insane. What is clear is that the signs of the king's illness were thought to be well understood and the progress it would take was also assumed to be predictable. It was perhaps also implicit that with fifty years on the throne and the House of Hanover fully established and an heir in waiting, it was not essential that George III himself should remain on the throne although the administration of Spencer Perceval would not have been expected to survive the imposition of a regent.

Political concerns for the survival of the Perceval administration may have been behind a curious incident on 1st November when the physicians to the royal household reluctantly agreed under pressure from the Lord Chancellor to call in Dr Samuel Simmons who arrived at Windsor the same day with a team of orderlies. Simmons was a specialist 'mad-doctor' at St Luke's Hospital who had treated the king in 1804 and had claimed the credit for curing his patient. Simmons demanded sole control over the patient, but this was refused by the regular physicians attending the king. Apparently unwilling to compromise, Simmons and his team immediately withdrew. The government were not finished yet for on 6th November the Prime Minister brought Dr Robert Darling Willis with him to Windsor. Robert Willis was the youngest son of Dr Francis Willis and an experienced 'mad doctor', but unlike Simmons was readier to compromise on the issue of exclusive control and so was accepted by the other physicians. Essentially what these manoeuvres signified was an early drawing of battle-lines between the specialists in treating madness and the generalists. For the moment a reasonable compromise had been reached, but the battle would be joined in earnest a year later.[15] In the meantime Perceval had a representative of the specialists in place. One who had, in concert with his brother Dr John Willis, apparently cured the king before in 1801. The Prime Minister may well have considered that he had done what he could to ensure the recovery of the king while also doing all he could to ensure the survival of his own political administration. He might even have congratulated himself in showing some sensitivity to the royal family's aversion to the specialists.

The queen had done all she could to manage the problem within the confines of Windsor but this was not simply a private matter for the family to deal with. Parliament was due to meet on 1st November unless it was prorogued before. At that point the illness could not be contained by the government as the king's fitness to exercise his constitutional role would become a subject for parliament to address. The Lord Chancellor visited Windsor on the morning of 1st November to see if the king was well enough to sign the necessary Commission for prorogation. He was not. The king had been very ill that night and so was very irrational when talking to the Lord Chancellor although he was apparently quite calm. Indeed the king had been so deranged the night before that he had had to be restrained.[16] In fact on 1st November the two houses of parliament were persuaded to adjourn until the 15th November against the expectation that the king would improve or even recover in the intervening period. On that same day the king had been overheard talking to himself about the causes of his illnesses. 'This' he said of his illness at the time, 'was occasioned by poor Amelia.'[17] The Government continued to monitor the king's condition and on 11th November the Lord Chancellor was able to visit Windsor and see him. The king apparently asked his physicians how long he had been ill and when he was told he remarked that it was the fourth blank in his life.[18] In a sense this marked an important improvement in the king's condition as he was able to contemplate his illness with the detachment almost of an observer.

The king's condition appeared to be improving and this was the basic message on the 15th November when Perceval addressed the Commons. He said he had been to Windsor that day and had been told by the physicians that the king was in a state of progressive improvement. Parliament was adjourned for another two weeks although this was not without considerable dissent from the Opposition which argued that immediate consideration of a regency bill was needed. The government's apparent optimism seemed to be justified. While progress was not entirely smooth or consistent, the king continued to improve so that on 26th November the Princess of Wales wrote to her friend Miss Berry to inform her that the storm had passed over their heads.[19] To make sure the difficulty was over; the physicians were examined before the Privy Council on 28th and 29th November. They said that, while the king was tired at that moment, they expected him to recover in body and mind. Sir George Rose commented that the physicians were confident about recovery but could not predict exactly when it would happen.[20] This confidence in a complete recovery in a short, if unpredictable, timeframe remained the view of the physicians until the end of the year.

In fact the questioning by the Privy Council had not been very searching and focused simply on the king's ability to fulfil his constitutional duties. The illness itself was, it was believed at the time, understood so there was no attempt to revisit the actual nature of the underlying diagnosis. The king was simply understood to suffer from very occasional and short-lived bouts of insanity. This latest illness simply appeared to be consistent with the king's two previous short crises in 1801 and 1804. The Privy Council did not question this understanding and the physicians did not offer any alternative view. In mid-December the nature of the king's illness was explored in greater detail when the royal doctors were examined again by separate committees of the Houses of Lords and Commons. The overall assessment of the medical team confirmed that given to the Privy Council, but there were some expressions of doubt about the underlying diagnosis of insanity which are examined in the next chapter.

The Opposition was increasingly against further adjournments as the international situation with war against France and the domestic situation of considerable social unrest meant that there had to be a fully functioning government. The Opposition also assumed that the institution of the regency would involve a change of government and so had a vested interest in a constitutional resolution of the king's illness. The Opposition was given additional ammunition for their concerns about the government's management of the king's illness with the discovery that in 1801 the king had apparently been declared well two months before he had fully recovered and that the king had carried out his constitutional duties as mediated by his physicians. As the period in question had involved naval actions against Denmark it was considered by the opposition with some justification that an alternative to a potentially compromised king was needed.

The story that the king had been declared well two months earlier became public knowledge on 1st February 1811 with an article in the *Morning Chronicle*. The focal point for the supposed deception was the Chancellor Lord Eldon and a campaign began to exclude him from the Privy Council. Of course there was much political posturing in the claims of the opposition, but the episode encapsulates the pressures the physicians were under. It was not enough to try to care for their patient, or even to cure him. They had to deal with the strongly competing pressures of the government and opposition with each wanting to use the illness of the king to their political advantage. With their control over access to the king this incident was a demonstration also of the political power which the physicians could exercise at times during his illness. In hindsight the king may have been allowed to resume his constitutional role a little early in 1801, but it is entirely possible that this reflected the variability of the recovery process and that the king was better on some days than on others. In 1804 the same difficulty of determining the point at which the king's behaviour returned to 'normality' meant that some observers saw a difference between the king's behaviour in a public or official context and his behaviour in the private context. Sadly it would appear that the king's immediate family bore the brunt of the difficulties in his behaviour at this transitional stage. In late 1810 the outward signs were that the crisis in the king's health was easing but this was not a straightforward business. It is therefore important to focus more closely on what was actually happening at Windsor and on the process of assessing the real state of the king's recovery.

Chapter Three

Specialists or Generalists?

'Three men attend our Monarch daily,
Willis, Herberden and Bailey.
They are all most clever men,
Bailey, Willis, Herberden.
Question, which him first will kill is?
Bailey, Herberden, or Willis.'[1]

> This doggerel appears in several versions
> and is usually entitled, *King's Doctors*.

The team of eminent physicians appointed to care for the king were all familiar to him. Indeed for the most part they were people he had chosen himself to be his physicians. Dr Matthew Baillie had, for example, been called in to help treat Princess Amelia in 1810 and had been appointed Physician Extraordinary by George III himself a few days before his relapse in October 1810. Baillie had been asked to assist in the treatment of Princess Amelia by Sir Henry Halford who was physician to the king and the royal family and who surely set an unbeatable record by being physician not only to George III but his three successors. Dr William Heberden was a very successful London practitioner and son of a highly successful physician of the second half of the eighteenth century. He was appointed Physician in Ordinary to the king in 1809 by which time he was already well known to the royal family. David Dundas was a Windsor apothecary and was essentially the GP to the royal family in Windsor and was the first point of contact for medical matters. Indeed he had attended the king during his first crisis in 1788. Dr Henry Revell Reynolds did visit the king and was examined by the Privy Council. Although he had attended the king during his earlier crises he was not to play a direct role in caring for the king this time as he was at the end of his career and died in 1811. The key point was that although the specialist 'mad-doctors' were represented by Robert Willis they did not have control of the king's case as had happened during earlier crises and as Simmons expected in November. This decision was to have repercussions later on and to lead to bitter wrangling, but at the onset of the illness there was relief for some prominent members of the royal family that the brutal methods associated with the specialists would not be automatically used on the ageing king.

The Duke of York wrote to Sir Henry Halford, who was the doyen of the medical profession and the senior doctor at Windsor, on the 31st October 1810 to express his relief that Halford had been responsible for setting up the regime to care for his father. Referring to the methods employed to 'cure' the king in the past, the duke commented, 'the very thought of which I confess for every reason makes me shudder and which nothing but the most urgent necessity could warrant'. The duke also added that he was pleased that Halford would oversee the king's care as this was what George himself would have wanted and referred to the 'confidence which he has placed in you'.[2] There was clearly a feeling of guilt within the royal family that more had not been done to protect the king during his earlier illnesses. The methods had been credited with curing the king, but this did not make them any more acceptable to the patient or his family.[3]

The perspective which the Duke of York was expressing was one which was beginning to gain wider currency in the country. This was that the mentally ill should be treated with greater humanity. It was an irony of the case of George III that he was normally treated with very great deference, but once he was ill much of that deference was put aside. The royal family were, at this point, like any other family in the land; they had to accept what the medical profession considered was appropriate treatment to secure the patient's recovery. All was done to enable the king to carry out his constitutional duties but the increasing reluctance to accept the full rigours of the treatment was clear though in the Duke of York's comments to Halford. The problem was that important elements of the treatment of the insane appeared to consist of punishing the patient. Physical restraint was the focus of concern. It was one thing to use restraint to control a patient experiencing a manic episode when he or she could be a danger to themselves or others around them. It was another to use it as a curative therapy. Significantly Dr Robert Willis set out the thinking behind this management of the patient. 'The emotion of fear is the first and often the only one by which they can be governed. By working on it one removes their thoughts from the phantasms occupying them and brings them back to reality, even if this entails inflicting pain and suffering. It is fear too which teaches them to judge their actions rightly and learn the consequences. By such means is their attention brought back to their surroundings.'[4]

The hallmarks of Robert Willis' father are clearly on this explanation. What Robert Willis was endorsing for insane patients was essentially to intimidate them back to health. Extended periods of confinement isolated in a darkened room wearing a hood and gag while strapped in a 'straight-waistcoat' to a fixed chair had been used on the king during his earlier illnesses as a basic part of the therapy. For the less exalted patient the situation was generally worse as the 1815 House of Commons Select Committee on Madhouses in England was to highlight.[5] For the Duke of York though, the prospect that his father would be humanely treated, by generalists whom his father knew, was hugely attractive and reflected a need which was felt more widely in society.

The royal family may have been happy to have familiar generalists managing the king, but ultimately the responsibility of government was to ensure that he could carry out his constitutional responsibilities. It was inevitable that the longer the illness continued the greater the chance that controversy would arise over the management of the patient. The king's illness was the focus of intense and sustained public interest, but it was also public property in the sense that a wide range of people considered they should offer their views and advice on the problem. For the most part the views of the ordinary people were confined to expressions of loyalty and concern as well as suggestions of homespun remedies. The king's 'insanity' acted as a great leveller and for many people the fact that the head of the first family of the nation was suffering in this way attracted considerable sympathy. Not all comments offered on the king's illness were disinterested. An important example was the letter which Lord Westmorland, who was Lord Privy Seal and therefore a member of the government, sent to the Prime Minister, Mr Perceval, on 8th November 1810.

Dr. J[ohn] Willis has been here and from the little conversation I have had with him and from what he has elsewhere heard he forms a very favourable judgement of His Majesty's case, so much as almost to doubt whether the disorder has taken positive hold, at least certainly not to the degree in former attacks – he considers all the preparation and anticipation as very favourable symptoms – the sense and prescience of Princess Amelia's death as it took place more so than in former commencements of the Disorder he would in no degree have been capable of any such sense or observations and the aberrations of understanding afterwards do not remove the favourable impression that circumstances gave him but delay in proper management was most dangerous and to be avoided. He thinks that [the] state of blindness must have a great effect in checking the increase of the disorder and giving the mind an opportunity of returning to itself – That he has not now had the opportunity of doing those things which in the commencement of the disorder would have increased its violence and confirmed the complaint – such as riding, walking hurrying etc – so much at least is favourable from a person who has not seen him but well knows His Majesty and these complaints.[6]

Dr John Willis was an older brother of Dr Robert and was a specialist 'mad-doctor' as members of the nascent profession of psychiatrists were called at the time. Although Dr John Willis' views were not based on direct observation of the king the comparisons he drew with the onset of earlier crises were important. The fact that there was an explanation for the king's relapse in the illness and death of Amelia was positive and John Willis also highlighted the fact that George had been able to discuss his daughter's death rationally as a pointer to the relapse being mild. However reassuring Willis' favourable prognosis might have been this was not the real thrust of his argument nor was it the reason he had spoken to Lord Westmorland. John Willis was engaged in a lobbying exercise which was strongly founded on self-interest. Willis' view was that the king's recovery had been jeopardised by the care being in the hands of generalist doctors. This was what he meant by the need for 'proper management'. Essentially Dr John Willis was pointing to the need, as he saw it, to limit the disorder of the king's mind by limiting the stimulation it received. This meant removing the patient from familiar surroundings and contacts and instead to seek isolation in both physical and mental terms. This is why John Willis commented to Lord Westmorland that the king's blindness was an advantage in limiting the extent of the relapse and as a potential contributor to a rapid recovery.

The discussion with Lord Westmorland was almost certainly made on the assumption if not the actual agreement that Willis' views would be passed on to the Prime Minister in the expectation that he would be called in immediately to oversee the treatment of the king. If that was the case John Willis would have been disappointed for what the Prime Minister did on 9th November was to pass Westmorland's letter to the physicians at Windsor with the following covering note. 'Mr Perceval, takes the Liberty of including a letter which he received that day from Lord Westmorland. Mr Perceval is sorry to believe that the opinion this contained is formed on a more favourable representation of His Majesty's complaint than what the present state of it would justify, although the circumstances attending its commencement seem to have been accurately stated.'[7] Perceval at least saw the crisis in the king's health was serious and seems to have been rather dismissive of John Willis' views and content to let the regular physicians remain in control. In any case he had succeeded in introducing Dr Robert Willis into the team so a specialist perspective of the case was available even if John Willis was not prepared to acknowledge it.

The regular physicians sent an immediate reply to Mr Perceval on 10th November and refuted what Dr John Willis was reported to have said.[8] They were understandably of the view that they had done all that they could and all that was necessary for the king. In a separate letter of response to Mr Perceval from Dr Robert Darling Willis he explained why he had not added his name to those of the other doctors. On Lord Westmorland's letter he says, 'highly as he [Dr Robert Willis] may prize the opinion of his brother generally speaking, his brother's opinion can be of little value in this instance, it being evidently formed upon an imperfect representation of the symptoms of the case'.[9] Robert Willis' views may have been somewhat disingenuous as there was evidence that he was in fact giving his brother some account of the progress of the king's case. What the flurry of correspondence did was to harden the battle lines between the generalist doctors attending the king and those who considered that specialist 'mad-doctors' should be brought in. This was a debate which was to recur with varying intensity during the succeeding months and as positions hardened the alternatives increasingly meant the exclusive control of one side or the other rather than a cooperative approach.

The confidence of the regular physicians must have seemed entirely justified at the time. After an initially severe crisis the king appeared already to be making significant progress. This was progress in which the patient was expected to take an active part. The team of physicians at Windsor formally addressed the king on 15th November in a written memorandum in which they made the following points:

'They have witnessed with great satisfaction His Majesty's amendment from a most severe fit of illness, but they are impressed with painful apprehension that the hurry they have lately observed in His Majesty's conversation and the various arrangements and multiple directions, which are apparently crowding His Majesty's mind, must infallibly produce a return of His disorder unless His Majesty can so far command himself, as, by stopping at once every beginning of business, and submitting to a regular arrangement of diet, and of medicine and general management, to preclude the sad necessity of employing again the most unpleasant means of restraint to which His Majesty's physicians would never recur, but under the most imperious sense of their duty.' The memorandum is annotated: 'His Majesty in answer was pleased to say that He would submit entirely to the Directions contained in the paper delivered by His Physicians. Signed, George R. 15th November 1810. A quarter [in figures] past 4'.[10]

This document is a fascinating insight into the situation of the king. He was clearly expected to be an active contributor to his own cure and he was assumed to have had sufficient reason and self-control to make this possible. At the time it was believed by some in the medical profession that even patients suffering from insanity had reserves of self-control which could be engaged to enable them to actively contribute to their own recovery. This practice came to be known as 'moral therapy' although it is questionable whether the doctors treating George III at this time would have used the term. Dr William Browne, amongst others, outlined the strategy later in his set of lectures published as *What Asylums Were, Are and Ought to Be* in 1837 in which he stressed the need to reject violence and cruelty in dealing with insane patients.[11] The document above is also interesting in that the royal doctors highlighted their unwillingness to use restraint on the king – at least not at this stage while recovery hung in the balance. This was counter to what Dr John Willis would have recommended no doubt, but the threat of its ultimate use was real nevertheless. Actually the document demonstrates a collective confusion on the part of the physicians attending the king. They were positive in trying to engage the patient in his own cure, but were unrealistic in expecting him to control his development of derangement. At the same time the positive engagement of the patient was intellectually undermined by the threat of violence. To which was added the irony that it was happening to one of the most powerful men of his age.

The limits to involving the king in his own cure were tested over the issue of whether to correct him when he displayed 'errors' or 'delusions'. The debate centred on whether he was capable of complying with correction or whether doing so would simply encourage the king to internalise the problem so that the physicians would lose an important check on his progress. The essential point though is that in dealing with the crisis the physicians had been confident right from the start of a successful outcome. Against that background engaging the king in the process of his own recovery would have seemed reasonable. The virtual contract with the king may also have had the additional advantage of implicitly formalising the idea that specialist 'mad doctors' were not needed. It is also possible that the doctors had an eye to the future and relations with their patient after his recovery. They were fully aware of the loathing the king felt for the 'specialists' who had treated him during earlier crises and so a contract of positive engagement with the patient might have been considered advantageous in preserving their positions once the king had recovered.

A month into the king's illness was also a time for taking stock. So on 28th November 1810 the Privy Council met to examine the physicians. Dr Reynolds was 'called in and sworn' and then questioned on the prognosis for the king. Although Reynolds took the view that George III was incapable of exercising his public duties at that time he had 'every confident hope of His Majesty's ultimate recovery'. Reynolds was asked if the majority of people with the king's disorder recovered. He replied that in his experience most recovered, but he would not put a specific timescale on the king's recovery as all patients were different. Reynolds pointed out that the time taken for the king to recover had varied during his previous crises. Again Reynolds emphasised that he was very confident of the king's ultimate recovery to the point of being able to carry out his public duties.[12]

Sir Henry Halford repeated the thrust of Reynolds' comments. 'I think it is in the highest degree probable that His Majesty will recover.'[13] Halford said that this view was founded both on the symptoms displayed by the king and general experience. Yet despite this, Halford was more guarded than Reynolds in his remaining answers. The other doctors endorsed these positive views and Dr William Heberden, while he claimed no special experience in 'mad doctoring', pointed to the fact that the patient retained his underlying faculties as a positive sign. Two weeks later on 13th December the physicians were examined by a committee of the House of Commons and a separate committee of the House of Lords.[14] Unexpectedly Dr Robert Willis chose this moment to question whether the king was actually insane.

In trying to assess the king's complaint as a whole, Robert Willis stated that it had 'never borne the characteristics of insanity; it never gets beyond derangement'. Willis went on to try to clarify his thinking. Essentially he spoke of there being steps in the process in which a patient could be said to have become insane. In the king's case he could become delirious in the early stages of a crisis and as the crisis deepened this could deteriorate further until the patient became deranged. Willis argued that this was as far as the process went with the king and that he never became fully insane. In summary Willis stated that 'His Majesty's illness, uniformly, partakes more of the delirium than of the insanity.'[15] This was an important attempt to refine the diagnosis of George III's insanity. In the king's case Willis' ruminations were not to have any definable impact on the way he was treated, nor on the eventual outcome of his case. Combined with the doubts and uncertainties expressed by the other doctors Willis' thoughts seem to reflect a real puzzlement over the king's illness and the sense that Willis was at the limit of his comprehension of the problem. Robert Willis did not return to his doubts as the case developed, but Dr Heberden was to return to the almost eerie sense that understanding of the case was just out of reach.

One impact for the modern reader in the story of George III's illness lies in the apparent normality and domesticity of his world in early 1811. He seemed to have recovered physically while he had also regained his reason. He lived in his own apartment on the north side of Windsor Castle where he received visits from Queen Charlotte every day and more often than not she would visit twice in a day. She was always accompanied by at least one of the princesses. George's sons were also frequent visitors. Senior politicians came regularly and some effort was made to keep the king briefed on political developments. He was even kept up to date on the progress of the bill to establish the regency. Actually the situation was more complex.

The crisis of 1788/9 had altered the relationship between Queen Charlotte and her husband. Throughout the period from her marriage in 1761 until the birth of Amelia in 1783 the queen had been pregnant or had recently given birth. Yet, as was set out in chapter one, she learned during the crisis that her husband had apparently preferred another woman all along. Queen Charlotte has generally not had a good press. She tends to be written off as cold and unfeeling and considerable blame has been levelled at her for the dysfunctional nature of her family. She has even been accused of abandoning her husband when he was ill; not least by George himself. All this is despite the more vulnerable and emotional picture of the queen presented by Fanny Burney in her diaries. It was not simply the delusions involving Lady Pembroke which became so real for George when he was in a deranged state. Allowance could be made for such behaviour when it was clearly the impact of serious illness. More difficult for Charlotte and her family to cope with was the stage between normality and derangement. The neat separation in words was not the same when it came to monitoring George's behaviour, yet for the physicians, assessing this stage of the king's illness was crucial in determining where the patient was in the process of recovery. For both Queen Charlotte and the king's physicians this was a difficult and to some extent a subjective problem to deal with and it was not one which was confined to the crisis which began in 1810.

At the beginning of March 1789 there had been an almost laughable and totally unscripted incident which potentially tested the concept of convalescence to destruction. The king had been tetchy for some days before 3rd March when a general ramble in the vicinity of the old Palace at Kew turned into an extended walk to Richmond by the king and a small group which included Dr Francis Willis and Robert Fulke Greville his equerry. George expressed a desire to see how things were progressing at the new workhouse at Richmond which he had generously endowed. 'The Master of the Workhouse having shewn the Appartments allotted to the Poor …. asked Him if he would see <u>their Madhouse.</u>' The visit followed and included conversation on the use of straight waistcoats. 'Fortunately HM heard this ill-timed conversation without the least agitation.'[16] The sheer unpredictability of the king's behaviour during convalescence is encapsulated in this incident when experience and understanding of the effects of his illness was still very limited.

There are pointers to darker behavioural changes in the king which bridged the extremes between outright loss of reason and complete recovery. These changes occurred during the convalescent stage of each of the crises which afflicted George III and created enormous difficulties for the doctors in managing the case. The changes were also particularly difficult for his immediate family, especially the queen, because they occurred when George was apparently rational but nevertheless appeared entirely unaware of his modified behaviour. Essentially the king became like a sexual incendiary ready to flare up at any moment and without inhibition. The subject is hedged around in the contemporary record. Those who would have been best placed to record manifestations of the problem used euphemisms, wrote around the subject, or simply ignored it. Fanny Burney was chased by the king round the gardens of Windsor in early 1789 and when he caught her he kissed her.[17] This incident appears to have been harmless if undignified, but the account will have been subject to censorship by Miss Burney who was intensely loyal to her friend the queen and to the king. Such behaviour was inconceivable when George was fully well.

George III's delusions about Lady Pembroke had been very damaging to the relationship between Queen Charlotte and her husband during the crisis of 1788. Worse was to come during the crises of 1801 and 1804. While the descents into 'insanity' were very short in both years, a matter of a few weeks of serious illness, the convalescence in each case was slow and extended so that the period when the king was rational, but displayed modified behaviour was very difficult to manage. By 1804 Queen Charlotte was resolutely refusing all intimate relations with her husband. She seemed to have conceived a loathing for her husband at this time. Despite pressure from close family members, senior politicians and clerics the queen refused to 'do her duty'. Princess Sophia, the fifth daughter, railed against her mother for refusing to sleep with the king while ironically complaining of unwanted attentions from her father.[18] A possible explanation for Charlotte's refusal to risk close unsupervised contact with her husband is that she had been subjected to some sexual assault by him. Whatever the explanation one can only have sympathy with the queen that one grotesque side-effect of her husband's illness was that the most personal and private aspects of the relationship with her husband became public property. Meanwhile all women about the court had to be protected from the attentions of the king during these periods of convalescence.

The evidence is limited and to some extent the result of rumours, but the concern for the king's behaviour indicates a further difficulty for those trying to manage the king's illness. Caroline the Princess of Wales complained of unwanted attentions from the king when he visited her while she was living at Blackheath and there is no doubt that in 1801 he developed an interest in the princess. Whether the princess was really saved from her father-in-law's embraces by a conveniently placed chaise-longue is open to conjecture. The point is that stories circulated and were believed at the time and were bolstered by some authenticated comments such as the Duke of Kent's in June 1804 that his father had recovered to the extent that he could be 'particularly kind, but in a proper and not in an outré way'.[19]

There are multiple references to 'indecent' and 'foul' language in the correspondence of the sons after they had visited their father and in the daily record kept by Robert Willis in early 1811.[20] An example of the nervousness about the king's sexual aggression when ill may lie in the note written by Princess Elizabeth to Robert Willis some time before 24th May 1811 when George III last rode in Windsor Park. 'Mama wishes you to know that the King is going for a ride and has desired to see her when he comes in, therefore she hopes you will be in the house.' The apprehension the queen felt about meeting the king is clear and it is implicit that she expected some behavioural distortion by her husband related to his illness.[21]

The obsessive delusion with Lady Pembroke is best seen as a separate issue in understanding the impact of illness on George III. In discussing the nature of the delusion when it first arose in 1788 the emphasis in chapter one was on its unreality. The same separation between the Pembroke obsession and the very real sexual aggression which the king displayed during convalescence after the succeeding crises is appropriate. While George talked about setting up residence with the sixty-seven-year-old Lady Pembroke in 1804 this and his threats to take a mistress were simply fantasies on which he never tried to take any action. For the physicians managing his case, however, the delusion about Pembroke proved to be a finely calibrated instrument for measuring the state of the patient's mental disturbance. Robert Willis noted in late 1810 that twenty-four hours could hardly pass without the king referring to his obsession with Lady Pembroke. As he improved in early 1811, Robert Willis was able to record on the 8th February, 'Some very slight allusions to E' but 'not dwelt upon'. While for the following day he recorded that the queen and princess Elizabeth had visited for over half an hour and the conversation had been 'very satisfactory'.[22]

Probably the best account of George III's modified behaviour during convalescence comes from 1804. He was not deranged but was living with his family and even attending to some official business. Yet in this sub-crisis state his behaviour was significantly modified but he was not manic or delusional. In fact he had few inhibitions, did not conform to social norms and his heightened sex-drive was very noticeable. Sir Robert Wilson, a soldier who had an exotic career involving many major campaigns of the early nineteenth century, visited Weymouth in early September 1804 where George III and his immediate family were on holiday. The king spotted Wilson as was doubtless Sir Robert's intention and invited him to join the royal party. Wilson had published accusations that Bonaparte had ordered the execution of prisoners during his Egyptian campaign in a broadsheet, *The Tender Mercies of Buonaparte in Egypt: Britons Beware!* George was interested in the account and discussed it with Wilson in some detail. As Wilson became more familiar with the king's behaviour over the succeeding days he became very critical.[23]

Wilson became exasperated by the king's seeming refusal to concentrate on serious matters for any length of time and his lack of discretion in nevertheless making comments on sensitive political issues within earshot of sailors and servants. Wilson was also appalled by the king's bad manners in criticising individuals in rough language in front of large numbers of people. Particular ire was prompted by George's lack of inhibitions on sexual matters. 'The King frequently threatens to keep a mistress several times has declared that since he finds Lady Yarmouth will not yield to his solicitations he will make love elsewhere.' The lady in question was not one of spotless reputation so could have provided a realistic candidate for his stated needs. The claim that she had rejected him complicates sure interpretation! During the timescale when any 'solicitations' might have occurred the lady was almost certainly living in Paris. What is clear is that this is not in the same delusional territory as the obsession with Lady Pembroke. A separate recollection from Wilson seems to suggest that the king was in the habit of inappropriate sexually explicit talk during this period of convalescence. 'On Sunday evening he (George III) was talking such ribaldry that Ld Uxbridge was obliged to leave the Lodge, being unable to witness this humiliating conduct.' This problem returned in 1810 and 1811 as is demonstrated by myriad references from those who were about the king at the time, to his indecent comments.

The worst incident perhaps was on 1st October 1804 on board a naval vessel on which the royal party was going to sail along the coast. George remarked to one of the party, 'Mrs Drax, you look very well, very well indeed, dear lovely Mrs Drax, how I should like to stroke you.' 'Stroke' was apparently a euphemism for sexual intercourse and Wilson described the impact of the king's uninhibited enthusiasm. 'The confusion of the gentlemen was so great as that of the ladies, but the officers of the ship & many of the sailors who heard the speech which was attended with peculiar emphasis and strength of voice could scarcely contain themselves.'[24] In hindsight George had been allowed into the public arena prematurely in 1804. At the start of 1811 the same questions were to be raised again in the process of determining when the king could be trusted to behave with safety and decorum without close management first with his family and then more widely.

Chapter Four

Regency

'To pronounce a man not mad, is much more difficult than to determine on the measure of insanity which should place him out of the pale of society.'[1]

A Treatise on those disorders of the brain which are usually considered and called mental. David Unwins, 1833.

In the political world the impending Regency was stoking up rivalries, but the rapid recovery threatened to upset the apparent certainties. It was clear, however, that there was a line of thinking that even if the king did recover now, a further relapse was inevitable and a regent would be required. Robert Plumer Ward, the MP for Haslemere, quoted from a discussion with a colleague, 'So the King means to put an end to all our discussions and arrangements by getting well, nevertheless we must have the Bill.' 'I said no not the Bill but a Bill to provide for a relapse.'[2] Ward walked home with Perceval from the Commons on the 15th January when the Prime Minister was recorded as saying, 'there was an excellent account from Windsor, but that the King's state could hardly prevent the Bill from passing.'[3] Ward commented in his memoirs that the Opposition – expecting to take over with the Regency – had been disconcerted by the king's improvement.[4] Indeed they might have been as the outlines of the office holders in the new administration were already being drawn up.

It seems to be an indicator of the intense concern over the progress of the Regency Bill that politicians used whatever means were available to determine the true state of the king's health rather than rely on official bulletins. Plumer Ward quotes discussions with an associate who had been to Windsor to consult Dr Heberden; ostensibly about his own health problems. This had provided the opportunity for encouraging Heberden to indulge in some erosion of patient confidentiality. Commenting on the king, 'Heberden said he went on as well as could possibly be expected, and almost as rapidly as they could wish; that he was for the most part himself – was as if his mind had been clouded with some confusion but cleared again.'[5] Just what the government would have wanted to hear of course, but an indication that George really was close to recovery.

The Prime Minister and the Lord Chancellor visited Windsor on 26th January and talked to the king for over an hour. Plumer Ward, clearly a government insider, recorded the Prime Minister's impressions of the king in his diary. 'His manner was hurried at first seeing (for he saw) them, but that soon went off, and in all other respects he was as much himself as ever. Whether anything and what passed politically, has not transpired, but he told them of his improvement in his sight with great pleasure. He said that Mr Perceval having small features, and standing with his back to the light, he could not have known him without hearing his name, but the Chancellor he should have known directly without being announced. He could not tell whether this was owing to the medicines he had taken during his present illness, or to his having left off the old regimen, but he could not help hoping that Providence had yet other blessings in store for him.'[6]

This was a poignant and ironic moment. In the midst of the concern for his sanity and all the constitutional implications his illness brought on, the king had apparently experienced a sudden and noticeable improvement in his eyesight. While not doubting the king's impression that his sight had improved, this does seem surprising given that he suffered from cataracts which meant that there was a physical barrier to his seeing. Nevertheless the king's joy at the improvement in his sight is almost palpable despite the account being third hand. It is also clear that the king's preoccupation with the improvement in his sight was not only a pleasure, but was also an indication that he considered he had recovered from his other illness. In fact all was not well as Lord Eldon's comment in a letter to Sir William Scott reveals, 'I saw the King on Saturday for much more than an hour. He is not well, and I fear he requires time.'[7]

Mr Perceval visited the king on 29th January to explain the progress of the Regency Bill through parliament. George III was noted in the daily log of the physicians as having listened to the Prime Minister 'with attention, and composure and occasional remarks'. The following day the king returned to the subject of Mr Perceval's visit and commented on it, 'in a proper manner'. In a very real sense the king was able to understand important issues which directly affected him and discuss them with detachment, but a 'cure' was far from complete. Again on 30th January 1811, the daily log includes the comment that the king, 'disclosed anecdotes of his family which had better been kept private'. It is possible that this rather coy comment is an indicator that the king had said something inappropriate about his wife. Certainly it is an indicator of the difficulty in determining when the king was recovered, even when he appeared well in many ways.[8]

On the 31st January 1811, Lords Eldon and Liverpool saw the king again to further explain the progress of the Regency Bill. He asked whether it was the intention of the Prince of Wales to replace the current ministers and was told that it was believed that was the Prince's intention. The king replied with apparent confidence that he would return the present ministers to their places when he was well again. Eldon and Liverpool said that the king was hurried, but entirely rational. There had been no delusions and no derangement.[9] The king also seemed to expect the Regency to be of short duration and this may account for his calm response when briefed on the progress of the Bill. Interestingly the issue of a possible change of government became the focus of a bizarre and apparently unnecessary piece of protective therapy. Queen Charlotte, assisted by Sir Henry Halford, successfully lobbied the Prince of Wales to agree not to change the government once he became Regent. The argument they used was that such a change would so enrage the king that it would potentially cause a relapse.[10] The *Morning Chronicle* chose this moment, when George teetered on the edge of recovery, to reveal that the world had been deceived about the state of the king in 1804 and that therefore Lord Eldon the Lord Chancellor then as well as in 1811, should not be made a member of the Queen's Council.[11] This exercise in political muck-raking was rapidly overtaken when the regency was authorised.

The Prince of Wales agreed, but, as he told Perceval on 3rd February, he did so reluctantly. In fact matters may have been more complicated. The Prince of Wales had already become more distanced from the opposition so it is possible that the initiative by the queen and Halford was more agreeable than he told Perceval. Certainly his father's illness made a convincing excuse for a change of intention by the Prince of Wales. On the 2nd February Lord Grenville wrote to the Duke of Cambridge to tell him that he was no longer required to draw up a list of new ministers 'lest the knowledge of any change should produce any effect in retarding H M recovery'.[12] The Regency Bill became an Act on 5th February when it was finally passed with the Royal Assent rather glossed over by the use of a Commission.

The management of the king's illness had thus far been the responsibility of the Prime Minister with the Lord Chancellor as well as the physicians and the queen herself. Queen Charlotte had been concerned by the constitutional implications of her husband's illness during earlier crises and had wanted to spread the responsibility for looking after him beyond the royal family. She had also been troubled by her husband's criticisms of her for not protecting him from the ministrations of the mad-doctors. The drafting of the Regency Act of 1811 was responsive to the concerns which the queen had expressed. The terms of the act envisioned the Regency 'to provide for the Administration of the Royal Authority' but also 'for the Care of His Majesty's Royal Person during the Continuence of His Majesty's illness'. The act brought into being a council 'to assist Her Majesty in managing the care of the King'. There were to be occasional tensions between the queen and her council, but there was no doubt that the council had the final word and that the queen accepted this and was grateful for it.

The Queen's Council was set up with statutory authority under the chairmanship of the Archbishop of Canterbury who was assisted by seven other eminent gentlemen including the Archbishop of York and the Lord Chancellor. On one level the constitutional responsibilities of the Council were discharged through the quarterly process in which the king's physicians were asked individually to give their written answers to a series of questions on their patient's illness and capacity. The primary aim of the questions was to determine whether the king was well enough to resume his official responsibilities. This was in fact only the formal manifestation of what was to become a very considerable and long-term commitment for council members who frequently became involved in the management of the king's illness on a daily basis. The Council sat at the centre of a set of relationships which included the political leadership of the country, several senior members of the royal family and the physicians who directly ministered to the king. The Council was responsible for managing these relationships in so far as they related to the king's illness. These relationships could work smoothly while it seemed that the patient was recovering. As doubts over the progress accumulated, however, the potential for friction became apparent and increased as the king suffered a relapse and was increasingly isolated from the outside world.

The daily medical log for the period of early 1811 when the Queen's Council came into being seemed to justify the confidence of the physicians that the king would recover and this impression was conveyed to the Queen's Council in the evening letters which were sent daily at this period to Lambeth Palace. The report of the physicians for 7th February for example, includes the statement, 'His Majesty seems to be making gradual progress towards recovery'. Yet behind the progress the king was undoubtedly making at this time there always lurked the indicators that all was not quite well. Dr Robert Willis summarised the problem in the entry in his notebook for 5th February. 'Before dinner He grew angry with his imaginary friends and demanded heavy punishments on several of them.'[13] If George inhabited another world at least in part, it was one which still held the appearance of reality to him.

The records, both official and private, are full of references to the king's 'errors' and 'delusions'. The infatuation with Lady Pembroke has been the focus of considerable interest because it appeared in all four crises. According to Jesse, 'the King had conceived a passionate admiration for a lady of spotless virtue and stately loveliness – Elizabeth Countess of Pembroke.'[14] Horace Walpole referred to her at the coronation of George III when she led the procession of Countesses as 'the picture of majestic modesty'.[15] The witty if rather waspish Lady Bessborough commented, 'In favour of his taste, she is the handsomest woman of seventy I ever saw.'[16] Whatever else it might mean to some observers, the obsession with Lady Pembroke was a clear pointer to the aberrations which illness signified for the king.

By the time of the 1810 crisis it was nearly fifty years on from the start of the supposed passion. The delusion is clear and unreal in the sense that George's infatuation was with the vision from when he first beheld the lady at the time of his coronation in 1761. According to Jesse the proof the obsession was with the early image lay in George's references to the lady by her maiden name of Elizabeth Spencer, a daughter of the Duke of Marlborough. However, this was not the case as the record in March 1811, for example, clearly shows not only the use of the lady's married title, but an extraordinary intensity of feeling. The king 'said to his son, the Duke of Sussex, is it not a strange thing, Adolphus, that they still refuse to let me go to Lady Pembroke, (the old Countess) although everyone knows I am married to her; but what is worst of all, is, that infamous scoundrel Halford (Sir Henry) was by at the marriage, and has now the effrontery to deny it to my face!'[17] Quite how this affected the king's perception of the status of his son is not clear! (There appears to be an error in Lord Grenville's letter as Adolphus was the first name of the king's seventh son, the Duke of Cambridge. The first name of the Duke of Sussex was Augustus.)

Arguably the 'delusions' and the behavioural ticks which the king displayed to some extent, even when he appeared to be cured, are important pointers to the problem the physicians were trying to deal with. Day after day there are references in the daily log to the king 'adjusting his bedclothes'. Similar obsessive behaviour occurred sometimes when he would spend hours in arranging the hair in his wigs. Generally such behaviour was simply noted without additional comment by the physicians. More often than not the king would wake well before the appointed time to get up and begin the routine of the day. For periods, sometimes of several hours, George would rearrange his bedclothes. The behaviour has the feel of a kind of obsessive compulsive habit although later in the illness George would throw off his bedclothes almost as an act of defiance and prompt a controlling response from the medical attendants.

Besides the imaginary friends, the king was in the habit of earnestly setting out plans which were entirely illusory. One striking example was his solemn account of the army which he claimed to have gathered at Weymouth and with which he expected shortly to embark for a military expedition to Hanover.[18] Clearly the king was concerned that his Duchy was in the hands of the French but the imagined solution disorientated visitors because it was advanced with such seriousness but was patently unreal. The king was also in the habit of announcing at great length the plans he had for improvements to the royal palaces or new orders of chivalry he planned. Yet even in hindsight the strategy of the royal doctors does not seem unreasonable at the time when George appeared to be recovering. The aim was to occupy the king. To channel his attention and thinking into more positive and realistic lines in the expectation that the delusions would gradually be supplanted by reality. Contemporary authorities such as William Hallaran at the Cork asylum and the Tukes at the Retreat at York would have endorsed the royal doctors' strategy.

The regime for the king's treatment was not arbitrary and was the subject of constant review. The physicians were after all reporting on a daily basis to the Queen's Council on the condition of the king. In February 1811 there was a distinct impression in the daily log that George was on the edge of recovery, but was not quite there. The physicians sensed that the king had improved so much that he just needed a nudge to help him get over the residual aberrations in his behaviour. They proposed changes which would, they hoped, make the transition from seeing the king as a patient to seeing him as someone who had recovered but still needed some convalescence. The physicians sent a proposal to the Queen's Council on 27th February in which they set out their thinking for how the king should be managed. The basic thrust of the proposal was, 'that the present medical attendance should be lessened and His Majesty gradually restored to his ordinary habits of life'.[19] In a further bit of fine tuning the physicians proposed on 9th March 1811 that George's management should be dependent on two principles: 'That His Majesty's time be occupied, so far as is consistent with his security, in his usual manner, and with his usual attendants.' The second principle was 'That the medical establishment, so far as is consistent with his security, be withdrawn.'[20] These proposals are very important as they demonstrate clearly just how close George had come to recovery. The physicians clearly viewed him as convalescent and much less as an actual patient needing active intervention. Dr Robert Willis recorded that it had been agreed that the king's delusions were not to be corrected.[21] The physicians did not want to drive this crucial indicator of possible recovery underground.

In terms of the early nineteenth century the king's treatment at this stage of his illness was remarkably sensitive. This sense is increased by the knowledge that George was expected to be a participant in his own recovery. In November 1810 the king had agreed to almost a contractual relationship with his physicians aimed at securing his recovery. This approach continued with the commitment to engaging the patient's consent to his management. The document for 27th February,[22] notes that the king had agreed not to use his attendants to send directions on his plans outside Windsor Castle. George had as part of his misplaced almost manic activity been in the habit of sending out instructions on alterations he wanted made to royal properties. In one sense he was only indulging his life-long interest in architecture, but the physicians feared that this activity served only to excite the king and make his symptoms worse.

It is fascinating to note how each little reverse in the king's progress was linked by his doctors to some external development thought to be preying on the king's mind. From the outset, with Princess Amelia's illness, emotional stress was seen as the driver of his condition. There have been modern attempts at statistical analysis looking for a correlation between politically induced or family induced stress feeding through to the king's mental ill-health. Of course George himself endorsed a link by acknowledging the relapse of 1810 was caused by the mortal illness of Princess Amelia. For this author the possible correlation between the politically induced stress and the signs of mental aberrations appear to be hard to justify. If there had been a direct correlation it would surely have come in the disastrous year of 1782 with the end of the American war rather than six years later when the king first displayed signs of mental illness? Family induced stress factors are interesting in theory as a possible driver for the timing of the king's mental difficulties. Doubtless the king was severely exasperated with his eldest son's debts but judgements on just what level of stress the king suffered by this and other tensions within the royal family are inherently subjective and in any case family based stresses would not necessarily have been recorded at the time and therefore be available now. The key correlation is that George did not suffer illness with recorded mental symptoms without attendant physical symptoms of illness at the onset of a crisis. While Dr Robert Willis, who was the expert mad-doctor amongst the team attending the king, could comment that the king's derangement fell short of insanity, he and his colleagues were unable to link the very real physical symptoms which the king displayed at the onset of each crisis and continued to display with his behavioural aberrations. It was an indicator of the limitations of medicine of the time that the physicians could not consider the possibility that the behavioural problems might be brought on by organic illness. Although had they done so there would have been very little they could have done.[23]

The daily routine recorded up to April 1811 shows that the king was in the habit of walking on the North Terrace at Windsor for extended periods with one of his sons. If they were not available then equerries like Generals Garth or Manners were available to see that George benefited from both exercise and sensible conversation. If they were not available then there was always at least one of the physicians to accompany him. Bedtime was early, but the record shows that the queen would sometimes visit in the early evening, but if she did not the king would often play backgammon with one of the physicians. It was a picture of apparently benign domesticity. Although George III was not completely better his physicians felt justified in reporting formally to the Queen's Council on 30th March in the following terms. 'We continue to retain the confidence we have hitherto expressed that His Majesty will completely recover.'[24] This statement of apparent confidence was not ultimately to be justified and for the doctors the issue increasingly was how long the confidence of eventual recovery could reasonably be sustained.

The process of recording and reporting the progress of the king's illness had many levels. There were statements made for the public which were published in the newspapers. These began as a daily process but moved to a weekly rhythm. The physicians drew up these statements and in hindsight they could be seen as masterly examples of bland obfuscation yet there is something impressive in the way that the public statements did convey a sense of the progress or reverses in the king's condition without intruding on his privacy. The daily reports to the Queen's Council were more detailed, but even these show a restraint which was in part probably driven by a discretion which considered it better not to include in the formal record insights into the king's illness which would potentially undermine his constitutional position following recovery or which would cause embarrassment to relations between the king and his family and official contacts. These reports therefore contained nothing of the detail of the king's sometimes outrageous utterances or actions. Instead such details were contained within the generic statements on continuing 'errors' or 'delusions' and indeed were allowed to pass into the public statements when it was thought appropriate. There was also an element of defensiveness, particularly as time went by, when the physicians seem blandly to have reasserted their confidence in ultimate recovery when the timespan for previous recoveries was long passed. Behind all these official communications on the patient's condition lay individual doctor's own notes of the case. These again were discreet about the detail of the king's behaviour, but nevertheless convey a very clear picture of the reality the physicians were dealing with. The daily notes in edited form provided the basis for the daily reports to the Queen's Council. There were also reports direct to members of the royal family. The Prince Regent asked for briefings from time to time, while Dr Robert Willis sent notes direct to Queen Charlotte at periods of particular sensitivity in her husband's illness.

The physicians' records have largely survived in the case of Robert Willis. They were probably the subject of some editing compared with the rough notes which were probably written in real time and then destroyed. These included contributions made by the keepers who attended the king on a continuous basis during his illness. An example of this most basic level of recording survives in the Lambeth Palace Library. The key point about the contemporary doctors' records is that they include the medication which was administered to the king. This is an important detail which is notable for its absence in the formal reports to the Queen's Council and in the public statements. The fact that anything was administered was reduced to the generic term of 'medicine'. Yet even here a potential trap lies for the modern reader. In the context of the treatment of the insane in the late eighteenth and early nineteenth centuries 'medicine' had a specific meaning. It signified variations in the application of the awful triumvirate of bleeding, purging and vomiting. George certainly experienced all these treatments with regularity, but in addition he was also prescribed remedies which were closer to a modern understanding of the term medicine. The actual details of what was being administered are not immediately accessible to a modern reader and would not have been accessible to a non-specialist reader even at the time. The record was kept in Latin with frequent, and at the time understood, abbreviations generally employed by the medical profession. What the record points to is that George III was given a daily a mixture of opiates, antimony and other substances including mercury which amounted to a toxic mixture with a potentially disastrous cumulative impact. The impact of this, particularly over time, could be an important element in explaining why the king did not recover as he had so confidently been expected to do when the crisis hit him in November 1810. A more detailed account of the treatment George experienced is set out in chapter eight.

The high point in the king's recovery seems to have come in the period of late March to early April 1811. For the most part the king functioned perfectly well within the confines of Windsor. As a private citizen in an affluent family he could probably have led a reasonably 'normal' life. As the king, he was subject to more exacting standards. As head of state he had an important public role and his constitutional duties underpinned the political process. The physicians who would take the responsibility for deciding whether George was cured needed to formulate a basis for taking this momentous decision. They also needed to be able to defend their decision if it proved to be wrong in the longer term. Two versions of an undated draft have survived which most probably relate to this moment when the king appeared to be on the verge of recovery. While the draft is quite short and simple the fact that it was drawn up at all seems to be another important pointer to just how close George came to being declared well.

The physicians were looking for basic criteria to establish that the king was well and that there was nothing of his madness remaining. Time and again the king's obsessions and delusions had been the basis for determining that he was mentally ill. It was logical that the absence of these obsessions should be the basis for determining he was well again. As before the physicians appear not to have wanted to act in isolation. George himself was to have been brought in again in almost a contractual agreement. The first point was that all allusion to 'a certain Lady' should end. The second was that the king should agree to undertake no alterations to royal buildings or other schemes for a period of twelve months after he had been declared to have recovered. Essentially this requirement lay outside the competence of the physicians. They had no locus in determining what changes should be made to royal residences or whether a new order of chivalry for women should or should not be set up. The physicians were clearly aware of this and in a move of some diplomacy they sought to engage the king in underwriting the condition. By endorsing the condition George would be endorsing the credibility of the Queen's Council and of the physicians' assessment that he had recovered. In other words it was in his own interest to agree to the condition and to abide by it.[25]

So while great progress had been made there was not complete confidence that the recovery could be relied on and as the weeks passed the sense of doubt grew. There were brief flashes of the problem. On 21st April 1811 there was a 'palpable reference to the Delusion' while Queen Charlotte and Princess Mary were visiting the king. This happened again when the Duke of Cambridge was walking on the terrace with his father. In this incident the king was guilty of 'some indecency'. The physicians meanwhile were searching for some way in which they could further engage the king positively in the hope that this would get him over the last hump before complete recovery. Colonel Taylor who had acted as George's private secretary was allowed to attend him again – much to the king's delight. In addition George was allowed his keys again which meant that he could have access at will to his desk and papers.[26]

For the most part the king was normal and interacted happily with his family and visitors. But there were flashes of irritability and stomach pains which were reminders that the crisis had not passed entirely and that the illness had physical manifestations. The contrast between the official statements and the reality could be marked. The official bulletin for 27th April stated, 'The King is going on well.' The doctors' record of the day states, 'the whole day has been hurried and unsatisfactory.' The recovery was on a plateau and despite days when a ride in Windsor Great Park seemed to invigorate the patient, by 21st May the physicians were forced to admit to the Queen's Council that, 'the general impression on our minds is less favourable than we have lately been able to express'.[27] What this meant was that the king was not deranged all the time, but his grip on reality was slipping. The question was what the doctors could do for their patient.

The timing of the physicians' admission that the king's condition was deteriorating was ironic. On the 21st May George rode in Windsor Great Park. The fact that he was going to do so had been well publicised and a crowd turned out to cheer him and there was even a salute fired by cannon. What should have been a mundane event had caused a popular sensation in Windsor. The people of the town had been accustomed to see their king regularly when he was in residence. His illness was the subject of popular concern and many wished to take the opportunity of witnessing his walks on the terrace or his rides in the park to make their own minds up about the progress of their sovereign. George was out for over an hour. It proved to be the last time he was seen by the public.

Chapter Five

Relapse

'In songs I have heard it several times – "Beauteous Queen" who shares my love shall share my Crown'.

Mr Penlington – July 1811.[1]

The admission that the care of the king was in trouble had come gradually and reluctantly. As late as 27th April Dr Robert Willis had declared to the Queen's Council, 'I entertain the most confident expectation of complete recovery on the grounds 1st of the material progress which His Majesty has already made towards recovery 2nd of the absence of any new unfavourable symptoms, 3rd of the probability which exists judging from the similarity of this and former attacks that His Majesty's health will continue to improve till the recovery is complete.' Willis suggested no change to 'the current regime'.[2] Yet the Queen's Council Report dated 11th May recorded that its authors would have liked to have stated that the king was so far recovered that he could take up his duties again. However, they could not. Reference is made to projects and plans which 'had the effect of making Him more excitable than was desirable'.[3] The formal account seems almost trifling in its concerns for the king's aberrations, but at this moment of great sensitivity the reality was that the king's condition, particularly the physical symptoms he displayed, had deteriorated significantly. The Queen's Council made it clear that they wanted the king to be made aware of the report in the hope that it would encourage him to exercise greater self-control. In fact a confrontation was developing. It was clear that the king had been of the view that he had recovered and that he could both dispense with medical supervision and resume his royal duties. The king had spoken 'in cold and deliberate terms of resentment against the Queen's Council' on 5th May.[4] With the report of the physicians dated 29th May 1811 it was clear the patient had deteriorated and the report includes references to 'hurried and unguarded discourse'.[5] Ominously there is mention that the king was suffering from a fever and agreement that there was a need for him 'controlling himself and of submitting for a time to greater restrictions in his intercourse with his family and attendants'.

The crisis was brought to a head in an interview between the Archbishop of Canterbury and the physicians on the one hand and George himself on the other. An apparent eyewitness account of the meeting survives in the archives although there is no indication of who actually wrote it.

'June 1st 1811,

On last Saturday the Queen's Council together with the five physicians waited upon the King and the Archbishop stated that he was to read to His Majesty the unanimous resolutions of the Council. The King received them with great dignity and being seated requested the Archbishop to proceed. The resolutions were that H[is] Majesty would not be declared well until he forbore all allusion to the subject of his illusions – until he changed his mode of conversation with his pages + attendants. The Archbishop paused + the King said with all the dignity of a King. "I can if it be necessary do even this – go on my Lord."

On the third resolution being read stating that it was necessary to restrain him from any communication with his family – the King said with much emotion, "I can bear even this also because I know that separated as I may be from everyone else I am always in the presence of the God whom I adore. I would my Lord (addressing himself to the Archbishop) that you adored him as I do". When the Archbishop had done the King rose from his seat with great dignity [and] bowed them out of the room.'[6]

This account of a crucial moment in the progress of the king's illness is fascinating. The account presents the king as calm, dignified and apparently entirely lucid when presented with what can only have been the most painful additional conditions and restrictions on his already circumscribed existence. The Archbishop of Canterbury's statement had come at a time when the king had considered himself to be well. Under the circumstances his calm controlled response seems extraordinary as well as moving. It is evidence that even at a time when his doctors considered that his condition was deteriorating he was clearly not deranged. His ready compliance is a testimony to his commitment to getting well and the confidence he appears to have had in the treatment he had already undergone as being in his best interests. The problem is that there seemed to be little in the way of alternative treatments although there was agreement that unanimity amongst the physicians was important.

There was not in fact a complete consensus. The isolation of the king from his family and usual attendants was a very significant step and represented a fundamental reversal of the regime which the physicians had tried to maintain thus far. Although no one was using the word 'failure' it must have felt like that to the physicians themselves. Increasing isolation of the patient which is what the changes meant was a fundamental shift towards the kind of regime which the specialist 'mad-doctors' of the time would have prescribed. While George's benign daily routine of the earlier part of the year was swept away not all the physicians were in agreement with so drastic a change. Dr Heberden broke ranks in a letter to the Queen's Council dated 14th May 1811.[7] In his letter he stated that the king had had his normal daily routine completely changed. Heberden argued that George should be allowed a regime which was closer to his normal pattern. He argued that much of the 'error' in the king's thinking and expression was born of frustration from his boredom, loneliness and isolation. In what seems to a modern reader to have been a remarkably sensitive letter, Heberden emphasised the impact of blindness on the king's behaviour. In direct contradiction to the views of Dr John Willis reported by Lord Westmorland, Heberden argued that blindness deprived the king of the main route for acquiring new sensations and ideas. It was no surprise that George had turned in on himself. Unsurprisingly Heberden hedged his letter round with statements that he was not implying criticism of his colleagues and that his views were, at least in part, shared by others of his colleagues. With the passage of time his letter now looks clearly like an assault on the increasing dominance of the Willis perspective for managing George.

On the 31st May 1811 Queen Charlotte had written to her Council complaining that Dr Robert Willis had been put in sole charge of George III without the other physicians being informed of the change.[8] She went on to argue that in fact Willis should have been put in charge much earlier. The attempt to recreate, so far as possible, the domestic routine of the king was at an end. With some discussion the Queen's Council had by 11th June arrived at an order for a wholly new regime. The key to this regime was that no one should communicate with the king except, 'with the consent and in the presence of Dr Willis. Only excepting the physicians and Mr Dundas no one to be admitted to the King's apartments without Dr Willis' consent'.[9] The humane regime recommended by Heberden only two weeks previously had clearly been overtaken by events. The queen's agreement to the harsher new regime may seem unfeeling, but it was based on the lessons of experience. Her husband had become deranged during three previous crises. On each of those occasions George had recovered quite quickly under the Willis endorsed regime of seclusion. This time the king had not recovered within the timescale of earlier illnesses. Therefore by endorsing a stricter regime Queen Charlotte was clinging to the only course which she thought stood a chance of curing her husband. It is also possible that the queen considered that an endorsement of Robert Willis, whom she seems to have come to accept, was preferable to risking a greater role for his brother Dr John Willis or other specialist 'mad-doctors'.

There had also been some incident which had obviously rattled the queen. In her letter, of 31st May,[10] she refers to scenes 'on Wednesday last' which the Queen's Council members had witnessed 'with delicacy'. The reference to the incident is a veiled offer of thanks and suggests that the king had done something which had involved some kind of unacceptable behaviour which directly affected the queen. One possibility is that he behaved with sexual aggression towards her or that he had again referred to his 'preference' for Lady Pembroke as he had during his first crisis in 1788/89. It is interesting, however, that the queen goes on to argue that a doctor should sleep in an adjoining room to the king to ensure proper supervision of Willis' men. Clearly closer supervision of the patient had already been deemed necessary and the king's usual attendants had been withdrawn. It is possible that 'the incident' simply involved the king exhibiting such excitable behaviour that it had been necessary to restrain him and the queen wanted to ensure that this only happened when it was absolutely necessary. At the time such a development would have been viewed as a significant set-back to hopes of a recovery. Although the physicians had stated that they would only contemplate restraint under the 'imperious dictates of duty', that dictate had come with a vengeance. In addition there are references to the king being given Dover's powder which meant that he was dosed with opiates in an attempt to sedate him.

The physicians were still focused on curing the king. There were those, however, who considered their efforts inevitably doomed to failure. How far people in general considered the king to simply have been insane is not clear, but there were those in the wider society of the United Kingdom who considered not only that this was the case, but that there was an explanation for it. A striking example survives in the form of a letter which was written to Dr Robert Willis on 27th June 1811 by a Mr Cottingham who was living in Liverpool.[11] In his letter Cottingham drew Willis' attention to the fact that the wet-nurse of George III had been 'the mother of the late Admiral Smith who died yesterday'. The letter goes on to say that one of the Admiral's sons 'was confined twice in the lunatic asylum in this place'. The writer also says that a daughter had the same problem before going on to comment, 'there is perhaps reason to suppose that His Majesty may have imbibed into his frame matter from his foster mother that may have been the cause of the deplorable malady with which He is now afflicted'.[12] A fascinating example of a misplaced belief in the mechanism for inheritance! George himself was in no doubt of the debt he owed to Mary Smith when he stated 'to her great attention my having been reared is greatly owing'[13] and he gave her the position of laundress when he became king. That she was also the mother of an Admiral is not clear.

A rough paper of scribbled notes in the Lambeth Palace library dated 6th July 1811 provides a glimpse of the day-to-day reality of the care of the king at this crucial stage of gathering crisis.[14] It is unclear what the status of this document was. There are no annotations to indicate why it was written and why it includes contributions from some of the attendants as well as a short piece by Halford. It reads like a real time record of a short period – perhaps only a day or two – in the care of George III. There is a directness and an immediacy in the account which is in contrast with the more measured record in the doctor's log let alone the formal daily reports to the Queen's Council referred to above. Other parts of the document act as a summary of some weeks in the responsibilities of some of the attendants. The account is full of abbreviations and non-essential words are left out so it was not intended to be read by the Queen's Council or other official bodies. It is also important as it provides two distinct and each apparently unique perspectives of the king's illness. Firstly some of the attendants offer their perspective of their august patient's behaviour and illness. Nowhere else is their direct voice heard. Most surprisingly though is that the patient himself is given something very close to his own authentic voice.

The account begins with a note by Mr Penlington who was the head of the attendants brought in to manage the king on a day-to-day basis at the end of May.[15] His perspective is important as he comments, 'I am with His Majesty constantly in [the] daytime except upon occasion when [the king] is walking and when Dr Willis [is] here'. Here then is the person with perhaps the best perspective of the king's behaviour at the crucial time when his recovery stopped and then went into reverse. 'The King has expressed at length nothing is the matter with him' states Penlington who adds that the king resents his confinement and those who impose it on him. He observes, 'as is frequently [the] case in insanity the King displays the Irritability of temper and want of self-command' which is a 'feature' of his 'disorder'. What we see is in fact something of George's delusions about 'Eliza' – Lady Pembroke. 'In songs I have heard it several times – "Beauteous Queen" who shares my love shall share my Crown'.

Exasperatingly it is not possible to tie down the time-line exactly, but Penlington recounts that on a day when the Queen's Council were due to meet and report on the patient's condition, George was so confident that he would be declared well that 'he has said I should not remain long with him'. The king's confidence was misplaced and Penlington remarks that 'The degree of irritation I have observed in His Majesty is such that in an ordinary patient I would mark it as a clear symptom of derangement.' Penlington records the patient's 'bitterness' against the Queen's Council and his constant complaints against Dr Willis. Penlington makes an important distinction, however, in stating that George made no complaint against the queen. The frustration with the Queen's Council is endorsed in a separate note by one of the other attendants who says that the patient 'is very angry about the Council'. The king's frustration and disappointment at not being declared well during June 1811 is assumed in the official record. The attendants give a more immediate sense of the king's feelings from direct observation.

Penlington comments, 'I can't give an opinion on his probability of recovery. His memory [is] extremely good.' While Peter Hendry one of the attendants comments, 'Have been five weeks about the king' and goes on to say that the 'hurry' and 'irritability' had increased as time went on. The deterioration in the king's condition over the time Hendry had been with him is interesting. Hendry's reference to being one of the king's attendants for five weeks is consistent with a date for the paper in early July. In discussing the patient's behaviour of throwing off his bedclothes on waking early, Hendry illuminates the conditioned behaviour which the king had already succumbed to. It seems that the mere threat of sending for a 'Willis man' was enough to secure the patient's co-operation. Elsewhere Penlington refers to a moment when the king was in a rage, but was calmed by the hint that he would be restrained. This conditioned response was precisely what Dr Francis Willis had aimed to achieve in 1789 and which other practitioners such as William Pargeter had recommended. Penlington's comments exemplified the importance of achieving ascendency over the patient which conventional medicine regarded as essential at the time.

A further example of the difficulty of dealing with the king comes in a comment by Mr Penlington that one day the king had seemed to be displeased with him, '... next moment he said he thought I was a bugger and that he was obliged to keep his bum from me'. In a delightful almost ironic comment Penlington brushed off the accusation with the comment, 'I considered it as disease'. The account goes on to describe George wandering about his apartment, chamber-pot in hand and fully exposed, apparently entirely oblivious to his surroundings. The comment is made by Sir Henry

Halford, 'How often [I have] heard decent patients talk indecently in disorders.' Yet even at this time of returning crisis George was not deranged all the time. Mr Penlington records that, 'His memory is extremely good' and notes the king's remark, 'He mentioned to-day that the Council would meet tomorrow.' Oblivious as he might have appeared to have been to his immediate surroundings, George nevertheless had some grasp on what was happening to him. Which makes his confinement and the inability of the doctors to give him real relief all the more tragic.

The Queen's Council were at one remove from the actual treatment of the king, but the august men who made up the council were conscientious in carrying out their duties. Initially they relied on and accepted the optimism of the physicians who surrounded the king. The physicians were eminent in their field and enjoyed the support of Queen Charlotte, not least because they were all familiar figures to the royal household. As time passed, however, the Queen's Council began to exhibit some impatience with the continuing outward optimism of the physicians. The activities of the council did not operate in a vacuum. All the members were public figures and were linked directly or indirectly to the government. Lord Eldon, for example, was the Lord Chancellor and was responsible for determining the constitutional implications of the king's condition. Clearly the king's condition was deteriorating and was increasingly critical. By mid-July it was believed the king was dying.

The public statement on the king's health issued by the Queen's Council on 10th July 1811 is important. It was one of the regular quarterly returns which summarised the king's condition based on questioning the doctors. What is striking is the separation it demonstrates for the first time between the council and the physicians. 'That His Majesty's bodily health is but little disordered. That His Majesty's mental health is represented to us by all the physicians as certainly improved since 6th April and they appear to agree that neither His Majesty's bodily health, nor His present symptoms, nor the effect, which the disease has yet produced upon His Majesty's faculties, afford any reason for thinking that His Majesty will not ultimately recover.' Even by the standards of the time this was a prolix statement. It was also a potentially dishonest one too. The king's mental health was certainly not better than it had been in early April. He was frequently manic and seriously deranged. Mr Hendry's comment on the deterioration of the king was just one of many recorded at the time.

A new tougher regime for managing the patient had been introduced. This represented a ratcheting up of the system of isolating the king from outside influences which it was thought would excite the patient. Dr Robert Willis' response to the questions of the Queen's Council, which formed the basis of their statement on 10th July, was probably an attempt to justify the new regime of treatment.[16] He summed up his views with the statement, 'My expectations of His Majesty's final and complete recovery are as confident as they were on 6th April last'. The statement of 10th July demonstrates the beginning of some impatience by the Queen's Council with the physicians who had had charge of the king up to that time. 'His Majesty's mental health is represented to us' it implicitly goes on to say, 'And we don't believe them.' The Queen's Council was effectively placing the blame, for the non-recovery of the king, on the doctors. It is possible that the Council members saw no immediate end to their responsibilities. Change was inevitable.

The Duke of Cumberland in a letter to the Prince Regent on the evening of 16th July 1811 described the king as 'totally lost as to mind, conversing with imaginary persons, as he is constantly addressing himself to Eliza'. [Lady Pembroke.][17] Princess Elizabeth remarked to Lady Harcourt on 18th July, 'The doctors think there is no amendment, which is wretchedness to us tho' they are right in telling the truth.' She goes on to describe her father the king as 'the mind is blank to surrounding objects'.[18] On the 25th the Duke of York gave a very pessimistic report of their father to the Prince Regent. 'Everything continues in the same melancholy way. His Majesty was very irritable in the morning, refused to put on his clothes when desired to get up and continued to reject all food until two o'clock, when he told Dr Heberden that if he offered any to him he would take it.'[19] It is possible that the difficulty over eating was a reflection that George knew that he was being dosed with drugs placed in his meals. The sense of failure felt by the physicians is reflected in the Duke of York's further comment to his brother, 'Dr Willis [Robert] who I saw just before I got into my carriage, seems very much cut down and told me that if anything the King was a shade worse to-day. In short, appearances continue as bad as possible.'

In private the confidence of the doctors was eroded until it was clear they faced failure and the probable loss of their patient. Dr Robert Willis was briefing Queen Charlotte with informal and very frank notes on an almost daily basis. He was also in direct contact with Lord Eldon. In the longer term it was perhaps even more significant that he was in close touch with his brother Dr John Willis and was giving him a detailed account of the king's case. Indeed it may be that the shift to seclusion of the king was influenced by Dr John Willis acting through his brother Robert. It was abundantly clear that the treatment of the king had proved ineffective and that the physicians were at a loss to know what to do. It is interesting and to their credit that the focus of the royal family was still on trying to find a cure. Perhaps the best description of George during the gathering crisis was in the letter that Colonel McMahon, the Prince Regent's Private Secretary, sent to the Duke of Northumberland on 29th July. 'The King is quite emaciated, peremptorily and angrily refuses all sustenance, is even with the aid of opium without scarcely any sleep, and totally gone as to reason. It is now thought he cannot possibly exist ten days longer without some miraculous change takes place within that time.'[20] George was clearly in a manic state and his behaviour was fundamentally changed from the dignified man for whom his family was so important. Princess Augusta in a letter to her friend Mrs Williams on 15th August was remarkably prescient about her father's future. She said that the physicians were only treating his physical ailments while doing nothing for his mind. Her father could therefore 'last a long while'. The fundamental change in the king's outlook is exemplified in Augusta's comparison between his current attitude to his family and what it had been during earlier crises. She describes how the king had previously enjoyed his family contact and been saddened when the group had to break up after each gathering. In August 1811 by contrast he was listless and indifferent to family contact; a fundamental change from his attitude of only six months earlier.[21]

A process of further change was under way. This was not simply a move of desperation, but a logical response to the worsening situation in terms of the knowledge of the time. Until July 1811 the care and treatment of George had largely been in the hands of familiar figures to the king. With the exception of Robert Willis, they were not, however, specialist 'mad doctors'. This had been an important element in the benign nature of George's treatment for most of the time up to this point compared with his treatment by 'specialists' during earlier crises and the way the deranged were generally treated at the time. In the face of what looked increasingly like failure, the Queen's Council therefore reverted at the end of July to the specialists and began the process of approaching Dr John Willis. Queen Charlotte was informed. In fact, the royal family and the physicians attending the king had already anticipated this development. On 5th June Princess Sophia had written to Sir Henry Halford and mentioned the possibility of Dr John Willis being brought in. 'In my presence Frederick [Duke of York] mentioned to Dundas his dread of John Willis ever being admitted and Mr Dundas did not hesitate in telling him the horror he had of such an introduction.' Having spoken of her blood running cold at just the thought of John Willis caring for her father, Princess Sophia ended her letter with an emotional plea, 'Oh! Dear Sir Henry save us if you can from such an attempt.'[22]

Sir Henry Halford's response appears to have been rather less emotional and rather more balanced, but the underlying reluctance to see Dr John Willis involved was clear. In an undated draft or a copy of a letter which he had sent, perhaps to the queen, Halford attempted to balance his distaste for Dr John Willis and his methods, Halford's own undertakings to do what he could to protect the king from the specialists and his own strong desire to do anything which might help his patient. The resolution he came to might intellectually have been intended as a fair and balanced one, in reality, however, it was astonishingly patronising and displayed his powerful disdain if not outright loathing for John Willis. 'If Dr John Willis should state to his brother that he believes as an honest Physician that he could propose a plan of treatment for His Majesty which could only be executed by himself attending personally upon the King and if he should make it clear to my judgement that his scheme would be productive of advantage which his brother is not able alone to extend to the King' then Halford would be ready to stand silently by while Dr John treated the king. The problem, as Halford was soon to find out, is that he was no longer the arbiter of the king's treatment. The Queen's Council was in the process of handing authority to others.

Halford justified his opposition to John Willis' involvement by claiming official endorsement. Speaking of the king's aversion to Dr John Willis, Halford commented, 'The grounds of that prejudice have been examined by His Privy Council in the year 1804 and were held valid enough to ensure the Ministers at that time' should look elsewhere for assistance in case of need.[23] The Privy Council enquiry referred to by Halford was almost certainly based on the events of the earlier crisis of 1801 because John Willis was not engaged in 1804. One late nineteenth century account of the reality of treatment managed by the Willis clan harks back to the crisis of 1801, 'evidence, supported by Mr Battiscombe, a reputable apothecary at Windsor, of the very unbecoming violence employed upon the King ... and in the presence of the elder Willis by a person in his employ'.[24] A variation of the story in which the king was felled by a blow by a medical attendant appears in a biography of Lord Eldon.[25] John Willis certainly felt uncomfortable enough about the past to raise the subject of his alleged mistreatment of the king in 1801 in order to promptly deny it. It is possible that this background had been a factor in Queen Charlotte arguing for a doctor to sleep in a room adjoining the king's to ensure that he was not mistreated.

The Queen's reaction to the proposal to consult Dr John Willis was immediate and hostile as her letter to the Prince Regent on 1st August reveals: 'They came with a proposal of making Dr R Willis consult with his brother John upon the dear Kg.'s present situation, but not with the idea of seeing him unless absolutely necessary. Knowing the Kg.'s dislike to the man and the promise extracted from me of never letting him come into his presence or again into the house, I felt a great reluctance upon the subject.'[26] Queen Charlotte nevertheless went on to say that the length of the illness and the lack of progress in the treatment so far had persuaded her to agree. Her reluctance is palpable, but her agreement was of huge significance. Dr John Willis was regarded within the royal family as having mistreated the king during his management of the earlier crisis in 1801 and so the queen and other members of her family had promised her husband that they would not let him fall into John Willis' hands again. Queen Charlotte's agreement to bring in John Willis was therefore the surest possible indication of her desperation at her husband's failure to recover. It is worth noting what had happened in 1804 in order to have a context for the emotional charge of her 1811 decision.

In February 1804 two of the doctors treating George III during his third crisis, Drs Millman and Heberden, had been unhappy at the methods they found it necessary to use in treating their patient. They had therefore petitioned the Privy Council arguing that they considered it their duty to recommend that the specialists Drs Robert and John Willis be brought in. It would appear that Millman and Heberden considered the patient was beyond their control and it is likely that the king had been manic for an extended period and required restraint. The Privy Council had agreed the request and the government of Henry Addington had authorised Robert or John Willis to take over treatment of the king.[27] The Willis brothers duly responded and called together at the Queen's House [Now Buckingham Palace] on 13th February with the intention of resuming treatment of the king. They were refused access to the king by the Dukes of Kent and Cumberland. After consultations with Addington, the Willis brothers were withdrawn. That evening the Duke of Kent wrote to Addington and set out the reasons why he and his brother had denied access to the Willises. Kent said that he and his brother had given solemn undertakings to their father after his recovery in 1801 that if he had a further relapse they would never allow any member of the Willis family to treat him again. The crucial additional point he made was that if the Willis brothers were allowed to treat the king there was a real danger that the queen would be blamed and that it would lead to a rupture in relations between George and his wife.[28] After some manoeuvring in which Addington tried to keep everyone happy the services of the Willis brothers were dispensed with and Dr Samuel Foart Simmons was brought in from St Luke's Hospital in London. The result was that the patient was to experience the same regime of aggressive use of restraint; the only difference being that it was administered under the Simmons name in the place of that of Willis.

In 1811 the same scenario as that of 1804 was ostensibly being re-run. There was one significant difference, however. Queen Charlotte was protected from ultimate responsibility for her husband's care because the Regency Act had determined that the Queen's Council had responsibility for the king's care. So although Queen Charlotte may have considered that if the intention was to keep the king calm then Dr John Willis' presence was likely to produce the reverse reaction there were more important considerations. She understood that her husband's case was in new territory and was more serious than it had been in the earlier crises and that all possibilities had to be examined. The queen therefore forestalled any possible conflict with the Council by suggesting that Drs Thomas Monro and Samuel Simmons should also be called in.[29] The overriding consideration for the queen was to do all that was possible to ensure the recovery of the king. The simple concern for the implications of George's ultimate recovery demonstrates a touching belief on the part of the queen that all could still be well in the end and that her husband would recover. There was a lingering fear that she might nevertheless be blamed in the future.

She therefore insisted, as her letter to the Prince Regent of 1st August demonstrates, that the Queen's Council should keep the wider royal family apprised of what was happening and why. The urgency with which the queen wrote and her emotional involvement in the awful problem she faced is clear in her signing off to her eldest son – 'Pardon this sad scrawl but I thought you could not get this too soon.'[30] Indeed the introduction of the specialists provides a poignant insight into the relationship between George III and his queen. They had faced the dreadful probability that George would suffer a relapse and the king had clearly sought a reassurance from the person he trusted most to try to protect his interests as he saw them and to keep him out of the hands of the specialist mad doctors. Queen Charlotte has been described as cold, aloof and unfeeling including by some of her own children. Infamously some commentators have put down George's insanity to sexual frustration caused by Charlotte's supposed ugliness and frigidity.[31] Fanny Burney's insights during the crisis of 1788/9 demonstrate the huge emotional burden which her husband's illness caused Queen Charlotte. They also highlight the extraordinary self-control which she considered it was her duty to maintain. Undoubtedly as she grew older her temper and outlook deteriorated and she turned in on herself, but during the king's last illness she did not abandon George. She visited him frequently when allowed to, even when hope of a recovery had been abandoned by most people; including the physicians. For extended periods in 1811 and 1812 she was excluded from visiting her husband as part of the medical 'treatment' based on 'seclusion'. This was not Queen Charlotte abandoning her husband.

The issue of the introduction of the specialists also underlined one political reality. Although it was called the 'Queen's' Council, Charlotte did not have the final say in the treatment of her husband. It may have been a relief to her as discussed above that the ultimate responsibility was not hers, but the issue of the introduction of the specialists highlighted the fact that family ties counted for only so much. Ultimately the king had a constitutional position in the country and this meant that his illness was not a private problem. The problem would therefore be arbitrated by members of the constitutional establishment. The care of the king during his illness may have been a greater additional burden to their other responsibilities, but humanity was still an important driver in Queen's Council thinking. The Lord Chancellor commented in a note to his colleagues on the common-sense arguments for considering the use of the specialist 'mad doctors'. 'There is not a family in the kingdom, which, ... would not feel it incumbent upon them ... To take the Chance of learning whether other skilful persons ... [might] suggest any thing likely to be useful'.[32] It is also probable that the members of the Queen's Council had in mind one clear and very widely held view. This was that the longer insanity lasted the less likely it was that the patient would recover. There was a belief in the medical profession at the time that a patient who had suffered from insanity for two years was highly unlikely to recover. Indeed Dr William Black made a statistical analysis of the outcome for patients at Bethlem which demonstrated that after two years 'without lucid intervals' the chances of recovery were one in fifty to a hundred.[33] Such thinking would have been a spur to the council to redouble efforts to cure the king while there was still, in contemporary thinking, a chance of success.

Chapter Six

Bringing in the Specialists

'I have just learnt from the Queen's Council that they are determined to take Dr Robert Willis to town to consult with his brother.'[1]

Sir Henry Halford. June or July 1811.

It is convenient shorthand to refer to the specialists as if they were an undifferentiated group, but the reality was that in their desperation, the members of the Queen's Council were really thinking of one man. It was John Willis the Council were thinking of when they decided it was time to bring in specialists and Willis himself considered the call was long overdue. Yet there was still hesitation over finally deciding and openly declaring that the king's fate would be placed in the hands of Willis. So the eminent men of the Queen's Council determined on a consultation process which would explain and justify to government and royal family their ultimate choice of who should determine the king's medical care. The views of the most experienced specialists available were to be canvassed and it was hoped that a coherent and agreed treatment for the patient would be found and agreed. The immediate task which the Queen's Council set the specialists at the beginning of August 1811 was to assess the king and to make recommendations for improved treatment. They were given a case summary which had been prepared, somewhat reluctantly, by the Windsor physicians[2] and a series of questions was appended. The authors of the case summary may have hoped that the specialists would have to report back to them so that they could maintain control of their patient. This was not the position of the Queen's Council as the regular physicians were to find out.[3]

Dr John Willis made contact with Lord Ellenborough on 3rd August in Hatfield while the latter was passing through the town. Ellenborough reported on his discussions to his colleagues in the Queen's Council in a letter the following day.[4] John Willis wanted to achieve a number of objectives which involved a rerun of his lobbying through Lord Westmorland the previous year. He wanted to assure a prominent member of the Queen's Council that he had not been guilty of mistreating the king during the crisis of 1801. He specifically denied having 'roasted the king'.[5] He also clearly wanted to let the Council know that it was about time that the experts had been called in; although in this instance he meant himself. Even allowing for his having received commentary on the king's case from his brother, Willis seems to have taken no notice of the fact that the patient had suffered a further relapse and had remained ill for much longer than during his earlier crises. Significantly Willis considered he was in the position to assess and make recommendations on the king's case without even seeing him again. Of course he had treated the king before, but his diagnosis of 'nervous debility'[6] and the recommendation of a tonic look glib and suggest that George's case was going to be prey to complacency – even if the actors were new.

John Willis' comments made to Lord Ellenborough was not the only occasion in which he had voiced his own strongly held views on the management of the king's case. In a letter to Lord Lonsdale on 30th March 1811, he had remarked that if he was called in then to assist in the treatment of the king he would be angry as 'mismanagement has all along beset the case I have not the least doubt'.[7] While Willis had had to wait some months before the call did eventually come, the fact that the call also involved Drs Monro and Simmons was cause for further outrage. Willis clearly saw that the specialist mad-doctors were only being brought in because the Queen's Council were desperate. As he remarked to Lord Lonsdale on 5th August, 'This case was never before reduced to such a horrid state as it is at the moment. Never before was it so difficult to know how to do good'. Perhaps most maddening for Willis was the direction from the Queen's Council that the specialists should submit a joint assessment of the case. John Willis told Lord Lonsdale, 'I must submit – not in perfect patience".[8] Essentially Willis thought that Monro and Simmons were amateurs.

John Willis and Lord Lonsdale were regular correspondents at this time and the surviving letters provide important insights on both the physician as an individual, but also a clear view of what he really thought about the king's case. The picture of Willis which emerges is of a highly ambitious and self-confident man who saw his relationship with the other physicians as intensely competitive. He was disparaging about those who had been responsible for the king telling Lord Lonsdale on 23rd September, 'It's as if they had been playing at the game of curing, but not understanding the point of the game. They are obliged to ask bystanders what cards they ought to play.'[9] This is a great 'sound bite', but it hides a certain disingenuousness on John Willis' part. He was after all a specialist in treating the insane and it was in that capacity rather than as a bystander that he was being brought in. Perhaps the call had come late, but at least it had come. If a cure for the patient had been the point of the game, John Willis, as it turned out, had little in the way of new cards to offer. His dismissive attitude towards the ordinary doctors was however to translate into their eventual exclusion from the direction of the king's case.

John Willis was not the only one who was engaged in direct correspondence with members of the Queen's Council. Dr Simmons wrote to the Lord Chancellor on 23rd August 1811 and his fundamental message was an expression of regret that he had not been allowed to have the management of the king in November 1810. Implicitly he was arguing, like John Willis, that 'proper management' would have seen recovery achieved. After the self-serving statement, however, Simmons was actually more conciliatory than he had been the year before. He no longer sought sole responsibility and seemed to acknowledge the need for cooperation with the other physicians. Essentially Simmons was acknowledging that the king's case had become difficult and that recovery would not be easy.[10] The brief exchanges between Lord Eldon and Dr Thomas Monro were rather less focused on criticism of past endeavours and more on achieving 'effectual aid in this truly distressing case'.[11]

The Lambeth Palace archives contain a fascinating example of a wider public concern that the king's case had not been satisfactorily managed or resolved. George had been ill for longer than he had ever been before and there was some frustration that this might simply be because the issue had been allowed to drift because the king was old rather than because a more humane approach had been adopted to deal with the problem. The Archbishop of Canterbury received a letter dated 20th August 1811 which addressed this issue in very direct terms. The author is 'EH' who apparently lived near Stevenage given the postmark of the letter. Essentially 'EH' accused the Queen's Council and the physicians of having given up on the king's case as a 'lost cause'. He points out that the king had been cured twice by 'Old Doctor Willis' with the aid of Dr John Willis but that for spurious reasons of wanting to avoid irritating the king Dr John had not been brought back. In disobliging terms Dr Robert Willis is written off as seeking employment and personal advancement and that he was 'putty' in the hands of the other physicians. Even the royal family came in for criticism for 'turning their faces to the rising sun' of the Prince Regent and abandoning George III.[12]

The letter was clearly written by someone with some insight into the tensions and rivalries at Windsor and the reluctance to bring in the specialists. On one level the writer expresses a frustration and perplexity which many must have felt both at Windsor and more widely at the time. Why was the king's recovery taking so long? The letter also neatly encapsulates the crucial debate that was central to medical thinking on the treatment of the insane at the time. The conditioning and intimidation which had characterised the regime of Dr Francis Willis during the crisis of 1788–9 was no longer seen as the automatic choice for handling any patient let alone for the king. 'EH' seems to represent the old orthodoxy in dealing with the insane and was not sympathetic to the movement away from cure by intimidation and restraint as necessary fundamentals. In putting these views forward, 'EH' may have reflected a shift in the balance of the Queen's Council which was moving towards a return to the more brutal methods used during earlier crises. 'EH' apparently was not aware of the increasingly desperate battle which the physicians were waging to achieve even a semblance of order as the king slipped further into crisis.

The focus for much of the discussion between the members of the Queen's Council will have taken place in face to face meetings. Much of the correspondence generated by the Council will therefore have reflected the conclusions of those discussions. There are exceptions, however, and an example is the letter which Lord Ellenborough wrote to the Archbishop of Canterbury on 20th August 1811.[13] The style of the letter is conversational and it is clear from this and other letters that the two were friends as well as colleagues. Ellenborough argues that Dr Simmons should be allowed to give his views on the king's case. He says that the proposal is not that Simmons should take over responsibility for the king, simply that he should observe the patient and comment. It is implicit in the way the argument is put, that Ellenborough had an eye to the hostility of the regular doctors against bringing in specialists. There is a reflection of the real responsibility which the Council members carried between them in the remark Ellenborough makes that having Simmons' endorsement of the current course of dealing with the king would be valuable. This sense of the responsibility would have been emphasised by the knowledge that the isolation of the king was not popular with the royal family. Lord Ellenborough concludes with a prescient comment that ultimately the actions of the Queen's Council would be open to public scrutiny and that it was important that it was clear that no stone had been left unturned in seeking a cure for the king.

While Queen Charlotte had been persuaded that it was necessary and right to bring in the specialist 'mad doctors', the physicians who had been responsible for the care of the king since the beginning of the crisis were not so easily convinced. On 10th August they sent a joint declaration to the Queen's Council arguing that the introduction of additional doctors was unlikely to benefit the king and the process of observing the patient and the inevitable changes they would want to make would only be beneficial when the patient was better in his mind. In an apparent reversal of logic the established physicians argued that the specialists should only be brought in when the patient was recovering. 'Until His Majesty's mind shall have made considerable advance from its present state', they argued, nobody new should be brought in.[14] There is an argument that change could work to unsettle the king further and doubtless there will have been some concern about bringing in rivals from a branch of medical practice which was viewed with suspicion by mainstream members of the profession. Henry Halford attempted to clarify the views of the regular physicians to the Queen's Council in his letter of 24th August. Halford considered there was no possibility 'of reasoning with Him' and that 'he must recover much of the ground which He has lost within the last two months'. He concluded that the king could only benefit from a regime of management 'directed almost exclusively to His personal safety'.[15] Halford's arguments were probably right in terms of understanding at the time, but pride, professional rivalries and a mix of personal relationships, which were both good and bad, were all factors in how the players responded at this crucial moment in the king's illness. Princess Sophia remarked for example, 'Dr R Willis smiles and grins and provokes me with his manner beyond what I can say'.[16] Doubtless Princess Sophia will have felt justified in her dislike for Willis, but her views will have added to the tension of the professional rivalries.

Contemporary notes made by Dr Robert Willis chart the decline in the king. At the beginning of August George had clearly been delusional with his determination to expel the Marlboroughs from Blenheim Palace so that Lady Pembroke could be installed. The obsession with Lady Pembroke continued with Robert Willis noting on 3rd August that the king had dressed with 'gloves on and his cane ready in his hand to go with her'.[17] There was a gentle almost genteel unreality in these examples of the king's devotion to the idea of Lady Pembroke. This was, however, at the benign end of the king's disturbed condition. By early September 1811 George was increasingly violent and uncooperative. The entry for 11th September gives a good feel for the difficulties of dealing with the patient: 'Slept four hours – very noisy and intractable when awake – restrained – conversation bad – to be himself emperor of Rome and Prince Octavius to be King – Dr Baillie reminded His Majesty that Octavius was dead, upon which He became extremely angry and insisted upon it that he was in the next room – the usual tirade followed and the conversation ended. Refused His breakfast and had frequent bursts of passion in the day – played on the flute and harpsichord – went to bed reluctantly.'[18] Octavius had died in 1783 but the separation from reality which seemed to characterise the king at this stage of his illness could take on an almost whimsical nature. For the 16th September 1811, Willis noted that the king claimed that he was going down the Thames with the intention of cutting off a neck of land at Shepperton so that he may pass more readily – going to Rome by Hanover. George I was to rule in His absence and to be accommodated at 'Col. Desbro's house and old Gascoign to wait on him'.[19]

The physicians were essentially locked in a battle with their patient. The king was subjected to restraint for long periods of time on a regular basis. Attempts were still made by Dr Heberden to retain something of the former humane order. He tried reading the newspapers to his patient and to engage him in conversations on new subjects but these were increasingly token gestures. The king could not respond and was only distracted briefly as he had apparently no powers to concentrate on any subject for more than a moment. He was clearly in a manic state and the physicians responded with heavy doses of opium and antimony in an attempt to calm him. In some instances the drugs were administered by force – 'medicine was given at half past eleven by force and with great difficulty'. Willis notes that after violent vomiting in response to antimony the king had been calmer and had been prevailed upon to take some beef tea.[20] The reality was that a grim, one-sided battle was going on with force, numbers and drugs on the side of the physicians. George had few resources. Willis refers to the king threatening to soil himself or to wet himself and actually doing so. He would also systematically throw off his bedclothes. How far he was aware of what he was doing is unclear, but the king's actions do look like a pathetic attempt to register a protest at his treatment. When there were moments of relative calm George was noted as relapsing into conversations with his 'imaginary friends'.

In fact the episode when Dr Heberden had read to the king from the newspaper had resulted in tale telling and recrimination which demonstrated that there was no consensus on the king's treatment amongst the king's physicians. Indeed the recriminations highlighted the divergences and went to the heart of the differences of interpretation of the impact of restricting the king's access to the outside world. Dr Robert Willis wrote to Lord Eldon on 10th September outlining the fact that Dr Heberden had read to their patient from the newspapers on the previous Saturday and Sunday.[21] The patient had initially responded with an interest and concentration which Willis had found surprising, however, as the reading continued the king had become 'more disordered and extreme'. Willis went on to say that the experiment had only been conducted in order to humour Heberden and would not be repeated. There is also the inescapable sense that Willis was asserting his authority over Heberden and the other physicians. His private record for the days on which the readings had taken place, records the fact of their taking place, but no suggestion that they had been wrong or had been disruptive.[22]

Dr Heberden did not share Willis' views and was not ready to let the negative report of the experiment with the newspapers go unchallenged. He may also have considered that unless he was to explain his thinking formally to the Queen's Council, the takeover by Willis would be immediate and complete. Heberden wrote to the Archbishop of Canterbury on 12th September,[23] but carefully avoided getting into a direct debate on the newspaper incident. Instead he argued that the seclusion of the king had become a problem in itself. Heberden again highlighted the king's blindness and said that he was deprived of the main source of real impressions of the world compared with most people. In assessing the king's derangement, Heberden focuses on the 'wrong ideas' which the king displayed. Rather than cut the patient off from all new experience which gave little alternative to the 'errors', Heberden argued that a plan for promoting 'right thinking' was needed for use whenever George was potentially receptive. For Heberden the sense that the king was tantalisingly just out of reach may have been a spur to a more active involvement with his patient.

Heberden's letter seems almost calculated to appeal to a modern reader. It is patient centric and tries to offer an alternative to the almost punishment regime which was being imposed on the king. Heberden comes over as sensitive, caring and ready to experiment. He emphasises the difficulties which the king's case presents, but there is no sense that he identifies the physical symptoms which the patient still displayed as significant in driving the mental aberrations. It is a pointer to the tensions within the physicians who had been responsible for the king's care that they reacted sharply to Heberden's letter with one of their own.[24] They argued that Heberden's letter had not simply been a difference of opinion on the king's treatment but a piece 'which it is possible to construe to our discredit'. Clearly the physicians were feeling defensive about the failure to cure the king. For the Queen's Council, the differences highlighted by the divergent views of Willis and Heberden may well have strengthened the resolve to secure a consistent and long-term regime to manage the king's case. If it was to have any chance of restoring the king this meant bringing in the specialists and probably meant a commitment to control by the Willises.

The physicians attending the king were not, however, going to give an easy acceptance to the involvement of the specialists. They chose this moment to mount a rear-guard action lobbying the Queen's Council. In a further letter signed by all the physicians with the exception of Heberden they launched into a criticism of the decision to bring in the specialists, '... we are still astonished that the present moment should have been chosen as that in which a consultation with the extraordinary physicians would be most useful'. The letter goes on to say that what can be achieved was being done by the physicians who were already in attendance on the king. Essentially the specialists had nothing new to contribute.[25] This is a pretty ugly piece in which the authors combine a powerful sense of defensiveness with an arrogant assertion that they knew best. Whether they were more concerned at the admission of failure which the introduction of outsiders implied or whether financial gain was a concern is not clear. The reality was that they had neither the knowledge nor the resources to treat their patient. Their fault lay in their inability to admit their limitations. Ironically Queen Charlotte drew attention to the one doctor who admitted his difficulties in assessing and treating the king. In her letter to the Archbishop of Canterbury on 18th September she strongly criticised Heberden's recent clash with the other doctors, but reserved special criticism for his admission to a Parliamentary Committee that he, 'did not understand the complaint'. The queen was clearly under pressure as she observed her husband's decline. It is unfortunate that she chose to attack the one physician who was actually questioning whether the king was really suffering from a straightforward episode of insanity and whether the doctors were equipped to treat him.[26]

While the generalist doctors who had attended the king from the start of his illness did not want to give way to the specialist 'mad doctors' they had nevertheless produced a case history to show to them. This history was dated 4th August 1811[27] and had subsequently been circulated to the specialists by the Queen's Council along with a series of questions which sought reactions and recommendations. The case history which does not mention the king by name gives a very brief account of the original onset of illness in 1788. 'A person of strong constitution and regular habits, had been afflicted about the age of 50, and twice since, with derangement of intellect accompanied by great nervous irritability which lasted several months before it entirely subsided.' The account then covers the onset and crisis at the end of 1810 when the patient had suffered a relapse.

Essentially the account is polite and rather bland and charts a steady progress, temporarily broken by paroxysms, towards recovery in May of 1811. At this point the patient retained some relatively trifling manifestations that he had not fully recovered so 'it was thought advisable to make a formal forcible representation to him of his errors'. This effort to engage the patient in his own recovery, which was witnessed in the account of the meeting between the king and the Queen's Council on 1st June, had the reverse effect to the one intended by the physicians and caused 'great irritation in consequence of which seclusion and confinement again became necessary'. The physicians credit their patient with a supreme effort of will which meant that during June he hardly mentioned 'his diseased notions'. The disappointment that he was not declared fully recovered in July was put down as the reason for the subsequent decline into delirium.

This is a carefully crafted document which seems almost to be written with at least an eye on the official record and posterity. The account seems to say that these people have done all they, or implicitly, *anyone* could have done for the king. It is almost as if it was written for the Queen's Council and that self-justification was the priority. There is the sense that because there was an explanation for the king's relapse his condition was understood and therefore manageable. The parallel with the original relapse and the death of Amelia is striking. The implicit conclusion is that the Queen's Council had panicked in calling in specialists. A section on the treatment administered follows which does at least demonstrate that there was difficulty controlling the patient's mania. The randomness of the treatment is betrayed by the paragraph in which the slightly unusual colour of the king's stools is discussed. Although the subject is raised as if it was significant there is no attempt to explain what the significance might be and how it might relate to the patient's illness. Ultimately the physicians conclude that the colouring was not outside normal parameters! The distance between the reality and the case summary is enormous. The physicians had after all expected their patient to die during July!

The responses from the specialists were to be no better. It was doubtless no accident that Halford showed the Duke of York the specialists' answers to the request for initial views on the king's case. It was in Halford's interest that the regular physicians should not be side-lined. Certainly York promptly relayed the specialists' views to the Prince Regent with the comment in his letter to the Prince of 28th September that the specialist's replies 'contain little or no information'.[28] The only thing they seemed to agree on, according to York, was to overturn the views of Dr Heberden. The rivalry of the specialist and regular physicians had been entirely visible at the time and had applied to previous crises. One historian summed up the rivalry as 'notorious'.[29]

The situation was desperate and Dr Robert Willis noted that the consulting physicians arrived at Windsor on the evening of the 9th October in time to see the king going to bed.[30] What was startling was the apparent cynicism with which John Willis appears to have approached his task. On the same day he wrote to Lord Lonsdale again and commented, 'the king is deranged – the Kingdom thinks themselves proper to sympathise'.[31] Drs John Willis, Samuel Foart Simmons and Thomas Monro began their formal process of observation the following morning. The process did not start well. A series of conditions were imposed on the consultants' involvement with the king. They were allowed, by appointment, to observe the king in his apartment. They were not, however, to make themselves known to the king and were not therefore to break the system of seclusion which was then in place. It was also implicit that the king would have been expected to react badly if he realised the specialists were present. The Queen's Council closely monitored the assessment process by putting questions to the consultants on a weekly basis. Interestingly the questions indicate that Heberden's concerns about the isolation of the patient and the impact of his blindness were drawn to the attention of the specialists. The responses are significant and echo over a much shorter period of time the mounting sense of disillusion and helplessness which had brought the specialists there in the first place. Initially the consultants exuded confidence. After their first observations they were able to combine an entirely reasonable statement that they had not had sufficient time to make a full diagnosis with, perhaps surprisingly, confident recommendations of changes in the medicines given or the management applied to the patient.

After a matter of days there was an implicit admission that the case was difficult. With refined disingenuousness the consultants claimed, after further observations, that they had had insufficient time to make an 'exact' diagnosis or to assess the 'full extent' of the illness. There was a tacit admission that George's case presented difficulties, but a determination to avoid admitting that they did not know what to do. The consultants' initial certainty, that their recommendations for changes in management or medicine would be effective, were fast eroded to the hope that they might be helpful. Ultimately they had to acknowledge that their suggested changes to medicine or treatment seemed to have done more harm than good. Even the sense that the consultants could claim greater specialist knowledge and might act unilaterally disappeared as they sought safety by arguing that decisions on the king's treatment should be taken in consultation with the physicians already in attendance.[32] The conditions imposed on the specialists were absurd, but in reality the specialists brought so little extra by way of expertise that it is doubtful that the limitations affected the likelihood of the king recovering.

Queen Charlotte chose 23rd October for a revealing letter to the Archbishop of Canterbury. She began by expressing her displeasure that Dr Simmons had broken some of the conditions placed on the specialists in their assessment of the king. She remarks that Simmons 'presumes to claim exclusive merit' in the treatment of the king, but goes on to point out that it is a matter of public record that the king recovered twice without any intervention by Simmons.[33] Simmons was obnoxious to the king and to the royal family, but Charlotte was not simply sounding off against the medical profession and the specialists in particular as a reflection of frustration at the failure to cure her husband. An element of fatalism was beginning to creep in. Noting that on previous occasions her husband would have recovered by that time and that no one could wish for his recovery more than she did, nevertheless the lack of a recovery could be 'Providence' rather than a lack of expertise in the doctors. This was not an admission that Queen Charlotte had concluded that George would not recover, but it was a tacit admission that this was a possibility.

Chapter Seven

Confinement

'Confinement thwarts every salutary purpose, and defeats every effort nature makes.'[1]

A Treatise on the real cause and cure of Insanity, etc.
Dr Andrew Harper, London 1789.

It is not clear from the official record how and when the Queen's Council decided that Dr John Willis should take the lead in the care of the king. At any rate Queen Charlotte was informed of the decision in a letter dated 4th November in which the Council argued that having John Willis work in conjunction with his brother Robert offered the best chance of restoring the king.[2] Charlotte agreed in a long letter dated 10th November[3] adding a postscript that if John Willis was to be appointed on a continuing basis then Drs Monro and Simmons need take no further part in the proceedings. In fact the two continued to observe and comment on the case for a short while, but essentially the Queen's Council had decided that if specialist help was required then the safest option was to return to the Willis clan. It was a decision in favour of the full rigours of 'seclusion'. It was also an implicit decision to marginalise the general physicians who had been attending the king since the start of the crisis. There was a further brief spat with Charlotte as Simmons continued to be engaged, but his involvement seems to have been a decision by the Council to be seen to leave no stone unturned in looking for a cure. The reality of the situation was clear, however, in the responses of the specialists to the questions put to them about the king's indisposition. Increasingly their responses reflected an ebbing of confidence that they could do anything for the patient.

There may be some doubt over the integrity of Dr John Willis in taking on the lead role in the care of the king. The Queen's Council had concluded that giving the lead to the specialists offered the best means for restoring the king. It would appear that John Willis actually doubted whether the patient could be recovered right from the start of his official involvement. In his letter to the Duke of Buckingham dated 28th November 1811, Sir W. H.

Freemantle included the following claim, '[Dr John Willis] says the malady is so confirmed that there is no hope of recovery or even of amendment; but bodily health as good as ever'.[4] Freemantle's comment may have been based on an exchange between Willis and the Duke of Kent on 25th November in which John Willis apparently told the duke that there was little point in his further attendance at Windsor.[5] It is possible that these negative views had an important impact on the Duke of Kent and prompted a search for alternative treatments for his father and to do so without reference to the Queen's Council.

In the midst of the increasing sense that both the specialists and the generalists had failed in their efforts to cure the king, a letter written by Princess Elizabeth may indicate that the Queen's Council were casting around for alternative courses of action. Princess Elizabeth's letter to Lady Harcourt dated 24th October 1811[6] contains the following section, 'the first question the Council put to Sir Henry Halford and Dr Willis was, "Do you think that by throwing buckets of water upon your patient's head he would be cured?" You may easily believe that they both answered these strange question and proposals the same; that no regular bred physician would venture such an expedient, particularly my father being blind; at his time of life they could not answer for the consequences.'[6] Elizabeth went on to say that the admission had been forced out of Dr Robert Willis by Queen Charlotte. What was going on is not clear. Part of the difficulty is that Princess Elizabeth's account is at least second hand. The idea that the possibility of some treatment involving water and surprise had been suggested or even was under consideration would have seemed reasonable at the time. Shock tactics were considered a valuable recourse in treating the insane in the late eighteenth century and usually involved sudden immersion in a bath of cold water. There is no reference to the questioning in the surviving Queen's Council record however. The surviving medical notes of Dr Robert Willis cover the period but make no reference to having been asked the question by the council. Despite the lack of evidence beyond Princess Elizabeth's letter the implication seems to be that the Queen's Council was looking beyond the immediate and obvious medical circles for more esoteric or experimental possibilities such as a cold water douche.

In Lady Bessborough's letter to her lover Lord Granville Leveson Gower dated 31st December 1811 she sets out the gossip of the day and includes a lively account of the reconciliation between the Prince Regent and the Duke of Cumberland following the spat over allegations the duke was reported to have made about the prince's own sanity. Lady Bessborough says, 'The Prince has quarrelled with his brother the Duke of Cumberland from hearing his saying that his brother's illness was higher than the foot, and that a blister on the head might be more efficacious than a poultice on the Ankle.' She then moves on to discuss the king and to relate her recent conversation with Sir Henry Halford. The account may actually set out something approaching Halford's private thoughts on the king's condition. Halford's account begins with a curious statement that 'His physicians [George III's] will be at liberty after next Saturday, when the last report will be given in, and so far as I can make out from him, is *merely* declaring the King incurable. Yet he says his *perception, memory and judgement* are as good as ever, but it is impossible to fix his ideas for five minutes to the same thing, as if ever he recovers enough to give any hope of material amendment, the consciousness of his situation throws him back again. This was the case in April last, when he seem'd to be as well as when he recovered in 1804.'[7] What Halford had been alluding to was the imminent marginalisation of the regular physicians and the imposition of the full rigours of seclusion. Halford's comments also highlight an important perspective of the king's mental faculties. George was clearly very ill, but Halford considered that his memory and judgement were intact and this suggests that the king was not senile or that he suffered from dementia at this point.

At the beginning of 1812 'seclusion' was in place. The regular physicians who were familiar to the king had been effectively side-lined. Their responsibilities lay solely with their patient's physical health, but even in this they were subject to control by the Willis brothers. They were allowed to observe the king but were not to speak to their patient or make their presence known. No one spoke to the king without permission from the Willises. The king was in an effective solitary confinement; exacerbated by his blindness. The purpose of 'seclusion', as has been explained, was to avoid the king becoming 'excited' by the stimulus of contact with family and friends. What was actually going on was a kind of sensory deprivation which today would be seen clearly as a form of torture. The Willises nevertheless claimed that seclusion had an immediately positive impact on the king's condition. Others disagreed and criticised the basic premise of the 'treatment'.

The impact of seclusion was not, however, the focus of the regular quarterly return to the Queen's Council on 4th January 1812. This return was important as the physicians attending the king as well as the two consultants Monro and Simmons who had continued to observe the patient were directly asked, 'Whether the disorder under which His Majesty Labours clearly amounts to insanity'. Despite Manfred Guttmacher's claims in *America's Last King* that the whole issue of insanity had been denied, here it was being addressed formally, officially and on the record.[8] The response was unanimous and unambiguous: the king was insane. Simmons even added that 'it is to be considered Incurable'. The other doctors were also pessimistic in their prognosis that the king was unlikely to recover. The responses on the question of the likelihood of recovery ranged from 'improbable' to 'very improbable'. During 1812 the only nuances in this very pessimistic assessment were in the movement towards the consensus that the case was hopeless by the end of the year. Dr John Willis perhaps jumped the gun when he used a little emotional language in describing the improbability of recovery in January 1812 and had rapidly to retract it in a letter to the Queen's Council.[9] 'Dr John Willis having recollected that he has unguardedly made use of an expression which he is apprehensive may carry a meaning far beyond what he intended to express would be happy if their Lordships would allow him to correct it. He begs to assure their Lordships that while he thinks the final recovery of His Majesty very improbable He by no means despairs of it.'

It was acceptable to officially determine that the king was mad. For the moment at least it was not yet acceptable to totally discount the possibility of recovery. John Willis nevertheless believed that there was no prospect of his patient recovering and it does raise the question why he was at such pains to retract the open statement of what he believed; not least because Simmons had openly stated that the king's condition should be considered as incurable. At this precise moment John Willis and his brother Robert were negotiating with the Queen's Council to take complete control of the king's case. Against that background his statement reads like a cynical attempt to avoid damaging the support of the Queen's Council and perhaps even indicates that his priority was to retain the income and prestige for 'treating' the king. He was to continue drawing the stupendous payment of over three thousand pounds a year until the king died in January 1820.

The regular physicians made one last attempt to counter their marginalisation by the Willis brothers. On the 8th February, Halford, Heberden and Baillie wrote to the Queen's Council complaining that they had been reduced to 'mute observers' of the king's condition and were not allowed to contribute to his treatment or comfort. 'We have sufficiently shown our willingness to bear the humiliation and indignity of being made spectators of H Majesty's condition without the power of contributing our services either to his recovery, or to his comfort.' They concluded that only a sense of duty precluded them from resigning.[10] Although the language remained restrained the very real breakdown in relations at Windsor between the general physicians and the specialists was complete at this time. John Willis gave his perspective in a letter to Lord Lonsdale. 'The violent kick back which we have some days been expecting has taken place betwixt the other three physicians and myself and my brother.'[11] The same letter contains the rather sinister statement 'the Council empowered us with disciplining power over the patient'. Restraint to control mania and paroxysms had been used when necessary on the king, but Willis' bald statement indicates that he and his brother were being given full authority in the management of their patient. This was precisely what some members of the royal family had feared when it had first been proposed to bring in the specialists.

While the Queen's Council had committed to the Willises they had not done so with the intention of excluding the other doctors entirely. So following a further intervention by Queen Charlotte[12] a series of Orders were issued setting up a roster for the regular physicians to attend at Windsor to deal with any concerns for the king's physical health.[13] The changes did nothing to soften the rigours of the king's seclusion however. William Heberden wrote to Sir Henry Halford on 12th February 1812 to recount 'a very long, friendly, and confidential audience[14] with the queen'. It was clear from the account that both the queen and Heberden were unhappy with a regime that meant that there was no-one around the king in case he improved and began to recover. Under such circumstances a sympathetic and familiar face would be invaluable. Crucially both were still thinking actively about possible recovery although it was equally clear that Heberden did not see the Willis regime as helpful. Heberden directly contradicted the Willis account of significant improvement during the first week of February. Instead Heberden saw this as the time of greatest irritability so far in the king. Any calming effect of seclusion Heberden thought was the result of dejection as the king withdrew into himself. Heberden's feelings were beautifully encapsulated in the postscript to his letter. 'Since writing the above, the K has talked more at his dinner, with some singing, much of his Queens, and not without grossness. Even this I like better than silent dejection.'[15]

It is possible that Heberden's discussion with the queen had reflected an indirect initiative to enable the regular physicians to regain direct access to the king. A direct approach simply demanding access independent of the Willises would have meant confrontation with the Queen's Council. Heberden's concerns about the king's isolation were not the dominant view, however, and this extract from Robert Willis' records while undated does seem to be a response to concerns expressed by the Queen's Council over the possible impact of the king's isolation. 'We believe that it has not been found by experience that deranged persons are apt to become imbecile from seclusion and the measure of amusement and intercourse with HM family which was ... to His Majesty was in fact found to be more than He could bear. It became not a matter of choice but of absolute necessity to withdraw the indulgences which were granted him.'[16]

As 1812 progressed a status quo and a routine were established. The Willis brothers had charge of the king's care and controlled access to their patient. They were nominally responsible for his treatment, but this amounted to management of his derangement and control of his mania. He was administered 'medicine', sometimes by force, but this was not given as part of a curative process. It was simply part of the process of containing the patient. His physical ills were ministered to by the three remaining regular physicians and the Windsor apothecary Mr Dundas. The process of regular public statements on the king's health was significantly scaled back. While neither the regular nor the specialist doctors totally excluded the possibility of the king's recovery, none of them actually believed it was now possible or that their ministrations contributed to the possibility of recovery. The structure which the Queen's Council had put in place represented a holding exercise in both a literal and a figurative sense.

For the most part the patient at the centre of the structure remains elusive. In both official correspondence and in the letters of family members he is generally referred to indirectly and rather remote terms. Dr Heberden provided a brief snapshot of the patient in a report he sent to the Queen's Council in March 1812.[17] In the report George briefly comes alive. Heberden explained that Robert Willis had been in London and that John Willis had suggested to Heberden that he might speak to the king if he wished. Heberden may have suspected a trap as he said he would speak to the king if he deemed it was necessary, but that while he did not approve of the system of seclusion, 'he did not desire wantonly to interfere with it'. If the system of seclusion was to be ended then he, Heberden, would be happy to co-operate. John Willis explained that he wanted to administer 'a powder', probably a laxative, to the patient. Heberden agreed to try to persuade the king to take it. It is worth going into some detail of Heberden's account of his exchanges with the king.

The king received Heberden with great kindness and said that he had not seen him for a long while. He asked after his family and referred to Heberden's sons by name. Heberden said that he had come from the queen's apartments and the king had responded by speaking warmly about his wife and his children. Heberden even mentioned that the Duke of Cambridge had been suffering from gout. So far the conversation had been warm and entirely rational. Suddenly the king spoke of Lady Pembroke and sang part of a song which he regularly applied to her. He then told Heberden that his sons were in the next room although Heberden did not know this. As the sons supposedly included Octavius who had died in 1783 the total irrationality of the king's assertion was obvious.

Heberden then introduced the subject of the laxative and a rational and compliant conversation followed in which the king said he would take anything which Heberden recommended. Just as quickly the king changed again and played the music of Psalms 100 and 104. He then drank Lady Pembroke's health while downing his 'medicine'. For a moment George comes alive and accessible again. In doing so this simple episode encapsulates the difficulties the physicians had in knowing how to deal with their patient. He clearly recognised Heberden and even recalled the names of his doctor's sons. So there was no serious deterioration in his memory. He was gracious in receiving Heberden and in doing so was true to his normal behaviour as a gentleman when well. Yet these manifestations of normality were paired with a sudden accession of energy during which Heberden took on the importance of a piece of furniture while the king played his harpsichord. A moment of calm followed in which the patient agreed to take his medicine, but did so with a toast to his imagined lover. Was this the king's way of mocking his doctor? These contradictions did not take in the violence and anger which were so often manifest in the king's behaviour and which required heavy doses of drugs containing heavy metals and a straightjacket to control. Essentially George was in a limbo where the pretence of a possible recovery had been abandoned and where a routine based on containment was systematically enforced. Heberden and Halford made one last attempt to have the rigours of seclusion relaxed in July, but nothing came of it. Conventional medicine of the age, both regular and specialist had failed. The Queen's Council which had been appointed by statute to care for the king had run out of obvious options. It was probably about this time when the king's family was coming to terms with the increasing likelihood that George would not recover that Princess Mary included the shattering comment in a letter to Sir Henry Halford 'No one who loves our beloved king can pray for his life if his mind is to remain as it is now.'[18]

Conventional medicine may have run out of options, but it was still well rewarded. Dr Mathew Ballie received over £3,000 each year for a decade for his care for the king.[19] Henry Halford received £2,700 for his contribution to the king's care in 1811.[20] and the other doctors can be presumed to have received similar sums. Over thirty thousand pounds a year were expended on the medical care of the king. For another seven years the king was kept in what was effectively solitary confinement. He did not suffer in the crude sense of the word and members of his family reported that he achieved a sort of contentment through his music and the inner world he retreated into.

Princess Augusta for example wrote to the Archbishop of Canterbury on 26th September 1812 and referred to the king as being 'happy in himself' and that he was sleeping well.[21] The relative calm which the king had retreated into may have given some of his family a degree of comfort after the earlier crises. This was not the same thing as recovery which is what the royal family had wanted and expected when the crisis began in late 1810.

At the end of 1812 George III remained officially insane with little expectation of improvement. The human being himself remained fleeting and elusive. There are many references to the king's memory, both short and long term, remaining effective while there were also several references in the contemporary correspondence and even in the medical reports to the king retaining his capacity for logical thinking. When he had, on increasingly rare occasions, access to external stimulus he took a sensible interest although his attention span was very short. The scope for any new initiative in the handling of the case was extremely limited; particularly from those charged with the patient's care.

With the passage of time it is not clear whether this was a rational accommodation of George III's limitations of illness and age or whether he was the victim of a stubborn adherence to a medical regime which while ineffective seemed at the time to have no alternative. It is noteworthy that he appeared not to have missed his family but after Heberden's account of his talk with the king it is possible that his feelings for his family had been internalised. Princess Augusta had remarked on the contrast with his behaviour during earlier illnesses. It may be that the king became institutionalised and unconsciously adjusted to the limitations of his existence at Windsor. However, the apparent acceptance of the situation was not complete within the royal family. There were those who were prepared to look for alternative ways of dealing with the king's illness, perhaps stimulated by the tantalising indications that in some ways his brain continued to function normally and that the personality he had always been was almost in reach.

The Queen's Council had brought in specialist mad doctors because the experiment of allowing the generalist physicians operating in a familiar environment had failed. For all the initial confidence in both diagnosis and treatment it became clear over time that the specialists had nothing better to offer in terms of diagnosis or treatment. By the end of 1812 therefore there was a recognition that George had made no progress towards recovery from his illness. Despite the promise of early 1811 when he had appeared to be on the verge of a complete recovery by the end of 1812 the patient was at best absorbed in a closed world of introspection, at worst he was subjected to extended periods of restraint and the forced administration of potentially damaging drugs. While the physicians understandably could not be categorical in their assessment of the king the language employed in reporting on their patient was a reversal of what they had used a year or more before. While the doctors said that recovery was not impossible, their approach to their patient was increasingly that of bystanders who no longer made any real claims that they could do anything for their patient beyond ministering to his physical needs. To paraphrase John Willis, if they had been playing at curing they had run out of cards.

The stage was therefore set for an alternative. Almost any alternative. And one was waiting in the wings which promised a cure for insanity.

Chapter Eight

What Orthodox 'Medicine'
Meant for the King

'The fate of a lately deceased illustrious and revered Sufferer, has offered an example, no less calamitous than awful, that neither pre-eminence in virtue, nor in rank, exempts us from the greatest of all earthly afflictions; mental derangement. Those feelings which so great a national misfortune excited, have since been repeatedly tortured by reports of abuses abhorrent from our nature, in the system of managing persons similarly afflicted.'[1]

An Inquiry into certain errors relative to insanity etc.
George Mann Burrows, 1820.

'It has been the general object of his Physicians to administer some tonic medicines, whenever he seemed to be in a state to bear them. With this view he has sometimes taken Cascarilla, sometimes the Calx of Zinc, sometimes the Bark, and for a considerable time took a compound of the extracts of Camomile and Poppy with apparent advantage. In the periods of excitement, it has been attempted to relieve the head by leeches, by cupping and by blistering, and to lessen the general agitation of the frame by tartarised Antimony and James' Powder, neutral salts and other gentle apericuts [sic] and sometimes by opium. He has likewise frequently used both a foot bath, and a general warm bath.'[2]

This concluding extract from the account by the royal physicians is a bland summary by any standards. It was produced under pressure from the Queen's Council and covers the clinical aspects of the case history which was to be used to brief the specialist mad-doctors who were being brought in to re-assess the case and to make recommendations on the treatment of the king. It did not acknowledge the increasing struggle the physicians had been waging to manage their patient and there is only passing mention of the regular employment of physical restraint. The royal doctors knew that they were facing failure and that the confident expectations of recovery had not been realised. Undoubtedly the royal doctors felt rather defensive in being called to give an account for their actions. They had opposed the introduction of the specialists and they continued to do so. To formally admit failure would have been enormously damaging to their reputations. It is also possible that there could have been political implications for the Queen's Council and perhaps even the government itself in such an admission. At the time it could have been argued that the specialists should have been put in charge of the case earlier if not from the start. Indeed this was precisely the kind of argument which the royal doctors feared they were likely to face. The document was therefore written with great care. The point was not really to give a detailed clinical history of the patient's case in the modern sense. Instead with the minimum detail the doctors were simply trying to demonstrate that they had done what was expected of them and had used all the recognised therapies available at the time for treating the insane.

For the most part medical treatment in George III's time did not involve particular remedies targeted against specific complaints. Treatments were generalised and relied on a mixture of 'cure-alls' like James' Powders, interventions such as bleeding the patient and tonics which were often rooted in tradition and were applied without any understanding of how they might be expected to have an effect on the individual patient's disease. Indeed much treatment by physicians in the late eighteenth or early nineteenth century was carried out in order to be seen to be doing something. Clearly this may have been in part a cynical way of justifying the physician's fee, but in part it was a way of giving reassurance to those close to the patient that all that could be done was being done. The very predictability of the physicians' interventions across a wide range of illnesses may even have been reassuring for the patient and had a powerful placebo effect.

Medical practice in the late eighteenth and the beginning of the nineteenth century was still heavily influenced by the theory of the 'humours'. Hippocrates is generally credited with systemising the theory of the humours although it probably predates him in its essence. Central to the theory was the idea that the four humours existed as four liquids in the body: blood, phlegm, black bile and yellow bile. These in turn were related to the four fundamental elements of earth, air, fire and water and the four seasons to produce a kind of universal set of relationships which explained existence. Good health was dependent on the right balance being maintained between the humours while an imbalance led to disease. Treatment of disease was therefore aimed at restoring the humoral balance. Some of this treatment could be benign, but some was not. The theory of the humours was of astonishing longevity and still underpinned much medical thinking 2,000 years after Hippocrates is credited with formalising it.

In the case of King George he underwent the treatment he did because that was the orthodox treatment of the day for the insane. The actual treatment which George received was focused primarily on containing his manic episodes. Tranquilisers in the sense that they are understood now, were not available so the physicians resorted to the almost mechanical options which were available at the time. Generically these were often referred to as 'medicine' and were the focus of attention during the hearings of the 1815 House of Commons Committee for Regulating Mad-houses. The horrible trio of bleeding, vomiting and enemas were routinely used as a crude sedative at Bethlem and other asylums and worked by lowering energy levels. Indeed the euphemism of a 'lowering diet' was often applied to the semi-starvation which was used to control manic patients in some asylums for the insane. Even the relatively enlightened naval physician Dr John Weir, who was an important expert witness for the Commons Committee and who will appear in later chapters, had recommended 'lowering diets' for naval lunatics at the Hoxton asylum.[3] So there was no doubt over the respectability of this treatment at the time.

While the impact of 'medicine' may have reduced George's energy levels, liberal use was still made of the straight waistcoat combined with a tight leather knotted gag in order to control the worst of his manic episodes. While the meaning of 'restraint' or 'coercion' would have been understood at the time and its use assumed in the treatment of the insane, not least in order to protect the manic patient from himself, it is perhaps worth quoting a single example of its application to George III. It should be emphasised that this treatment of the elderly blind patient was a regular occurrence as his relapse continued. The king was forced into a straight waistcoat and a leather gag with a 'large knot in the mouth tied tight behind the head over the face and eyes – remained in this state seven hours'.[4] Restraint was, at the time of George's final illness increasingly the focus of criticism and the target for reform, it was nevertheless still seen as an essential part of the therapeutic process itself by most practising physicians. A key example of a prominent practitioner who regarded restraint as essential in the management of the insane was John Haslam.

John Haslam was the medical officer at Bethlem Hospital for many years and was ultimately to be forced out of that position following the House of Commons enquiry in 1815. Nevertheless he was one of the most experienced practitioners in the treatment of the insane and in many ways one of the most thoughtful. His *Observations on Insanity etc* of 1798 was a seminal work on insanity while he is generally credited as first identifying schizophrenia. He was one of those who argued for the therapeutic value of restraint although his concluding comment seems to indicate limited aspirations. 'Restraint is not only necessary as a protection to the patient … it also contributes to the cure of insanity … habits of self-control are established in the sane and the insane by the same agents. That the fear of punishment or degradation which deters the rational being who exercises his reflection, from the commission of a crime, would in due time and properly administered check the outrageous sallies of the lunatic.' Haslam goes on to argue that this conditioning would 'curb his propensity' to act on his diseased thoughts 'although the derangement of his intellect still continues'.[5]

However carefully Haslam argued his case for the therapeutic value of conditioning the patient's behaviour, the underlying use of threats was obvious. It is not clear whether a similar therapeutic effect to that identified by Haslam was in the minds of the royal doctors treating the king. Certainly the threat of the use of restraint was made in November 1810 as part of the effort to 'persuade' the king into reformed behaviour. In reality though, the actual use of restraint by the royal doctors and practitioners more widely was the reflex response to the need to control mania rather than a carefully calibrated measure to return the patient to reason.

The House of Commons enquiry of 1815 was to expose the customary nature of much of the treatment at the Bethlem hospital with the reliance on bleeding, purges and vomiting. This was highlighted when the Commons Committee cross-examined Dr Thomas Monro who was visiting physician at Bethlem Hospital. Lunatics in Bethlem were bled at certain times of the year *en masse* and the spring was a notable time for this mass blood-letting. The MPs asked Dr Monro whether the seasonal impact of bleeding patients in the spring was important and whether patients were chosen specifically because they were expected to benefit. Monro's reply was to admit that the bleeding was done indiscriminately to the patients and that there was no expectation that it would help any individual patients. Monro's response was almost laughable if it did not conceal astonishing human suffering. It was also symptomatic of some professional thinking at the time that Monro simply did not see the significance of the question and it's potential to strike at the foundations of his clinical administration of the asylum. Essentially Monro admitted that it was done in the spring because it always had been done then and because it was too cold during the winter. As the third generation of his family to have occupied the position of physician at Bethlem Dr Monro could have been expected to have a respect for tradition.[6] George underwent a similar regime although in his case it was not combined with the systematic neglect which could be found in some of the public asylums of the age nor the shattering chaos which has meant that the popular rendering of Bethlem has passed into the English language as the encapsulation of chaos – 'Bedlam'.

Traditional tonics would not have been directly harmful although they would not have affected the king's supposed insanity. The physicians claimed 'apparent advantage' for the tonics, but there is no indication of what the advantage had been. This is unsurprising as there had been no attempt to identify the effect that the physicians were looking for in applying the tonics. Generally, they would have been innocuous and would not have represented a significant danger to the patient. Most tonics of the day would have been based on turmeric, saffron, cinnamon, nutmeg, cloves, cardamom and plenty of sugar and would have been drawn from one of the *pharmacopeias* which were a standard resource of the medical profession at the time.[7] Quinine, or 'the bark', is an obvious exception to the innocuous tonics. It is the traditional treatment for malaria, but in the early nineteenth century had in many societies acquired broader application in the treatment of fevers. Quinine can have serious side effects, particularly in the crude ground form that would have been administered to George III, which is one reason why it has been replaced by a synthetic which causes fewer problems. Ironically many of the side-effects of quinine are analogous to the physical symptoms which the king's physicians were trying to manage. Nausea, constipation and restlessness were relatively benign compared with the danger of increased heart rate or damage to the kidneys.

The mechanical treatments such as bleeding, blistering and cupping were again rather general weapons in the armoury of Georgian medicine, but were rather less benign than the tonics. Cupping, which has recently undergone something of a celebrity vogue, is of ancient origin. Current practitioners trace the origins to the ancient Chinese although it was probably used first in ancient Egypt. For George III's physicians the justification for use lay in the endorsement by Hippocrates. This was not a treatment which was regarded as specific to the treatment of the insane. It was, however, associated with the idea of removing poison by drawing out impurities from a patient with an assumed benefit. There is no evidence that cupping has any value although the explanation for its use which the Georgians would have given has proved remarkably persistent.[8] The problem for the case of the king was that cupping frequently caused skin irritations and could cause open wounds, particularly if it was combined with scarification which involved puncturing the skin at the site with a needle or fine scalpel, which could become the site of infection. This was particularly the case as the king was cupped many times and often in the same place. Even if the Georgian practitioners believed that cupping drew off toxins, they must have known that the process caused irritation which was not going to contribute to the tranquillity of the patient.

Bleeding, or the use of leeches, was applied to a wide range of ailments. Again it was a practice which had ancient origins in Egypt. Taken up by the Greeks, blood-letting fitted with the belief in the need to keep the four humours in balance and that much illness was caused by an excess of blood. It was believed that one cause of insanity, particularly for sufferers with manic tendencies, was an excess of animal spirits which was associated with an excess of blood in the brain. The removal of some of the patient's blood was therefore thought to reduce the excess of such spirits. This was particularly so in the use of leeches around the temples of a patient's head which it was believed would reduce the excess of blood in the brain. There was also a sense that as with cupping the blood-letting could draw off some toxins. The danger was that the process would weaken the patient and in the case of many illnesses it could be directly harmful. With manic or deranged patients that weakening was a primitive sedation and a means of control. Therapeutic use of blood-letting in Georgian times often involved taking so much blood that the patient would faint. William Pargeter recommended, 'copious and repeated bleedings in the jugular vein will be the most advisable'.[9] The familiarity of bleeding patients with the lancet or leeches in Georgian Britain meant that the practice was accepted uncritically when used on patients almost whatever their complaint might be. If nothing else it was a sign that the doctor was doing something. Once again its use by the king's physicians owed more to custom and the need to be seen to be doing something rather than some direct therapeutic effect. Ironically George Washington died in 1799 from a throat infection for which he was treated in much the same way as George III was for insanity. In Washington's case he underwent multiple blood-lettings in a short space of time, enemas and a blister on the neck.

Blistering again harked back to the Hippocratic theory and the need to balance the humours. By creating an area of blistered skin using a natural irritant like mustard and then draining off the resulting blisters the expectation was that the bad humours would be drawn off out of the body. In reality the process was extremely painful and the sheer discomfort would surely have added to the aggression of some patients. An apparently routine reference to the use of blistering gives some idea of the actual application to the king, 'blistered him 4 times on the same place on each leg – twice on the same place on the back. Emetics and purges, two … On each side high in the neck are now open etc.'[10] 'Open' meant in this case that the site was probably suppurating. The awfulness of this single entry into the record of the king's treatment is staggering from a modern perspective when its potential effect is imagined on a healthy person. And this entry was routine! But in applying blisters the king's physicians once again were simply following the customary treatment of the day. From a modern perspective the idea of a 'treatment' which involved the real danger of creating the ideal conditions for an infection seems eccentric in a pre-antibiotic world. The general nature of this 'treatment' and its severe impact is demonstrated by the case of the king's granddaughter Princess Charlotte. In 1813 she complained of pains in her left side and was treated by Sir Henry Halford. He applied a blister. A week later the abdominal pains had gone, but the site of the blister was causing the Princess distress. 'Princess Charlotte is better than she was last week – tho' Her Royal Highness has suffer'd severely from her blister.'[11]

At least George III did not have to endure the use of setons. Setons were strips of material, often of silk, which were introduced into an artificially created wound and then agitated regularly so that the wound would not heal. As before the process was thought to result in the expulsion of toxins from the patient's body. There were many contemporary practitioners who considered setons should be used with patients diagnosed as suffering from insanity, as Joseph Mason Cox demonstrated in his *Practical Observations on Insanity* of 1813 and as William Pargeter had in 1792, claiming that they drained 'morbid serum'. Princess Amelia suffered two in her back in 1810 as she gradually succumbed to consumption so again this was a treatment used for a wide range of complaints.

The use of 'neutral salts' again falls into the category of customary medicine. It meant the application of purges which were a reflex treatment for the insane, particularly if they suffered paroxysms or mania. Purges, or the application of an enema, were, however, the normal treatment for a whole range of ailments so again this was generalised treatment applied to a specific illness. The idea behind purging was the general one that it provided a mechanism for expelling toxins from the patient. As with the lowering diet and bleeding, purging would result in lower energy levels and therefore could in principle have an impact on the manic stages of an insane patient, but it was an imprecise tool at best.

Control of mania was the key to the management of the king. The earliest signs of the approach of a crisis, as reported in earlier chapters, were signs of hurry in which his normal behaviour was subjected to a process of acceleration. In 1810 he had been overtaken by a frenetic and destructive energy which deprived him of sleep and involved talking uncontrollably for days and nights at a time. The recurrent element of 'medicine' which the king was subjected to was administered as antimony and was intended to provoke vomiting. Antimony is a highly toxic heavy metal. Its toxic properties were used until recently to kill or control the parasites involved in *Leishmaniasis*. The impact of antimony was relatively short-lived as it is water-soluble and is therefore excreted quite quickly in urine.

However, the antimony used medicinally in the early nineteenth century was not pure but was contaminated with arsenic with which it is usually associated as an ore. Refined antimony as administered to George III would have been contaminated with between 3 per cent and 5 per cent arsenic. The danger was exacerbated by the additional administration of James' Powders which had antimony as its 'active ingredient' if one can use that term about a quack remedy. The point is that the king would have been given additional arsenic through the James' Powders. Arsenic has a direct impact on the production of haemoglobin so if, as the main current hypothesis suggests, George was a porphyria sufferer, the regular administration of antimony contaminated with arsenic would have exacerbated the porphyria and increased its impact and extended the overall length of his illness.

The adverse impact of George's treatment would not have been dependent on his having been a porphyria sufferer however. The antimony-based medicine with which he was treated would have meant that he would have become ill, over time, with chronic arsenic poisoning in addition to whatever brought on the crisis in October 1810. Analysis of a sample of hair taken when George was on his deathbed has revealed arsenic at a level of 17ppm. (Note. 1ppm might be considered a normal level in hair of a person not exposed to direct arsenic ingestion.) Arsenic is accumulated in the body over time and is excreted only slowly. During the last twilight years of his life George withdrew in on himself and the need to treat his mania was lessened so that antimony-based medicine was not administered so regularly during the last five years of his life. It seems inevitable therefore that the level of 17ppm from 1820 was much lower than would have been found if a sample of hair from 1813 were tested. During the period from late 1810 until well into 1813 George was administered high doses of contaminated antimony on a very regular basis. On 21st April 1811 when George was as close as he came to a complete recovery, he was still dosed with antimony and opium. There were several weeks in which he was given it several times on a daily basis. This would be enough to have an impact on a healthy person. On an elderly man suffering a crisis in his health this dosing could have had the impact of extending his illness.[12]

Even if George was not a genetic porphyria sufferer the amount of arsenic he was administered could have been sufficient to cause spontaneous porphyria attacks. There is anecdotal evidence from the US of 'moonshine' drinkers suffering spontaneous porphyria attacks as the result of ingesting arsenic from their illicit distillations. Prosaically the arsenic is thought to come from solder used in the construction of car radiators which are subsequently recycled as condensers in the amateur still. The level of arsenic administered to George would almost certainly have exceeded the levels achieved by even hardened drinkers of 'moonshine'. The evidence of chronic arsenic poisoning is in the analysis of the king's hair sample. As with the effects of quinine noted above, the immediate symptoms associated with arsenic poisoning are difficult to separate from the symptoms of his illness. Stomach pains, diarrhoea and stomach cramps were all suffered at times by the king and were noted by the doctors, whereas discoloration of his skin or white lines across his finger nails would probably not have been noted as they would have been too benign to be of immediate concern.

The administration of contaminated antimony was not the only highly dangerous treatment which was used on the king. Opium was also administered on a regular basis, often in combination with antimony. An entry in Robert Willis' log for 7th October 1811 for example records. 'At twelve took Ant[imony] Tart Gr I. It produced no effect – at eight in the evening took another grain [of antimony] with 40 drops of laudanum.'[13] During the eighteenth century opium had been regarded and used as something of a cure-all, but by the start of the nineteenth century its use had become somewhat more targeted. The opium used on George III would not have been refined and would have contained noscapine which would have acted as a strong emetic. This would have fitted with the scenario of bleeding, vomiting and enemas set out above. In fact it was the sedative qualities of opium which were prized in its use with maniacs in the early nineteenth century. It was used to aid sleep and to reduce irritability. However, opium is less well tolerated by older patients and is highly addictive. Although opium can produce euphoria, this is usually overtaken by depression and withdrawal from social interaction is common with repeated use. Dr Heberden commented with sadness on George III's depressed and withdrawn state in a joint letter to the Queen's Council. Heberden's postscript commented that he was happier when he heard the king sing rude songs and talk about 'his Queens'.[14] It is possible that the use of opium contributed to the king's withdrawn state. Certainly mood swings are associated with opium use and with elevated or long-term use can produce considerable restlessness. Constipation was an on-going problem with the king and again the use of opium would probably have contributed to this problem. Opium did have serious drawbacks which were known at the time. Andrew Harper, a specialist in treating insanity, was troubled by the impact of opium on mania. His experience was that it could

aggravate mania rather than sedate patients with long-term use. His view
was to 'condemn the use of opium in mania as being exceedingly improper
and pernicious, not withstanding, I know it to be conventional practice to
administer it very liberally in this disease'.[15]

The summary of the king's case and treatment provided for the specialists
was not comprehensive however. He was regularly dosed with the innocuous
sounding calomel. This was actually mercury chloride and despite being one
of the most widely used medicines at the time was highly toxic. Humphrey
Davy identified the chemical composition of calomel in 1810 and warned
of its toxic properties while at the same time commenting on its potential
as a medicine. The comment was at the core of the balance which needs
to be applied to all medicines between the therapeutic effect and the side
effects. Calomel was the reflex treatment for syphilis by the end of the
eighteenth century. It was also very widely used in Gowland's Lotion to
remove skin blemishes. Calomel was also to have a career in treating the pain
associated with teething in infants during the nineteenth century and on
into the twentieth. A clear case where the possible therapeutic effects were
outweighed by the dangers! In the case of George III it was valued for its
purgative properties. Robert Willis' record for 12th October 1811 reflects the
regular use with the king. 'Antimony daily one grain and extract of calomel
twice weekly.'[16] The combination of antimony and calomel is again noted
in Henry Halford's letter to Dr Mathew Baillie dated 9th October 1812.
'I have ordered for purposes which Princess Sophia will explain 1 grain of
Calomel and two of James' powder every night and omit the bark at present.
I hope you will think this right.'[17] Not only was George III in danger of
chronic arsenic poisoning from the regular treatment with antimony, but he
was simultaneously in danger of chronic mercury poisoning. The possibility
of damage to kidneys, brain and intestines would have been very real and
would have been permanent.

Put bluntly, the treatment which George III experienced at the hands of
his doctors, almost all of whom he knew, liked, trusted and had appointed
would now be viewed as systematic torture. The obvious irony is that it was
happening to one of the most powerful men in the world at that time. The
royal doctors were not incompetent or sadistic however. It could not have
given them pleasure to have imposed treatment on their patient which caused
him such discomfort and which did not produce a cure despite the suffering.
George III was humiliated and demeaned. He was trussed up for hours while
doubtless feeling the excruciating aftereffects of cupping or blisters. He was
slowly but systematically poisoned. He was denied contact with his family
and familiar attendants and was subject to increasing isolation in an effort to

lessen the potential for outside stimulus to aggravate his mania. It is possible to look back 200 years with the knowledge base of the twenty-first century and to determine that the actions of the royal doctors were never going to have a positive impact on the king. The royal doctors, however, and the specialists who took over from them acted on the basis of the knowledge level which had been achieved at the very beginning of the nineteenth century. What is abundantly clear is that the therapeutic options available to practitioners in the treatment of the insane at the time were negligible.

Dr Heberden had broken ranks by questioning whether it helped or hindered recovery to remove the patient from his familiar surroundings. He had raised the issue of the king's blindness and expressed his fears that isolating him would simply make him withdraw in on himself. Heberden even questioned whether the king was actually mad at all. Essentially he was questioning whether the knowledge which he and the other royal doctors had was sufficient to justify their clinical actions. Heberden was clearly examining the impact of the treatments which were applied to the king and questioning whether they were all effective or appropriate. His doubts were echoed more widely in the medical profession. Others were pushing against the limitations of the therapeutic resources available for treating the insane and were trying to develop better alternatives. Of direct use might have been Edward Sutleffe's advocacy of ground ivy (glencoma) in the management of mania[18] while electricity was under active consideration by some practitioners. The fundamental concern emerging within the medical profession at the time and overwhelmingly among family and associates of those suffering from insanity in its various forms was over the use of restraint and seclusion.

What would undoubtedly be seen as torture in the twenty-first century was increasingly seen as unacceptable in the early nineteenth. Lest there be any doubt about the unacceptability of restraint, John Connolly described the reality of placing a patient in a straight waistcoat. 'There was a violent struggle; the patient was overcome by main force; the limbs were secured by the attendants, with a tightness proportioned to the difficulty they had encountered; and the patient was left, heated, irritated, mortified, and probably bruised and hurt, without a consoling word; left to scream, to shout, to execrate, and apparently to exhaust the whole soul in bitter and hateful expressions, and in curses too horrible for human ears.'[19] It should also be made clear what was actually involved in the employment of the straight waistcoat which was the relatively humane and more expensive alternative to chains. George III was confined for long periods of time. Eight or twelve hours of confinement were regular occurrences. This was nothing compared to the timespan which Haslam at Bethlem could contemplate with apparent equanimity. He commented in his evidence to the Commons Committee that he could tell by the hands of a lunatic how long he had been confined in a straight waistcoat. He would examine the state of the nails and had come across cases where the nails had come to resemble the claws of an animal because the patient had been confined so long.[20]

The patients Haslam described confined in straight waistcoats for extended periods of time were hopefully rare cases, but as Mann Burrows had remarked in the quotation at the beginning of this chapter enquiry into the treatment of the insane seemed to throw up just too many examples of abhorrent abuse whether it was physical or mental abuse. Andrew Harper was a kind of transitional figure in the treatment of insanity. He subscribed to the orthodoxy of the medical treatment of the age, but on the seclusion of the Willis regime he was entirely scathing. 'Confinement' he wrote 'thwarts every salutary purpose, and defeats every effort which nature makes.' Writing in 1789, Harper assumes a close personal interaction with the patient to be a prerequisite to any hope for successful treatment.[21] The royal doctors had written their case summary confident that in pursuing orthodoxy in their application of treatment to the king they would have done their duty. Increasingly this was not enough. '… since the time of Dr Willis, the once successful attendant on royalty. Low diet and coercion … have formed a favourite system of practice; and the patient, worn out by these means, has regained a state of imbecility; shewing occasional dawnings of recollection and thought of a temporary nature, supposed indicating a cure.'[22] Clearly orthodox medical treatment for the insane was increasingly seen as synonymous with abuse.

For the Duke of Kent and the Duke of Sussex the reality of contemporary treatment of the insane was unacceptable; not least because in the case of their father it was unsuccessful. They, like many others, sought more humane and effective treatment for those they cared about. This meant that they were prepared to look for alternative practitioners and experimental therapies; even if this meant going outside the realms of formal medicine for help. They were simply after an alternative to what they thought was bad treatment which didn't work. If that meant risking what would be called quack medicine they were prepared to accept that risk.

Chapter Nine

A New Approach to Insanity

'The doctors think very, very ill of the case, and give it a term which is a dagger to our hearts; yet we ought to be grateful that everything has been done that could, and that he does not suffer.'[1]

Princess Elizabeth to Lady Harcourt 11th October 1811.

The *Morning Post* of 24th August 1811 carried an open letter entitled, 'State of the King', addressed to Queen Charlotte. The letter, from a Mr James Lucett, was an offer to make a cure for insanity available for possible use on the 'Royal Sufferer'. Lucett stated in his open letter that he had tried to interest the physicians caring for the king in his curative process six months previously and to have invited them to investigate the process further. As a loyal subject of His Majesty, Lucett proclaimed his hope that the process would now be investigated. While clearly his first approach to the royal physicians had been ignored, Lucett now claimed he addressed the queen 'with the firm persuasion, that its adoption would be the means of restoring our beloved Sovereign once more to the society of his august family and loving subjects'.

Each of the king's previous illnesses had led to a popular outpouring of sympathy and concern and had prompted many to offer their often homespun remedies. The crisis of 1810 had been no different and remedies which reflected the kind of country lore which was rooted in ancient superstition and mysticism were offered. Windsor was inundated with suggestions of cures and offers of help and most will have come from concerned individuals from all levels of society. It is also likely that contemporary mystics and cranks made up some of this barrage. It is also probable that some physicians with an eye to possible professional advancement put forward possible cures in the hope that they might be allowed to treat the pre-eminent patient in the land. It was an over-crowded market which Mr Lucett sought to enter with his open letter in the *Morning Post*. If he was going to make headway in a crowded market and to overcome the obstacles of security round the sovereign and the resistance of the physicians who were already treating the king he would have to have something exceptional to offer, be very lucky, or both. The question is whether there really was anything to separate him from the crowd? He had by his own admission already failed once.

The claim that Lucett had already been in direct contact with the physicians treating the king is significant. His claimed chronology would take his action back to February 1811. This was precisely when it had appeared that the king was rapidly recovering. It is likely that at that time the physicians would have considered they needed no outside help, let alone the unsolicited help of someone who made no claim that he was even a qualified doctor. As has been seen, the regular physicians had strongly opposed the introduction of the specialist mad-doctors in mid-1811 when the king had actually suffered a further relapse. It is almost certain therefore that they would have ignored any initiative by Lucett or anyone else in February or March 1811 when they felt confident that a little time and a final effort was all that was needed to complete the recovery of their patient.

Judging by the open letter in the *Morning Post* of 24th August it is unlikely that any earlier offer by Lucett to the doctors treating the king would have been put in a way which was calculated to attract serious attention. In the open letter he claimed he had access to 'a process that had been successfully practiced by a foreign physician on a Hanoverian officer who was labouring under a similar malady to that of His Majesty'. On the professional level there would have been no evidence that the unidentified foreign physician actually existed or was qualified, while the assertion that the Hanoverian officer suffered from a 'similar' complaint to the king would have been easy to dismiss as an unprofessional 'diagnosis'. The fact that the only evidence for the success of the curative process was apparently a single undocumented and therefore uncheckable case related by a third party would probably have enabled the physicians to easily dismiss any initiative by the unknown Lucett in early 1811. Lucett's commentary might at best have been seen as the offer of a quack, but more likely it would have been seen simply as a nuisance if it was noticed at all. In August 1811 Lucett's offer in the open letter still had little to recommend it even after the king had suffered a relapse. It should have sunk without trace.

Lucett was made of sterner stuff than most of those who offered their advice or remedies to help cure the king however. On 27th September 1811 in a further open letter to the editor of the *Morning Post*, Lucett increased the pressure. In the place of a remote claim that the process had been used by an unnamed foreign physician on a foreign patient at some unstated time in the past, Lucett claimed that he had very recently cured insanity in a man who had been assessed as incurable by the medical profession. In a breath-taking show of confidence Lucett claimed in the open letter that he would bring relief to the king in twenty-four hours and a complete cure in a fortnight. Lucett was not quite so vulgar as to demand immediate access to the king, but he did clearly express the hope that the physicians could be induced to 'inquire into the process'. While Lucett's claimed initiative in February would almost certainly have been mistimed, September was a potentially more propitious moment as the physicians' confidence in a full recovery had suffered considerable erosion. Indeed, the quotation from the correspondence of Princess Elizabeth at the start of this chapter indicates that the doctors were privately indicating that the king would not recover. Lucett's claim for attention was also better made in September than it had been even a month previously. It was also made publicly and so was available to family and friends of the king not just the doctors who were treating him.

The open letter was reprinted in the *St James' Chronicle* on 28th September but contained what was in effect a blunt warning to Lucett of the barrier of scepticism he was up against. The text of the original letter to the *Morning Post* was replayed, but was followed by a statement from this newspaper. 'We should recommend that Mr Lucett be sent to St Luke's, where, with the consent of the Medical Gentlemen, he should try his process on the patients, and if he does not succeed that he should be treated as a patient himself.' The newspaper's comment was undoubtedly correct. Lucett would have to be able to prove his claims. That much was obvious, but the newspaper's comments contained the germ of an idea. He could prove the effectiveness of the 'cure' by testing it on real patients in an asylum; implicitly with the medical staff overseeing proceedings.

It is worth asking who the target audience actually was that Lucett had in mind with his open letters. He was unlikely to attract the interest of the professional physicians who were already engaged in the king's care and he probably understood this. Despite Lucett's claim that he simply wanted those physicians to evaluate his treatment there is some evidence that this was not his aim. In the second open letter he claims to have cured a patient of insanity. Clearly an important claim of itself, but perhaps the key point is that the patient had been someone that the medical profession had assessed was incurable. Lucett was in fact trying to appeal over the heads of the medical profession to the royal family directly. The letter is addressed to Queen Charlotte and in a literal sense she was the target audience because she was the most directly affected by the king's illness. Targeted with her were the immediate family members, especially the king's children, who were clearly appalled by the further relapse of their father and the return of the specialist mad-doctors. Lucett's message would not have been lost on the wider audience of the people of the United Kingdom who would also have noted the king's relapse and the failure of the medical profession to recover him. This wider audience would be important to Lucett in due course, but from the start he really seems to have been aiming for the top. He aimed to treat the king.

The timing of Lucett's intervention had not been the result of chance. The deterioration in the king's condition set out in the earlier chapters had been widely if not fully reported. The *Morning Post* of 15th July 1811 reported the king's deterioration and mentioned that he had suffered 'paroxysms' and that the 'indulgence which had allowed His Majesty of walking on the terrace [at Windsor] has been withheld'. On the very day that Lucett's first open letter had been published, the *Caledonian Mercury* of 24th August talked of the king suffering from water on the brain and clearly suggested that his life was in danger. The report even spoke openly that the physicians had to use restraint in order to protect the king from himself. This was the period when the Queen's Council was moving towards the introduction of specialist 'mad-doctors' in the hope of restoring the king. This too was reported in the press as the example of the *Morning Post* of 11th October demonstrates with its reference to the arrival of Dr John Willis at Windsor.

So who was this James Lucett who had so confidently claimed he could bring relief to the king in twenty-four hours? He had demanded publicity for himself and made extraordinary claims for his cure for insanity with his open letters. He had also invited controversy and he was soon to find it and it was to pursue him for most of the rest of his life. The *Examiner* for 26th January 1812, a popular weekly aimed at the educated elite, carried a statement which clearly reflected the views of Lucett. Indeed it is probable that this *Examiner* article was based on a letter to the editor written by Lucett himself and which had only been lightly adapted by the paper.

'Mr James Lucett, of the Bank of England, says he possesses the recipe of a foreign physician for the cure of madness which has hitherto proved infallible. By its operation the patient is thrown into a sound sleep: relief is obtained in 24 hours and the cure performed within a short period.' The statement goes on to set out that Lucett had drawn his cure to the attention of the physicians attending the king. With a touch of bitterness Lucett added that the lack of response reflected the physicians 'not thinking it necessary to enquire into the merits' of the cure. Lucett then adds what seems an extraordinary claim. This is that he had written to the Prime Minister to draw his attention to the cure and the apparent unwillingness of the physicians to take it seriously. Lucett even quotes the response he claims he received from Mr Perceval.

'Sir

Mr Perceval desires me to observe to you, in reply to your letter, that he cannot venture to recommend His Majesty's physicians, to permit any experiment to be made with regard to His Majesty's health which they do not themselves approve of,

 I am sir your obedient servant.' [No Signature.]

There is no indication in the article of what Lucett had actually written to the prime minister, but a fair assumption would be that it was essentially criticism of the physicians for their unwillingness to consider new ideas in the treatment of their royal charge as well as a restatement of the value of his own 'cure'. In fact, as it was to emerge later, Lucett had actually begun to treat patients with the help of a qualified doctor and the report of their treatment of one patient was included with the letter to Perceval. The Prime Minister's response was predictable. From Perceval's perspective everything possible was being done for the king and he was not in a position to intervene in the actual clinical treatment of the king. An entirely different version of the correspondence with Mr Perceval was to appear from Lucett in 1815 when he must have considered that following the Prime Minister's assassination, the new version was unlikely to be challenged. For the moment, however, Lucett's account was to continue its focus on the unwillingness of the physicians to examine the curative process which, he claimed, would bring relief to the royal patient. The *Examiner* article continues: 'Mr Lucett remarks that the Physicians aught [sic] not to approve or disapprove till they have examined the nature of the remedy of which they are now in complete ignorance.' The article finishes by saying that 'the King's physicians are not doing their duty in their refusing to attend to any other course than their own, which has by their own acknowledgement proved unsuccessful'.

The statement in the *Examiner* represents an extraordinary ratcheting up of the pressure of the earlier open letters formally addressed to the queen. It also represents a direct populist attack on the physicians for being closed to new ideas while manifestly failing to cure their patient. The argument that they were condemning a treatment without actually testing it would have had a popular appeal to natural justice. The focus was still primarily on the king and the need for new forms of treatment following the failure of conventional medicine. There is a sense though that the statement is also an advertisement, although it stops short of directly soliciting patients. It seems to mark a shift towards Lucett becoming a practitioner in the treatment of the insane although the focus is still firmly on the case of the king. It does give a little more information about the curative process than in the original open letters with the statement that patients were put into a deep sleep as the first part of the process. Against this though, the reference to Lucett being 'of the Bank of England' seems a puzzling inclusion to make for someone with pretentions to cure the most exalted patient in the land. Why would someone include information which seems to emphasise they were not qualified to deal with patients at all? Was it perhaps an inclusion by the *Examiner* itself?

The *Examiner*, which was resolutely independent at this time, soon went to work on the apparent inconsistencies in the Lucett perspective. An editorial dated 2nd February countered Lucett's claim of an 'infallible' cure for insanity advanced in the previous week's edition. Instead the paper referred to the case of a Mr Morgan whom Lucett claimed had been cured. The *Examiner* article states firmly that Morgan had not been cured although no supporting evidence for the dismissal of Lucett's claims is provided. Although a detailed account of the case, written by a third party, was to appear two years later which tended to support the Lucett perspective it could be of no help in 1812. Where Lucett appears to have been vulnerable to criticism was the reference to his having worked for the Bank of England. The *Examiner* did not, however, return to this passing reference. This was an important oversight by the newspaper and suggests that it must have been Lucett himself who mentioned the fact in contacting the paper. The reference would have provided the basis for enquiring into the background of this person who had pretentions to cure the king and perhaps for determining his suitability for the role.

Lucett was indeed a member of staff of the Bank of England and at the time of the *Examiner* exchanges was actually working in the stock office. The records show that he had joined the bank, or been 'elected', in 1797 and had been nominated by the Lord Mayor.[2] Candidates for employment by the Bank of England required the nomination of a director of the bank unless they qualified for the cadre drawn from the immediate relatives of serving clerks. The fact that Lucett had secured the nomination of the Lord Mayor suggests that he was from a prosperous background and that he had had a reasonable formal education; although not one which would have included any medical training. Given the lag between election and actually serving as Lord Mayor and because the date on which the application for election to the bank was submitted is not recorded, it is not clear who the actual mayor was. Sir William Anderson was elected in 1797, but it is perhaps more likely that Lucett's sponsor was the rather colourful Sir Brook Watson who was the subject of 'Watson and the Shark' a painting which records Watson's loss of a leg in his youth.[3] Watson had been the Lord Mayor of London in 1796 but was also a director of the Bank of England for several years. Watson had also had a role as a loyalist during the American Revolutionary War and his wife was awarded a pension in recognition of this service when Brook Watson died in 1807.

At the time Lucett joined the bank it was undergoing rapid expansion in response to the demands placed on it by the government in underwriting the war against revolutionary France. Between 1790 and the year Lucett joined the number of 'clerks' who carried out the work of the bank at all but the most elevated levels, had doubled. Candidates were tested for numeracy and literacy and their background was examined to ensure political and religious orthodoxy and presumably an assurance of reliability. Lucett's candidacy papers have not survived so there is no direct record of his family background or a perspective of him as an individual. His birth was later recorded as having been in 1771.[4] Lucett's career in the bank up to 1811, when the first open letter to the queen was published, appears to have been unremarkable. There is a record of him getting the normal salary increases which were customary and by the time he wrote to the *Morning Post* he was paid about £140 per annum in basic salary, although he may have received some additional allowances which were intended to help mitigate the effects of inflation brought on by the war.[5] What the record from the bank does not provide is any clue as to how or why a 40-year-old bank clerk, who was an apparently stable family man, should have considered that he was in any way an appropriate person to deal with the king's illness when the best medical practitioners of the age had failed.

Lucett and his wife Catherine Olivia Lucett had two sons and a daughter between December 1806 and September 1810. All were baptised at St Pancras Old Church which suggests that the family had lived in Somers Town for several years before Lucett approached the *Morning Post*. The two open letters to the paper gave Lucett's address as 5 Charles Street, Clarendon Square, Somers Town. At the time this was an up and coming area of new developments aimed at a solid middle class clientele. It was also apparently popular with French emigres and it is interesting to speculate whether his family fell in that category given Lucett's rather French name; it is sometimes recorded as Lucette. Ironically the area was to degenerate following the construction of Euston Railway Station in 1830.[6] There is nothing in the bank records to suggest that Lucett's intentionally public interventions on the king's case had been picked up by the management of the bank. This was despite the fact that the staff of the bank were required to declare their outside interests. Crucially the *Examiner* did nothing to pick up on the fact that Lucett was entirely unqualified medically or to raise any questions about the origins of the curative process.

Princess Elizabeth's letter to Lady Harcourt of 24th October 1811 had referred to the Queen's Council asking the physicians whether they considered that throwing buckets of water at their patient would be helpful.[7] No documentary link survives which points to the Queen's Council having responded to Lucett's open letters. Indeed it became clear later that the senior members of the Queen's Council were not aware of Lucett's existence in October 1811. Princess Elizabeth's letter does suggest, however, that they might have been actively casting around for alternative remedies and had apparently focused to some extent at least on water based treatment as a possibility. So while Lucett's offer was not the basis for Princess Elizabeth's comment, it did suggest that the care of the king was becoming a little more open to outsiders; potentially even including someone like Lucett. It may be that the formal declaration by the Queen's Council on 4th April 1812 that George III was not only unfit to carry out his official duties, but that 'his complete recovery is improbable'[8] may have acted as an additional spur for members of the royal family to seek alternative options for treating the king's illness.

While the medical establishment treating the king may have ignored Lucett, his persistence was to be rewarded. The records of Bethlem Hospital include that one William Harrison, a sergeant and bandsman in the Duke of Kent's former regiment, the Royal Regiment, was admitted to the hospital by order of the War Office on 19th August 1809 having previously been confined in the Hoxton asylum. On arrival at Bethlem he was assessed 'as an incurable lunatic' by Dr Monro and as 'one of the most outrageous patients in the hospital'. He was subsequently formally discharged uncured on 11th August 1810 and the sub-committee of the Bethlem Royal Hospital considered he was not a suitable candidate for admission to the hospital's small 'incurable' department. The intention was that Harrison should be returned to the Hoxton asylum. At this point the hospital received an intervention from the Duke of Kent who petitioned for Harrison to be admitted to the 'incurables' department. The hospital agreed to the request and Harrison was put on the list of incurable patients. Letters of notification were sent to the Duke and the War Office. The record is silent on Harrison until 19th September 1812 when the sub-committee on admissions of Bethlem considered a request, from the Duke of Kent, that Harrison should be granted leave of absence from the hospital. The request was rejected.

On the 26th September 1812, the sub-committee considered a further request from the Duke for permission to remove Harrison from the hospital. The sub-committee agreed on the understanding that the release was 'for the purpose of receiving other medical treatment'. The additional and rather important condition was imposed that Harrison would not be readmitted to Bethlem. The Duke of Kent therefore became formally responsible for Harrison. More significantly, Harrison was passed to Dr Charles Delahoyde and a certain James Lucett for treatment.[9]

The Director's Minutes for the Bank of England record that on 23rd October 1812, Lucett absented himself from the stock office and did not return. Indeed the management of the Bank only caught up with Lucett's absence in 1814 when a meeting of directors on 30th June decided that he should be sent a letter requiring him to return to his duties at the bank. Lucett had been receiving his salary throughout his absence! Interestingly, Lucett's response was to request permission to leave the bank's service which was granted. The fact that Lucett continued to be paid by the Bank of England, provides an interesting backdrop to the developing relationship with the Duke of Kent and to Lucett's eventual reinvention as a practitioner specialising in the treatment of the insane. Essentially the Bank of England had unwittingly been underwriting Lucett's career change and his involvement with the Duke of Kent.

Dr Charles Delahoyde meanwhile was recorded in 1799 as a surgeon and apothecary residing at 37 Mortimer Street off Cavendish Square in London. Insurance records show that he had been established in the area for some years and that he was reasonably prosperous.[10] The only account of the formation of the partnership is one written by Lucett in 1815 in which he explains that he rapidly realised that if he was to promote his cure for insanity he would have to do so in combination with a qualified physician.[11] Only then would his cure be taken seriously. There is certainly a logic to such an argument from Lucett's perspective; what is less clear is why such an arrangement should have appealed to Delahoyde. He was, after all, a qualified doctor and surgeon who was apparently well established in metropolitan practice some years before Lucett came on the scene. Three possibilities immediately present themselves: that there was something in the process which Lucett was promoting which suggested that it really would have a beneficial impact on the insane, that Delahoyde was not in fact so well established in 1812 and that he was on the lookout for any means which might improve his fortune, finally there is the possibility that Lucett was a silver tongued manipulator who simply persuaded Delahoyde to join him in an audacious plan to treat the king.

The *London Gazette* dated 21st September 1811 provides a possible pointer to what might have happened. 'Charles Delahoyde formerly of Alpha Cottage, Paddington and late of Mortimer Street in the County of Middlesex, Gentleman' was cited in a third notice as an insolvent debtor. The first notice had been on 14th September 1811. If this is, as it would appear to be, the same Charles Delahoyde then it would appear that however prosperous he may have been in 1799, a decade later he was in some difficulty. It is probable that he would still have needed some persuasion to join Lucett in promoting a relatively untried process. Clear evidence is not available but it is possible that Lucett was able to provide some financial help to resolve Delahoyde's immediate difficulties.

Lucett's account of 1815 does not explain how he and Delahoyde came to be partners although Lucett does repeat that he believed it would be advantageous in promoting the cure to have a medically qualified partner.[12] What is interesting is the confirmation that Delahoyde was a dependant when the partnership was formed and that Lucett had had to support Delahoyde's family as well. Some care is needed in taking Lucett's account entirely at face value as it was written after the partnership had ended and includes comments on Delahoyde's financial unreliability from the start. Nevertheless it provides some endorsement for the idea that financial difficulties explain Delahoyde's willingness to ally with the unqualified Lucett.[13] Lucett also claimed that Delahoyde had immediately seen the potential of the curative process. Whatever the truth was about the formation of the partnership the claim that Delahoyde had seen the value of the cure was one which Lucett could have been expected to ventriloquise. Delahoyde seems to have written nothing on the association with Lucett and his perspective of why he should have allied himself with an unqualified practitioner. It later became clear that Delahoyde was not the only qualified physician who had worked with Lucett and he had not been Lucett's first choice.

There is no evidence that Delahoyde brought specific experience in dealing with the insane to the partnership when it was formed. He was to work at an insane asylum after the relationship with Lucett ended, but it is possible that he was able to secure that job as the result of experience gained during his association with Lucett. Demarcation lines in medical practice were not very clear at this time. Lucett makes no statement about Delahoyde's medical capabilities, but modestly observes that he would not have been in a position to judge. All he does say is 'He seemed, however, to be exactly the man I wanted, and we quickly agreed.' Thereafter 'Our first care now was to establish the efficacy of the remedy.'[14] For that, as the *St James' Chronicle* had suggested, they needed patients.

In less than a year from an open letter in the press, Lucett had secured a medical partner in Charles Delahoyde and together they had managed to convince the Duke of Kent to support their efforts and to entrust a patient to their care as the chronology of the discharge of Harrison from Bethlem shows. Securing royal patronage could form the basis for a successful business venture in the early nineteenth century for any practitioner whether 'regular' or otherwise. This is before considering the potential impact of any involvement in the king's case. The Duke of Kent clearly had a direct personal involvement in Harrison's case which predated the relapse of the king or James Lucett's open letters to the queen. He therefore had a genuine desire to help Harrison if he could. Ultimately though, the involvement with Lucett was firmly focused on the possibility of finding relief for his father. Harrison would have presented an opportunity to directly test Lucett's claims while offering a chance of relief to someone for whom the duke clearly felt some obligation. A growing consideration for the Duke of Kent and other members of the royal family as well as for the members of the Queen's Council was the knowledge that the longer a patient suffered from insanity the less likely it was that they would recover. Although the recovery rate for people diagnosed with 'insanity' at the beginning of the nineteenth century was high, this was only during the first two years. Thereafter the recovery rate fell off until it became an unlikely development. This would have been a factor in the Duke of Kent's willingness to engage with Lucett and may also have been an element in the thinking that Harrison would be a good immediate test for the Lucett process. Harrison had been ill for more than two years.

Publicity for his curative process as the result of newspaper articles criticising the Windsor physicians for not examining Lucett's process may have prompted the Duke of Kent to make enquiries about him and ultimately to make contact with Lucett. This would probably have been through an intermediary in order to gather some insight into the practitioner and the claimed cure. While security would have been more relaxed than it is today the social separations of Georgian society would have imposed formidable barriers between Lucett and his target audience. It is possible that the first moves were made in late 1811 when the specialist mad-doctors were brought in to assess the king's case and the Willis brothers were given control of his treatment. However, it is more likely that the contact developed during the first half of 1812 when the Willis brothers had had control of the king's case for some time, but when it was becoming clear that these specialists had little expectation that their patient would recover. At that point members of the royal family might well have actively looked for alternatives. Uncertainties over Lucett and his claims would have argued for the Duke of Kent to say nothing to the Queen's Council initially. It is also possible that in the early stages of such enquiries the Duke of Kent would have been reluctant to be seen to second guess the Queen's Council.

Lucett was later to claim in a letter which he wrote to the Prime Minister, the Earl of Liverpool in March 1820, that he was able to cure Harrison over the succeeding three months.[15] What was actually going on was more complex and more important. There was a developing discreet relationship between Delahoyde and Lucett and the Duke of Kent which centred on the evaluation of the Lucett curative process. Initially it was a rather personal process, but in 1813 a transition began towards a more institutionalised and public relationship. Initially the Duke of Kent seems to have used his personal influence and military connections to secure the release of two members of the armed forces so they could be treated by Delahoyde and Lucett. It had been discreet and very small scale, but had shown promise with patients whose symptoms bore similarities with those exhibited by the king. In April 1813 came a fundamental change. The discreet testing shifted towards a more organised, methodical, even scientific evaluation of the curative process.

The *Oxford University and City Herald* of 12th June carried a reprint of a letter from Delahoyde and Lucett to the Duke of Kent dated 25th April which reported on the successful treatment of a patient called Moon and thanking the Duke for the introduction to a third patient named as Mrs Lancaster. 'Your Royal Highness will permit us to express our gratitude for your goodness in affording us another instance of bringing to the test of public experiment our peculiar mode of treatment in the care of insanity.' The letter concludes, 'We beg your Royal Highness to make such use of this letter as you may think proper and hope you will not be displeased at our giving copies of it among our friends (for which Mr and Mrs Lancaster have freely given their approbation) who cannot fail being gratified at our success in this instance as well as others that have come under your Royal Highness' notice.' The source of the letter in the Oxford paper was an article from the *Monthly Magazine* dated 1st June 1813 which had included a commentary on the curative process. The *Monthly Magazine* reminded its readers that it had been the first to report the success of Edward Jenner in using cow-pox as the basis for a vaccine for small-pox and then expressed the hope that this 'alleged discovery to cure the most heart-rending malady that afflicts human nature' will be proved equally successful. Whether Lucett and Delahoyde had had the Duke of Kent's prior permission to publicise their involvement with him is unclear. What is clear is that once the focus of the relationship was made public it immediately began to attract further publicity with replays and commentary. The comparison in the *Monthly Magazine* between Jenner and Lucett is an indication of the high level of expectation which had been created within the press at least.

The benefits to Delahoyde and Lucett of the publicity are obvious. If the pair intended to develop their own private practice then such publicity and the implicit endorsement of a senior member of the royal family would provide an enormous boost to such aspirations. The advantages to the Duke of Kent are less obvious. The royal connection would automatically have highlighted the case of the king in the popular consciousness and it is possible that it would be assumed that some agreement had been reached for Lucett to treat the king. It is possible that Delahoyde and Lucett's expression of concern that circulating the correspondence with the Duke of Kent might involve impropriety on their part could have been genuine. It is also possible though that the publicity actually reflected agreement with the Duke of Kent as a necessary part in the transition to a more formal evaluation of Lucett's curative process. An experiment along scientific lines implied greater organisation and finance than the discreet testing on a single patient at a time involved. This meant bringing in others to provide the necessary support. The shift to an open evaluation of Lucett's 'cure' clearly reflected real enthusiasm based on the initial trials. To test the cure more fully and scientifically required a much wider experience of the process and greater expertise in assessing the results of the trials. This was especially the case if the ultimate objective was to use the process on the king. Essentially if the Duke of Kent was serious about the trial and assessment of the Lucett process he had no alternative than to seek wider support and to acknowledge publically what was going on.

The Queen's Council had been set up under a provision of the Regency Act to ensure the care of the king while he was 'indisposed' and to take the ultimate responsibility for the head of state from his immediate family. Yet the Dukes of Kent and Sussex gave no notification of their involvement with Lucett and Delahoyde to the Queen's Council. The dukes were not trying to hide their activities as they did not deny their involvement or break off their contact with Lucett and Delahoyde following the publicity in the press. The reality is that the involvement of two of the king's sons in the evaluation of what was claimed to be a cure for insanity was driven primarily by concern for their father. The wider concern for the insane was secondary at this stage. Later correspondence revealed that it was assumed that if the evaluation of the Lucett process was successful then it would be used at Windsor. What the Dukes of Kent and Sussex knew was that there were formidable barriers against the use of any novel treatment with the king. The time to engage with the Queen's Council would be when the dukes could prove they had a better alternative to offer in place of dogged persistence with 'seclusion' and the use of restraint which undermined the dignity of the monarch.

Chapter Ten

Concern for the House of Hanover?
The Involvement of the Royal Dukes

'The proudest praise that man can give to thee
O KENT! Like thee may thy daughter be.'[1]
                The last two lines of *Monody on His Late*
                Royal Highness the Duke of Kent
                by Margaret Sarah Croker. 1820

The sense that the king was a prisoner of his illness and that his mind and personality were engaged in a struggle to escape captivity must have been very real to those around him and to his immediate family in particular. Fleeting glimpses of 'normality' came and went while flashes of insight suggested that George was to some extent aware of his circumstances; particularly during the earlier years of his extended decline. One of these moments of insight seems to have prompted the desperate pessimism expressed by Princess Mary when she said that she could not pray for her father's continued life when his mind was so diseased. In June 1811, when the patient teetered between recovery and relapse, he seems to have had a moment of astonishing clarity in which he was able to assess his own situation. That assessment was recorded by Princess Elizabeth for Sir Henry Halford. 'Poor dear man' she wrote. 'He said this morning very naturally, that could he have foreseen the length of this fever, he should have wished himself dead – it was very affecting – this passed in the presence of both Dr H[eberden] & Dr W[illis] but they say it came naturally, without anger or hurry.'[2]

Tantalising moments such as this when, 'without anger or hurry' George was able to put aside his illness for a few moments or when he was able to engage as a friend in conversation with Dr Heberden emphasised to the king's immediate relations that the man they knew so well still existed – even if he was just out of reach. In practical terms these flashes of normality will have acted as a powerful incentive to examine all possible avenues which might bring relief to the king. There are pointers to another important incentive to find a cure for insanity which was not acknowledged publicly. This was the possibility that a cure for insanity might be needed for other members of the Hanoverian dynasty.

Before George III himself suffered from 'insanity' his views on the illness were mixed. On the personal level he showed himself to be gentle and sympathetic when directly confronted by the manifestations of insanity as the widely reported incident of August 1786 when Margaret Nicholson attempted to stab the king demonstrated. Nicholson fell into the hands of the mass of people gathered outside St James' Palace and could have been very badly treated, but the king intervened directly shouting to the mob, 'The poor creature is mad! Do not hurt her! She has not hurt me!' George specifically ordered that Nicholson should be taken away and treated well.[3] George III's wider perspective was much more negative before his own first crisis in 1788. Indeed his firm belief that insanity was hereditary was a factor in the choice of his own wife. Princess Caroline of Hesse Darmstadt was George's first choice after the initial elimination process of candidates was completed. However, when reports on her character and immediate family were received the picture changed. The lady's father was described as at best very eccentric while the Princess was assessed as being ill-tempered and contrary. The language was veiled, but the meaning was clear. The sanity of the princess and her family could not be guaranteed and this candidate was dropped by George immediately.[4]

How far the disastrous marriage in 1766 of his youngest sister Princess Caroline Matilda to Christian VII of Denmark reinforced his view that insanity was hereditary is not clear, but the destructive insanity of the Danish king not only destroyed the marriage but ultimately led to the death of George III's sister. It was certainly a dire warning of the potential dynastic implications of insanity and one which had particular impact because Christian VII was Caroline Matilda's first cousin and therefore George III's as well. It seems ironic that care was exercised to avoid a connection with possible insanity in the case of George himself, but the same care was not taken with the choice of his sister's husband and no reports of Christian's probable schizophrenia apparently reached London.

George III was dismissive of 'nervous conditions', a common euphemism for insanity at the time, which he regarded as largely psychosomatic and which in his view reflected emotional instability; especially in women. It was not a subject which he was ready to discuss widely, but Lady Harcourt was an important exception. George III had been dismissive of the case of Lady Harcourt's mother who was diagnosed as suffering from some form of mental illness and was treated by Dr Francis Willis. Yet 'he had a greater horror [of insanity] than any person I have ever conversed with' according to Lady Harcourt. His conviction that insanity was hereditary within families was crucial in the intensity of his thinking. Ultimately George III considered it was better for an insane person to be dead than to suffer the disease.[5]

The understanding of heredity by George and his contemporaries was limited. People had long understood that characteristics were passed from one generation to the next in most living things. There was, however, no understanding of the mechanisms involved. Mr Cottingham's belief that George III might have been 'infected' with insanity through the milk of his wet-nurse was not an uncommon idea at the time. Understanding the mechanisms of heredity would have to await first the work of Darwin and Mendel but ultimately for the work of Crick and Watson. It is difficult to be certain how educated Georgians viewed a subject like heredity, but it seems reasonable to think that there was a tendency to assume the simple worst. The view of Dr George Mann Burrows can perhaps be taken as representative of an informed perspective on heredity and its implications at the time. In the introduction to his book on insanity published in 1820, Burrows commented, 'There is certainly no error in accounting insanity hereditary'. He went on to indicate that it was 'commendable foresight' for people who were considering marriage to enquire about the mental history of their potential partner and their family before making any commitment. Burrows' comments not only confirm the hereditary nature of insanity as an abstraction but indicate the clear contemporary view that people should act to ensure that they did not risk carrying the problem into future generations. Burrows' view was certainly a clear contribution to stigmatising those with any 'taint' of mental illness.[6]

In the case of the king, once it was acknowledged that his illness involved insanity, the assumption, in the thinking of the time, would have been that his offspring were potentially vulnerable. The spat over the ill-health of the Prince Regent which involved him and his brother the Duke of Cumberland was recorded by Lady Bessborough as an intelligent and thoughtful observer. In her letter to Lord Granville dated between 8th and 13th December 1811 she observed, 'The Prince is, I believe, very ill. Farquhar [the Prince Regent's physician] says he suffers such agony of pain ... that it produces a degree of irritation on his nerves nearly approaching to delirium. What will become of us if, as well as our King, our Regent goes mad? It will be a new case in annals of history.'[7] George III's physicians had distinguished between delirium and derangement as important in determining whether someone was insane. So Farquhar's comment was not a clear statement that the Prince Regent was in danger of becoming insane. The point about Lady Bessborough's comment is that she was articulating concern from outside about the possibility that insanity might touch other members of the royal family.

Joseph Mason Cox in the preface to his book *Observations on Insanity* comments, 'Insanity unfortunately is not only frequent but said to be peculiarly endemial to England.' The view that insanity was particularly common in the UK was a widely held view for a time in the early nineteenth century. Cox's explanation for the supposed incidence of insanity was also typical of thinking amongst the members of the medical profession. He blamed, 'promiscuous marriages where one or both of the parties have hereditary claims to alienation of the mind are sufficient to explain the lamentable fact'.[8] The timing of Cox's work to 1813 was probably coincidental but there is an uncomfortable sense that it would have hit readers hard coming as it did when the idea that the king's insanity was incurable was widely assumed.

The question is whether there was any sense within the royal family that insanity was a problem which could go wider than the king. Given the rather limited and literal understanding of heredity at the time it would not be a surprise if there had been such a concern. Sickness was a commonplace at the time. Infant mortality ran at between 25 and 30 per cent by the age of five while life expectancy over all was consequently pulled down to around 42 years. In the pre-antibiotic age death came suddenly and often from what would now be considered trivial complaints or accidents. Even allowing for all this there was considerable even chronic ill-health in the offspring of George III and some of the symptoms were strikingly consistent. Bilious attacks, stomach pains, even spasms were not the exclusive preserve of George III as adjuncts to his insanity. Drs Macalpine and Hunter highlighted these recurrent physical symptoms amongst members of the royal family in *George III and the Mad-Business*. They did so as part of their thesis that the king had suffered from porphyria and that as a hereditary genetic disorder it was bound to recur in other members of the family. In pursuing evidence for the symptoms of porphyria both in George III's contemporary family members and his ancestors, they highlighted just how many of his offspring suffered chronic ill-health with markedly similar symptoms. On each occasion that George III became ill and this developed into derangement and insanity it served as a reminder to the rest of his family and beyond that the physical manifestations of illness could develop into mental manifestations as Lady Bessborough had concluded.

How far people at the time noticed the similarity in the symptoms and assumed that this denoted that the risk of insanity could potentially affect others besides the king is of prime importance. Several of George III's sons spent extended periods of time in Hanover. Amongst them were the Dukes of York, Kent and Sussex. While they were in Hanover all were ill, with York and Sussex recurrent and severe sufferers. The Duke of Sussex apparently began to be ill when he was 15 and ironically this coincided with his father's own crisis in 1788. The symptoms which concerned Dr von Zimmermann and his colleagues in Hanover were paroxysms and dark amber discoloured urine. Having treated two of Sussex's brothers, Zimmermann was in a position to draw the following conclusion in a report to George III, 'It has come to our knowledge that several members of the Royal Family and in particular His Royal Highness the Duke of York and Prince Edward [Duke of Kent] are subject to the same paroxysms [as the Duke of Sussex] and this arouses our suspicion of a hereditary predisposition.[9] This was a most serious issue to raise with the king and it can safely be assumed that Zimmermann felt very sure of his ground when he did so.

Whether the Duke of Kent was prompted to consider the familial similarity of symptoms highlighted by Zimmermann is not clear. He would, however, address the subject directly soon after he left Hanover and to his father. In 1790 when Kent was a young man of 23 stationed in Gibraltar with the army he wrote to his father after suffering chronic ill-health, exacerbated by the heat of the summer. Kent's letter was a petition to be relieved of his posting and he argued, 'my health has so materially suffered during the immoderate heat of last summer that the Surgeon General of our Garrison, who has constantly attended me during the frequent bilious attacks from which I have felt the most violent and serious effects, has given it as his positive opinion that by my remaining here [Gibraltar] another summer season my health would be exposed not only to the most prejudicial but perhaps the most fatal attacks of a complaint, the severity of which, is, I believe, not unknown to your Majesty.'[10] In addressing the subject of the commonality of symptoms between himself and the king and implicitly the wider similarity with other members of the royal family, Kent was breaking an apparent taboo. An absolute discretion seems to have been maintained in the correspondence which has survived and is available.

As Lady Bessborough was prepared to do in late 1811, Sir Robert Wilson was prompted to set down his perceptions during George III's third period of derangement. In September 1804 he had visited the king and his party in Weymouth where George III was convalescing. The visit coincided with a period when the king was well enough to travel and had been able to attend to some business but when his recovery from the relapse of 1804 was not complete. Indeed it appeared likely that his condition would deteriorate again. Wilson wrote a long memorandum which recorded his impressions of the impact of illness on the king's behaviour.[11] His version of events presents a picture in which the outrageous behaviour of the king was tolerated and managed so as to keep up the pretence that all was well. Wilson was not so accommodating. His verdict against the government was 'that from mistaken attachment or love of present employment abuses the nation by dressing up George III in the regalia when he can no longer independently exercise the Royal functions'. Wilson concluded that 'the Throne is usurped by the King's Ministers'.

The sensitivity of Wilson's comments on the way the monarchy was undermined by the king's illness was nothing compared to the sensitivity of his comments on the impact of illness on the wider royal family. He addressed the subject head on; the fear that the king might not be the only member of the family who could become insane and that some of George III's offspring were in danger of losing their reason. 'I fear from what I learn that the King is not the only one of his family likely to be affected by this grievous malady.' This apparently was not a case of Wilson in isolation drawing a conclusion from his own observations. Rather this was a case of Wilson in guarded conversation with a confidant in the royal entourage. Wilson relates comments from his source, but does not identify the individual. Whoever it was, this person had the seniority or confidence to give his views to the king's physician at the time, Sir Francis Milman. Wilson comments that he fears 'A younger Princess subject to spasms was the object of my friend's lamentation to Sir F Milman.' Professor Arthur Aspinall, editor of much of George III's correspondence as well as the correspondence of the Prince of Wales, identifies the sufferer as Princess Sophia, the king's second youngest daughter. Wilson has not finished, however, as he goes on to relate a further confidence from his friend. 'I fear,' said this friend, 'in one of those attacks, she will lose her life – say rather, her senses for ever, for to that misfortune is more than one of these Royal personages doomed, & I know an eminent surgeon who is of the same counsel.'

Sir Robert Wilson's confidant was therefore not alone in fearing that insanity was a familial weakness which had been passed on to some of the king's offspring. Wilson's account demonstrates that discreet conversations were had on the subject even within the royal household. It is hardly surprising that there was concern and speculation about the king's intermittent descents into derangement or insanity. The constitutional implications were manageable if they affected a single individual as the establishment of the regency in 1811 demonstrated. The possibility that the problem went wider and could affect the succession was a much more difficult problem to deal with. Wilson was a polemical figure who seems to have courted controversy throughout his life. He had recorded with disdain the heightened sex drive of the king while he was still convalescent. On the subject of the danger that members of the younger generation of the royal family were at risk of becoming insane, Wilson's account contains none of the moral outrage in his comments on the king's sexualised behaviour seen in chapter three. Instead the account of his confidential exchanges on the danger to the younger generation of the royal family is expressed calmly and with some sympathy and has greater impact as a result.

It was inevitable that with each relapse and every period of derangement there should be a mounting concern over not only the future of the king, but also for his successors. The single crisis of 1788/9 could be dismissed as an aberration and the succeeding decade of good health would have made the problem seem like a one-off at the time. By 1804 with two further relapses anxiety would have increased. With the crisis of 1810 and the apparent failure of medicine to recover the king the anxiety about the succession would have been greater. As the king's offspring reached maturity, the chronic illness in several of them and the similarity in the physical symptoms meant that it was inevitable that there would be speculation that the problem of insanity would not be restricted to George himself.

The beginning of the nineteenth century was a period of continual crisis. From the start of the century until 1815 the United Kingdom was constantly at war. The strain on the economy was immense and was exacerbated by the fact that both Bonaparte and the British government used control of trade as a weapon of war. There was considerable social unrest in the UK during the wars and if anything the situation became worse with the eventual return of peace and the difficult social and economic transition this brought with it. The court and the upper echelons of the political class were insulated from some of the impact of the wars but they were concerned that the government should continue to function effectively. Any doubt over the succession had implications for political stability. At precisely the time when the regency was brought in the Regent himself suffered a series of serious illnesses. The future George IV has had a worse press than his father and is largely written off as lazy, self-indulgent and profligate. This populist assessment may well have a strong element of truth in it, but this should not distract from the fact that the future George IV was extremely ill during 1811 and 1812 and that at times his personal doctor was concerned that he would die. The surviving correspondence within the royal family points to a real concern for the safety and survival of the Prince of Wales. The Duke of Northumberland for example wrote to the Prince Regent's private secretary Colonel McMahon in December 1811 to express his concern at the reports he had heard that the prince was suffering from 'spasms'.[12]

Illness was to pursue the future George IV throughout his life. He was too intelligent not to have seen and understood the similarities in illness between himself and his father and immediate family. Discretion was very strong within the family. The Duke of Kent's observation to his father in his letter written from Gibraltar was an exception. So too was the enigmatic comment made by George IV to Sir William Knighton a physician turned courtier and close associate of the king. In a personal letter dated 15th November 1825 he says, 'As to bodily health, I am certainly not as well as I ought to be, ... but as to that which is more and most essentially (as it is the main-spring to everything, and the only security for health) the state of my mind and feelings, I shall reserve all I have to say till next we meet.'[13] Discretion is maintained, but the exact context of the correspondence is lost. The *Memoirs* were edited by his wife and the focus was to present Knighton in as impressive a light as possible. In this instance the fact of the king's confidence in Knighton is key for the editor rather than the context of that confidence.

Discretion in reference to possible mental manifestations of familial illness in the royal family was inevitable and at the time quite natural, but the tragic death of Princess Charlotte in childbirth served to jolt some commentators out of such reticence. The death of the heir to the throne following the still-born birth of a male baby caused a strong reaction in the country and the need to identify those imagined by the press to have been responsible for the disaster. So while the press blamed the doctors responsible for the princess' care before and during the delivery there were alternative views. Writing in the *London Medical Repository* on 1st December 1817, Dr Anthony Tod Thompson picked up on the symptoms which Princess Charlotte was recorded to have displayed some hours after the birth. She apparently became nauseous and was thought to be having a bilious attack and began talking with great rapidity. These were all symptoms which her father the Prince Regent and her grandfather George III had displayed in the run up to spasms. Thompson clearly was familiar with these symptoms and wrote, 'We have been informed that the whole of the Royal Family are liable to the spasms of a violent description, and to this hereditary predisposition, and the increased excitability of the amiable Sufferer ... are we left to ascribe an event which has destroyed the flattering hopes of a nation.'[14] While robustly defending the physician who had been responsible for caring for Princess Charlotte during her delivery and who subsequently committed suicide, Thompson addressed a medically interested audience on the assumption that they would be aware of the hereditary problems of the royal family and that only the briefest description of the symptoms would be necessary to be recognisable.

The evidence of widespread illness in the royal family and concern that insanity might touch others besides the king is clear despite the tremendous discretion with which such concerns were understandably held at the time. It seems possible that the search for a cure for insanity could have been driven, at least in part by concern for the succession and for the wider royal family. The Committee set up to investigate the Lucett process may have been driven by this wider concern as well as some self-interest on the part of the Dukes of Kent and Sussex. They too had suffered during health crises from similar symptoms to their father. The involvement of the royal dukes in the work of the Committee was not a token one. Instead it was consistent with a deep personal commitment to the experiment. It seems reasonable to consider that the Lucett curative process could have been seen as a potential backstop for the Hanoverian regime as well as a possible cure for the king.

Chapter Eleven

Psychiatry's First Therapeutic Trial

'It has been observed in my *Treatise on Hysteric and Nervous diseases etc*, that mental disorders have never been scientifically considered, nor judiciously treated.'[1]

William Rowley in *Truth Vindicated etc*. 1790.

The transition to a formal, public and ultimately scientific mechanism to evaluate Lucett's curative process came in mid-1813 with the establishment of a Committee to 'investigate the Merits due to the Process, practised by Messrs Delahoyde and Lucett for the cure of insane persons' and 'to defray the expense of such enquiry'. The inaugural meeting of this ambitious project took place at Lord Dundas' London house at number 19 Arlington Street on 31st May 1813. It is probable that the actual gathering took place in the Great Room of what was a grand aristocratic town house built in 1732 which had had improvements carried out later by Robert Adam.[2] The minutes of that meeting survive in the papers of Earl Fitzwilliam one of the senior committee members and they set out the objectives which the formation of the Committee were intended to achieve and the mechanics for doing so.[3] All that was missing was the fundamental reason for the whole business; there was no mention of the king.

It was noted that press reports of the activities of Delahoyde and Lucett had come to the attention of the public and that it was this publicity which had led to the formation of the Committee. 'The instances of cure of Insanity performed by Messrs Delahoyde and Lucett, and which have come to the knowledge of the public, have induced the under-named to form themselves into a committee, for the purpose of ascertaining the efficacy of their process, and to promulgate to the world the result of their experiment.' This wasn't quite true as the publicity for Delahoyde and Lucett's activities was not simply the result of spontaneous reporting of their independent activities. As has been clear, the Duke of Kent and others had been engaged with Lucett and Delahoyde on a discreet basis for some months and so the formation of the Committee was the logical next step given that the initial trials of the Lucett curative process had shown significant promise.

Nevertheless the claim that there had been widespread publicity was calculated to stimulate public interest in the Committee's activities and to attract additional support. The Committee was set up under the joint chairmanship of the Dukes of Kent and Sussex who were joined by a group of men which included some of the most illustrious figures of the day. [See Appendix for brief background on the Committee members and supporters.] It is not clear how the men who subscribed to the project were identified or how they were approached. Some would have been carried over from the early stages of the contact with Lucett and would probably have come from the Duke of Kent's immediate circle of associates. The need for expansion when the more ambitious formal committee was set up would have involved going beyond that immediate circle. Although it was never stated publicly that the trial was to test a therapy, which if it was successful, was intended for use on the king it is almost certain that Committee members and subscribers were told of this intention from the start. It emerged later that others may have been approached and one was later to claim he had refused to support the experiment. It is also highly probable that some other members of the royal family were informed of the activities of the Duke of Kent and even of the detailed treatment of Harrison, Moon and Lancaster.

A plan of action was agreed during the inaugural meeting of the Committee which centred on the sponsoring of a 'receiving-house' where Delahoyde and Lucett would treat patients. This was subsequently referred to as 'Sion Vale' in correspondence and while it's exact location is not on record, Lucett himself said that it was in Brentford to the west of London. Ten patients drawn from the Hoxton asylum were to be selected by the Committee under the guidance of their medical advisor Dr John Harness and placed under the care of Delahoyde and Lucett for a period of three months, although there was scope for the patients to remain longer if it was considered they needed further treatment 'for their restoration'. The arrangement was to be 'free of expense in every way' for the patients and their families. In a sense the agreement at this first meeting of the Committee to set up the receiving-house simply confirmed activity which was already under way. The first disbursement of £200 had already been made on 24th May and is a pointer to the urgency with which the project was being pursued.[4]

Dr Harness was formally appointed to assess the effectiveness of the treatment, but Lucett and Delahoyde were to expect additional monitoring. Members of the Committee were guaranteed access to Sion Vale to see the patients unless Delahoyde, as the qualified medical man, considered it would be against the best interests of the patient at that time. So while Delahoyde had discretion over admitting Committee members it was clearly implicit that he would have to have a very good reason for not allowing a particular visit. In the records which survive there is no indication that there was ever any difficulty over Committee members having access to Sion Vale. Indeed the indications are that Harness had unsupervised access to the patients while they were with Delahoyde and Lucett and was able to form an independent and accurate impression of the effect of the process. This was a crucial element in validating the whole trial as it ensured that the results could not be manipulated or falsified by the practitioners. It is ironic that in setting out these arrangements the Committee were creating precisely the system of close inspection which was increasingly seen as essential for the effective management of insane asylums.

As a further element in the process for monitoring and assessing the treatment of the patients at Sion Vale a system of 'accounts' of the patients' progress were to be provided for the Committee members. No specific timetable was proposed and there was no determination on whether they would be published in the press although this possibility was raised at the meeting. These accounts were published in abbreviated form with the report of the activities of the Committee dated 27th September 1813, but the records of the Committee activities which survive indicate that reports of the patients' progress were provided under the signature of Delahoyde alone. Looking back it was perhaps a weakness of the system that these were not simply chronological accounts of treatment and how the patients responded, but rather that they also represented opportunities for Delahoyde and Lucett to promote the success of their treatment. More dispassionate accounts were provided by Dr Harness and copies of several of these were sent direct to Earl Fitzwilliam and have survived.

The financial arrangements which were put in place were intended to be proof against maladministration and a bank account was set up with Messrs Child and Company to receive the subscriptions of the sponsors. These varied from a maximum of fifty-two pounds and ten shillings in the case of the Duke of Kent and the Duke of Bedford to ten guineas in the case of Dr Fleming and James Alexander MP. Lucett and Delahoyde did not have direct access to the money. Instead three members of the Committee were appointed to be trustees of the fund and to make disbursements as directed by the Committee in response to the expenses of Delahoyde and Lucett in running Sion Vale. As was common at the time, it was agreed that three members formed a quorum of the Committee. The minutes of the inaugural meeting are actually dated 8th June and were professionally printed. It seems likely that they were intended for distribution to Committee members, subscribers and probably to other interested individuals. Certainly the subscribers list which was included, along with their contributions, is a longer list than the Committee members.

Although Lucett claimed proprietorship of the curative process, in setting up the parameters of the therapeutic trial the Committee gave precedence to Delahoyde. This was not accidental. He was after all the 'regular educated surgeon'[5] and therefore provided reassurance against possible charges of quackery. The resolutions make it clear that while the Committee would have a role in selecting the patients who would be sent to the receiving house, it was Delahoyde who had the last word on which patients were actually accepted to be part of the experiment. It is to the credit of Lucett and Delahoyde that they seemed to relish taking on the most difficult cases. Nevertheless the fundamental point is clear. Delahoyde was clearly seen as the senior partner and was expected to take the lead in all matters related to the treatment and welfare of the patients. Lucett is only mentioned in the context of the administrative aspects of the experiment. Ultimately the Committee was being careful about the image of the therapeutic trial presented to the outside world. If the Lucett treatment was to stand any chance of being used on the king or more widely then it was vital that there was a clear separation from possible accusations of quackery. In hindsight the missing element in the establishment of the trial was that there should be full disclosure of what the curative process involved. It is probable that disclosure was assumed to be inevitable as the trial progressed. In fact this oversight was to become the subject of some contention.

The enquiry, under the auspices of the Duke of Kent's Committee, has been described as 'psychiatry's first therapeutic trial'[6] and it was the first attempt to evaluate the effectiveness of a therapy to treat mental illness on a scientific basis. Dr Francis Willis when called in to treat George III in 1788 had made an important psychological step forward in attitudes towards insanity by asserting that it was curable like any other illness. Willis was subsequently credited with curing the king, but no real assessment had been made of the process by which Willis' treatment of the king had achieved a 'cure'. The patient had recovered, but there had been no attempt to determine whether the patient had simply recovered spontaneously, or as the direct result of Willis' interventions. There had been no attempt to establish causality between any specific intervention and an improvement in the king's condition. The evaluation of the Lucett curative process represented a practical step towards establishing an objective assessment of the impact and value of a treatment which it was claimed would treat insanity

Although the trial was set up with the immediate view of determining whether the Lucett process represented a potential treatment for the king, the ambitions of the Committee were much wider. It is clear that those involved in the experiment were also motivated by a desire to improve the human condition by finding a cure for an illness which was regarded with great fear at the time. So whether the beneficiary was to be George III or humanity in general there was no question of so august a patient as the king being involved at the experimental stage. It was also essential that the trial established a credible scientific basis in order to achieve respectability and to overcome the widespread revulsion felt for mad doctors and their methods.

After setting out the framework within which the trail of the curative process was to be evaluated the Committee made the following statement of intent.

'In case the experiment about to be made, under the present plan, should be the means of establishing the success of the process, and a permanent society should be formed, the subscription of £20, and upwards to be considered as life governors of such society.'[7]

The longer term ambition was to evolve from a temporary grouping formed to evaluate a curative process to a permanent Society which would underwrite a centre to provide treatment for the insane. The ambition and enthusiasm implicit in this statement is enormous and encapsulates Enlightenment thinking that the human condition could be improved through science and technology. Not only was it intended to recover the king but also to make treatment for insanity available to those of his subjects who needed it. It is an indicator of just how convincing the Lucett process seemed that the Duke of Kent and the other Committee members were prepared to publicly commit to the project for the long term.

The trial of the curative process was based on the use of patients drawn from the ranks of naval lunatics held at Hoxton or Bethlem. A letter and inventory dated 21st April 1813 survives in which Dr Weir, the Inspector of Naval Hospitals, provided a list of the naval lunatics then held at the two establishments and his assessments of their cases.[8] The inventory had been requested by the Lords Commissioners of the Admiralty and it is likely that this document was used in the initial stage of deciding which patients would be suitable for the experiment as most of the names of the patients involved in the therapeutic trial appear on the document. From a modern perspective there is an automatic revulsion at the idea of people being the subject of medical experimentation without any possibility of their giving informed consent to that involvement. The Nuremburg Code of 1947 put in place a framework of medical ethics for human experiments in response to some of the perversions of medical practice carried out in concentration camps during the Second World War. In the early nineteenth century there was not the same concern over ethical issues such as informed consent; particularly for those at the bottom of the social scale. They did not have the vote in the political sense and probably did not expect much consideration from their 'betters' more widely. Dr Thomas Monro giving evidence to the House of Commons Committee in 1815 highlighted the way social status conditioned the treatment of patients suffering from insanity when he remarked that chains were fit only for pauper patients at Bethlem, 'if a gentleman was put into irons, he would not like it'.[9] For the members of the Committee a serious concern in setting up the experiment would have been over possible fraud so there was no question of Lucett and Delahoyde providing their own subjects who could then be shown to have undergone miracle cures. Formally the committee wanted subjects who had a history of insanity and who had been assessed by the medical authorities as incurable. These criteria mirrored the current assessment of the king's case.

It is perhaps worth noting that the concept of 'incurable' has a clear meaning today which is centred on the likelihood of a patient recovering from a medical condition. The meaning of 'incurable' was not necessarily the same in the early nineteenth century when applied to individuals who were assessed as insane. Mr Haslam defined the contemporary meaning in testimony before the House of Commons Committee Enquiry on Madhouses in 1815. As the long serving medical officer at Bethlem Hospital he had a direct professional knowledge of the term's significance at the time. He defined an incurable patient as, 'After a residence of twelve months if such a person has exhibited symptoms of malevolence, or is mischievous, and it is considered necessary that society should be delivered from them, they are declared incurable, which declaration is subsequently confirmed by the Governor.'[10] So the definition of incurable applied to the patients used in the trial under the auspices of the Duke of Kent meant that not only were such patients unlikely to recover medically, but that their condition meant that they were so violent that they could not be allowed to mix in society. The contemporary definition therefore meant that the trial of the Lucett curative process involved considerable potential risk in taking on such disruptive and potentially violent patients.

In a further effort to ensure scientific rigour in the trial, a medical assessor was appointed to monitor the impact of the treatment on the patients and its value as a potential cure. Clearly a prime concern was that at the end of the trial it should be determined whether the process was safe and whether it could be used at Windsor and elsewhere with the expectation that it would be effective. This meant that a balance had to be achieved in the choice of assessor. The assessor had to be a man not simply qualified medically, but a person of complete discretion and integrity as well as someone who was potentially open to new ideas. The person chosen was Dr John Harness who at the time of the formation of the Committee was the Medical Commissioner of the Royal Navy and the medical member of the Transport Board which, despite its rather prosaic name, was responsible for the sick and injured members of the navy. He had also been involved in the preliminary trials involving Lucett and Delahoyde before the formation of the Committee to manage the trial.

Harness was a serious choice as scientific and medical arbiter for the Committee. He had a number of relatives who had been eminent physicians including a more distant one who had been physician to George II. He had had a serious medical training by the standards of the time which had been both academic and practical before he became an assistant surgeon in the Royal Navy in 1776. He had had an important role in eradicating scurvy from the Royal Navy and had insisted on the systematic consumption of citric acid by sailors in the Mediterranean fleet under Admiral Hood. Harness had subsequently promoted the professionalism and status of naval surgeons. Unsurprisingly Harness was a man of his age. When called upon to give evidence to the House of Commons enquiry of 1815 he compared the space allowed to 'patients' at the Hoxton asylum favourably with the space an individual might have had on board a Royal Navy ship. Clearly these were not comparable situations and the reasons for individuals being in either location were rather different. Harness also told the Commons enquiry that the use of mechanical restraint was inevitable and that he had low expectations for medical intervention in cases of insanity.[11] Dr Harness was therefore an assessor who was definitely not predisposed to be sympathetic to the claims for an effective cure for insanity; especially one which claimed to dispense with the need for restraint. He was a reasonable balance of scepticism and commitment to scientific enquiry with the additional practical advantage that he knew many of the potential patients and their histories from direct experience.

The Committee was made up of extraordinarily eminent people of the day. In addition to the two royal dukes there was Lord Dundas, Earl Fitzwilliam, Sir Joseph Banks, Lord Melville and the Hon. John Spencer. The full list of committee members and supporters encompassed both sides of the political divide and included political as well as social and health reformers. The composition of the group also reflected society in change. There were the representatives of the old landed aristocracy working in concert with the new elite of entrepreneurs and scientists. With Richard Troward, a lawyer who had been a member of the prosecution team in the trial of Warren Hastings, appointed as the committee secretary and John Dent the renowned glove maker as the accountant this was a well organised undertaking by serious minded people.

It was of course important that the Committee should be well founded and run. The members of the Committee and their supporters were risking more than their money. They were also risking their reputation if anything went wrong. It was implicit that success in the trial would involve the release into society of individuals who had been under the most severe restraint as they had been thought to be violent and dangerous. It needed only one of the patients to have a relapse and to kill or maim someone for the Committee and its members to achieve notoriety. The Georgian press was capable of the kind of exposures which are common today and the cartoonists would have immortalised any scandal. The Committee were to come quite close to such a disaster.

In the opening statement of the first meeting of the Committee reference had been made to the impact of the publicity surrounding the activities of Delahoyde and Lucett and to their success in curing patients. The account of the first Committee meeting published on the 8th June included three case histories which provide a context for the confident tone of the proceedings. William Harrison was described in this account as having a 'complaint of the most violent and outrageous kind; he had been occasionally sullen for months together'. On his release from Bethlem he was apparently taken to Delahoyde's home at Westham in Essex on 30th September 1812 where the treatment began. Having examined their patient Delahoyde and Lucett began the process and within 24 hours it was no longer necessary to restrain the patient. In three or four days Harrison had apparently become 'perfectly rational in his behaviour and conversation' and took an interest in books and began to play musical instruments again. On the sixth day Harrison not only went to church where he behaved with 'perfect decorum', but also met his wife whom he treated with marked affection. This was in strong contrast to the hostility he had treated her with during his confinement. By the twelfth day he was able to accompany his wife on a visit to their children while on the 15th day he visited the Duke of Kent at Kensington in order to express his thanks for his intervention on his behalf. Apparently Harrison met several of his former comrades while he was in Kensington and received their congratulations on his recovery. The account of Harrison's case ends with the statement that he had been well ever since.

Clearly this account will have derived from Delahoyde and Lucett's record of the case and it is true that in later years Lucett would advance a version which produced an even more rapid recovery by Harrison. Nevertheless Delahoyde and Lucett cannot have had free reign to create whatever fictional account they wished. The Duke of Kent had been directly involved in the release of Harrison and seems to have taken a close interest in subsequent developments. Others too were involved so that this account, which was used as part of the evidence for taking the Delahoyde and Lucett process seriously, would have been open to challenge if there were obvious untruths in it. What is clear is that Harrison was not simply isolated in some secret location in a state of extreme derangement from which he was later to emerge recovered as if by magic.

The other two cases used as evidence for the effectiveness of the Delahoyde and Lucett process were those of John Moon and Elizabeth Lancaster. Moon was a former marine who had been confined in Bethlem for over twelve months and had been considered so violent that he had been chained and handcuffed in order to control him. Following the success with Harrison, Delahoyde and Lucett had requested another patient so they could demonstrate the effectiveness of their process. Again the Duke of Kent intervened with the Lords of the Admiralty through the Transport Office and Bethlem records indicate that he was 'Delivered to the Transport Office' on 12th December 1812.[12] Moon would as a marine, who was still formally on the navy list, have been the responsibility of the Admiralty. Interestingly the account mentions that some gentlemen had witnessed Moon's 'outrageous' behaviour while at Bethlem and that these were gentlemen 'who interested themselves about the experiment'. Essentially they seem to have represented a nucleus of what later became the Committee. The key point is that their involvement is a clear indicator that Delahoyde and Lucett were not able to operate without some outside supervision even before the Committee came into being.

The case history again indicates that the effect of the process was almost immediate as the violence was subdued within 24 hours while on the twelfth day he apparently revisited Bethlem to meet his former keepers. Their astonishment at the change is noted. More important, however, is that Moon was taken to the Transport Office where he was examined by Dr Harness and the other Commissioners. This was significant as Harness would have been officially aware of Moon's case and would have been in a position to judge whether Moon's condition had changed significantly. The account ends with the claim that Moon had been transferred to Woolwich in May 1813 preparatory to being returned to his division.[13]

Records held in the archives at Lambeth Palace demonstrate that Moon's case was the subject of considerable scrutiny and that others besides Delahoyde and Lucett were involved in assessing the impact of the treatment. These were in some instances professionals with a formal involvement in the case. A letter to the Transport Office dated 1st June 1813 from the hospital ship *Batavia* at Woolwich gives a summary of Moon's former symptoms.[14] He displayed agitation and very rapid speech as well as extreme irritability. He had been assessed as deranged. The similarity between these symptoms and the warning signs that George III was entering a crisis is uncanny. It raises the possibility that he was chosen as an early subject for the experimental treatment precisely because of that similarity. The record is silent on this, but it would explain the Archbishop of Canterbury's focus on Moon once he became aware of the activities of the Committee.

For someone of his low social standing Moon has left a quite detailed account of his life thanks to the medical experiment sponsored by the Duke of Kent. There is a remarkably sensitive letter about Moon addressed to Dr Harness in his role as 'Commissioner of His Majesty's Navy' and dated 10th June 1813. The letter was written by a certain Captain Boyle as part of the process in the discharge of Moon from the navy. From humble beginnings in Wiltshire Moon had begun his working life in the cloth trade before joining the marines. Boyle comments that Moon was probably not suited to the marines and that 'the oddities of his behaviour may have accounted for the problems he encountered'. Problems he certainly encountered. He was apparently flogged three times during his career in the navy receiving forty lashes on one occasion and fifty lashes on the other two occasions. These were serious punishments and would have been potentially life threatening. It is easy to imagine that the rigid discipline of the navy was entirely incapable of dealing with the eccentricities of Moon. Captain Boyle implied as much and stated that Moon was no soldier and should be discharged. In an interesting additional comment Boyle said that he did not think Moon represented a threat to society and that he would benefit from 'a fair trial' with 'Mr Delahoyde's corrective measures for insanity'. Moon was transferred to the keeping of Mr Delahoyde on 16th June 1813. Thomas Robertson a naval surgeon noted that Moon was 'much agitated on seeing Mr Delahoyde and at first unwilling to go with him'.[15]

Moon appeared to have been a clear cut case of success for the 'process'. He was to return, however, with a different chronology and outcome in the later record of events. He was also to become the focus of attention for the Archbishop of Canterbury when he, as chairman of the Queen's Council, became aware of the activities of the Committee and the Delahoyde and Lucett experiment. The last case of Mrs Lancaster had a more abbreviated history. Unlike the other two cases this lady was not recorded as an inmate of Bethlem and there was no connection with the military. In her case not only was the Duke of Kent involved in her placement with Delahoyde and Lucett, but also his brother the Duke of Sussex. In fact she was the wife of Joseph Lancaster the educationalist and pioneer of mass literacy.[16] The date of 14th April 1813 was given as the date on which her treatment began and again recovery was rapid so that by the date of the first Committee meeting she had returned to her home and family in Tooting. This apparently straightforward case was to come back to haunt Lucett and to make him temporarily at least a target for attack in the media.

Dr Harness was closely involved in the crucial next step by the Committee. The private asylum at Hoxton was the asylum which the Admiralty used most frequently when servicemen became mentally ill. In the selection of patients for the trial this implied an advantage as the history of service patients would be well known and could be easily verified. As the Admiralty was still responsible for such people release to Delahoyde and Lucett could be facilitated by Harness. With these ideas in mind the Committee arranged during its first meeting, to reconvene at the Hoxton asylum on 7th June 1813 to make a selection of patients for the experiment. It is an indication of the sense of urgency in the Committee that the move to the selection of patients was arranged so quickly.

This follow-up meeting was no nominal affair in which a few representatives were sent to the asylum to deal with the practical implications of the enthusiasm of the first Committee meeting. Both the royal dukes as well as Earl Fitzwilliam and Lord Dundas descended on Hoxton. Dr Harness attended as might have been expected along with John Dent and Thomas Smith. In keeping with the first meeting this follow-up session involved a formal record and this shows that there were 146 former marines or seamen in the asylum and that 94 had been assessed by the Naval Inspector, Dr Weir, as incurable. The former naval service patients deemed incurable were seen by the Committee members and ten were selected as 'proper for the experiment'. The criteria on which the selection was made are not recorded beyond the general point that they were 'incurable', but it is tantalising to consider the possibility that the patients selected might have had symptoms similar to the king. Mr Delahoyde had been required to attend the meeting and he was given a list and history of the ten patients and asked to select those he considered most suitable for treatment. In keeping with the sense of urgency which seems to have applied to the activities of the Committee, four patients were selected and arrangements made for them to be immediately transferred to the receiving house of Delahoyde and Lucett.

A letter written on 9th June 1813 by Dr John Harness to Richard Troward, the Committee secretary, which survives in the Royal College of Physicians archive, is a pointer to the professionalism in record keeping which was to be expected of the Committee experiment. It was also a pointer to Harness wishing to keep the Admiralty fully informed of developments. In the letter Harness asked Troward to send him a list of the patients whom Delahoyde had selected from Hoxton on 7th June. This was despite the fact that Harness had been present. Harness went on in the letter to suggest that Troward should send a copy to Lord Melville at the Admiralty in addition to the list which he would be sending to Mr Angerstein. The impression is clear; all the senior members of the Committee should be informed of developments fully and quickly.[17]

A determining characteristic of the whole of the Committee's activities in the assessment of the Lucett 'process' was the positive use of publicity. Current sensibilities might assume that what would now be regarded as an exploitative use of the patients by a group of prominent members of society would have required discretion if not outright secrecy. Perceptions were different at the time. Indeed there was a widespread and undoubtedly justified belief that there was too much secrecy in the treatment of insane patients and that the attendant lack of accountability meant that abuse was rife. The Committee members clearly considered their activities to be worthwhile and publicity was seen as a way not only of establishing public confidence in the ethical standards of the experiment, but of ensuring that the results were considered reliable and valid. A resolution of the inaugural meeting states that it was resolved to send copies of the plan 'to enquire into the effect of the process practiced by Messrs Delahoyde and Lucett' to all the members of the two Houses of Parliament. There really was no question of the Committee superintending a trial of the 'curative process' behind closed doors. The primary purpose was clearly to settle confidence in the trial but it is likely that the publicity was also intended in part to attract additional funds through donations. Finally the wide circulation of the Committee's activities reflected a confidence at the beginning that the experiment would be successful.

Lucett and Delahoyde were engaged in what they hoped ultimately would be a successful commercial exercise so for them publicity would also have been desirable. On the 16th June 1813 the East Anglian newspaper the *Bury and Norwich Post* carried a full report of the cure of the three original patients as well as the background story of how the 'process' had come to James Lucett. The involvement of the Duke of Kent is reported although the establishment of the Committee is overlooked. There are additional details on the patients, their background and response to their treatment which are not in the Committee record, so this account was clearly the result of briefing from someone close to the treatment process. It is probable, given the prominence given to him, that Lucett was responsible for the briefing. Delahoyde is not mentioned but Lucett is specifically referred to as the person with knowledge of the 'cure'. What is clear is that there were no reservations about acknowledging the Duke of Kent's role publically and the story was replayed in other newspapers in the following days.

The next step was a crucial one and may have been brought about by the publicity in the newspapers. The Queen's Council and the Committee headed by the Duke of Kent were to be linked even if it was tangentially and temporarily. On 30th June 1813 Lord Ellenborough wrote to the Archbishop of Canterbury to draw his attention to 'the method of one Delahoyde, supposed to have recently had very considerable success in the cure of insane persons'.[18] Ellenborough was a senior member of the Queen's Council and in writing to the Archbishop of Canterbury as chairman of the Council he referred to two other members, Lord Eldon the Chancellor and the Duke of Montrose. Ellenborough indicated that Eldon and Montrose considered that the Queen's Council should meet to discuss the subject of Delahoyde before the next scheduled meeting on the following Saturday. While Ellenborough gave no detail of the Delahoyde 'cure' and did not mention the Committee or the Dukes of Kent and Sussex, the sense of urgency in the letter is obvious.

The Queen's Council moved quickly. Some of the urgency may have been driven by the impending quarterly meeting with the Windsor physicians. On 3rd July 1813 they were asked the questions which had by then become routine about the king's health, his ability to perform his royal duties and his likelihood of recovery. The physicians were formally asked an additional question, however, which directly reflected the Queen's Council's new knowledge of the activities of Delahoyde and Lucett. The question put was, 'Do you have any knowledge of the circumstances, related in the paper, now shown to you, respecting the cases of insanity by Messrs Delahoyde and Lucett therein represented, and, if so, does such knowledge enable you to offer any suggestions, which may be useful with respect to His Majesty's case.'[19] Clearly the Queen's Council was looking at the Delahoyde and Lucett process as potentially useful in treating the king. The paper referred to in the question was in fact the Duke of Montrose's copy of the Resolution of the Committee dated 14th June which had been extracted from the inaugural meeting at Lord Dundas' house. This was the copy sent to the Duke of Montrose as the result of the Committee decision to circulate the two Houses of Parliament.[20]

The responses of the physicians are fascinating. In their different ways they were all conditioned by the possibility that the Queen's Council was considering the involvement of Delahoyde and Lucett in the treatment of the king. Unlike the Archbishop of Canterbury or Lord Ellenborough the activities of Delahoyde and Lucett did not break in on the physicians as some kind of revelation. The responses were careful and the physicians would have seen the consideration of an alternative treatment as a threat to their positions and reputation. No doubt the thought that the responses were on the record will also have contributed to the care exercised. Dr John Willis simply stated that he had 'no knowledge of the circumstances related in the paper alluded to'. Dr Robert Willis' response was a rather more nuanced version of his brother's response. He had 'no actual knowledge' and was therefore 'not enabled to offer any suggestions with respect to His Majesty's case'. Interestingly there was no allusion by Dr Robert Willis to having received a communication from Lucett in 1811. The brevity of the Willis brothers' responses do absolutely nothing to encourage any further enquiries about Delahoyde and Lucett's treatment. Indeed the responses seem intended to close down further discussion of the subject.[21]

The Willis brothers had dominated the care and treatment of the king for over a year by this time. They could not have been expected to acknowledge let alone welcome an alternative treatment which just might have proved more effective. It is perhaps a little surprising that they had apparently not come across any of the publicity surrounding the supposed cures of the insane. Given the tension which had been involved when the Willis brothers gained the ascendancy over the regular doctors it is surprising or perhaps to their credit that the generalist doctors did not use the question about Delahoyde and Lucett to encourage further examination of the process in order to discomfort the specialists.

The other physicians were either better informed than the Willis brothers or felt they had the freedom to be a little more expansive although they were no less careful in framing their responses. Dr Matthew Baillie said he knew nothing of the cases related in the paper, but he admitted that he knew something of the activities of Delahoyde and Lucett. 'I have occasionally heard reports about them in conversation' but Baillie claimed that this did not extend to knowledge about 'their process' and that he was therefore not in a position to say whether it would be appropriate for use on the king. Interestingly Baillie added a rider, '…. from the little I have heard I am dispos'd to think that His Majesty is not likely to derive benefit from it'. This is a guarded response which seems to suggest greater knowledge than Baillie would admit to. He is too careful to indicate what he had heard in conversation, when this had been and with whom he had been in conversation. If Delahoyde and Lucett had been discussed in medical circles as frauds or charlatans then why not say so? He was being consulted professionally as a physician. It is also interesting that Baillie should claim that conversations had not given him knowledge of 'the Process' yet he considered he knew enough to suggest the king would not benefit from it. There is a clear inconsistency here which is probably resolved by Baillie having heard something about the background of Delahoyde or Lucett.

Mr David Dundas, the apothecary based in Windsor, admitted to greater knowledge of Delahoyde and Lucett. 'I have no knowledge of the circumstances alluded to respecting the cases of supposed cure of insanity by Messrs Delahoyde and Lucett excepting that of Mrs Lancaster. But having never seen her till she was reported to be cured (when she appeared to me not recovered) and knowing nothing of the history of her case but from the imperfect and unprofessional relation of her husband I do not feel myself competent to form any opinion of their cure.' This careful response amounts to a bombshell although it raises more questions than it answers and it would be fascinating to know what the response of the Queen's Council was. The record gives no indication of any attempt to clarify Dundas' commentary. Yet clearly Dundas had actually met one of the three patients whose cases had provided the impetus for the formation of the Committee and which had caused such excitement in the Queen's Council. Not only had he met Mrs Lancaster but he had concluded that she had not been cured at that time. Although he had had access to the patient Dundas gives no indication of knowing about the curative process itself in his answer to the Queen's Council and makes no direct recommendation on whether it might be useful in helping the king. One can speculate about the circumstances of the encounter and it seems likely that he had a greater knowledge than he admitted to. But Dundas' use of the term 'supposed cure of insanity' is actually an eloquent contradiction of the enthusiasm of the Duke of Kent, the core members of the Committee as well as now the Archbishop of Canterbury too. Dundas clearly did not think the cure was effective.

Sir Henry Halford was physician to four British monarchs. The necessary discretion and the instinct for survival which this long career of royal service suggests are plain to see in his response. He claimed to have 'no exact knowledge of the circumstances' of the three cases of supposed cure of insanity, but goes on to say that what knowledge he does have, 'gives me a great distrust of the pretentions of Mr Delahoyde'. Lucett would have been an easier target as he was not medically qualified and had a profile which would have made it easy to dismiss him as a 'quack'. However, Halford shifts his focus to the actual curative 'process' and indicates that he has good reason to believe it involves the application of cold as the key element and that cold had been used as part of the king's treatment. Therefore no outsider would be needed to administer the Delahoyde treatment. Halford ends with almost a challenge to the Council. He states that employing the Delahoyde treatment 'or any other medical experiment would require a temporary departure from the present system of exclusion'. It is interesting that Halford should be so committed to exclusion; a treatment which he implicitly did not believe would work and which he had originally opposed when he tried to keep out the specialist mad-doctors. It is possible that Halford considered that Delahoyde and Lucett were simply crooks but felt that it would not be tactful to state this openly to the Queen's Council and indirectly to the Duke of Kent and the newly formed Committee.

The most complex response was the one given by Dr Heberden. He had stood out against seclusion when it was first introduced as a treatment for the king and he had fallen out with his colleagues in 1811 over trying to engage the king's interest in current events in order to counter possible deterioration in his mind. In these earlier encounters Heberden had come over as someone who thought beyond the conventional precepts of his time. In response to the Queen's Council's question about Delahoyde's curative process, Heberden states that he has no knowledge of the cases in the paper shown to him. However, he had done some investigation of Delahoyde and Lucette [sic] and his words are worth repeating: 'Such information as I have been able to procure respecting their process makes me believe that it is nothing new, excepting that it is set off with a new assurance; and my enquiries respecting the persons who administer it, make me rather inclined to believe what they can prove, than what they may assert.' This is a devastating critique delivered with total assurance. His conclusions are in direct contrast to those of the Committee members at this time. With continued assurance Heberden went on to say that he would not recommend using the 'process' on the king. 'I am of opinion that it probably would be hazardous, and certainly would be highly imprudent, to subject His Majesty to such practice and such practitioners at least till their characters, and their remedies are better understood.'

Heberden had at least answered the Queen's Council's question. He had said so much more than his colleagues, but it is a frustration that he did not say still more. With an almost casual urbanity Heberden suggested that Delahoyde and Lucett were not to be trusted. The comment that the 'process' would probably be hazardous is in direct contrast with Halford's conclusion that it was the mere application of cold and that a variation had already been tried on the king. It is not clear whether Heberden's concerns about possible hazards in the 'process' were fed back to the Committee, but in late September Delahoyde and Lucett explained sufficient to convince both the royal dukes and Dr Harness that their treatment was safe. In the end though Herberden was not totally dismissive of Delahoyde and Lucett and recommended further investigation of the claims they made for the process. What should have been of on-going concern for the Queen's Council was Dundas' comment that he had actually seen one of the patients and did not consider that she had been cured.[22]

Over all the response of the physicians had been negative and this raises the question of why the Queen's Council appear not to have curbed their enthusiasm to receive reporting on the progress of the Committee activities. It is possible that the Queen's Council members were concerned by the physicians' qualified rebuff and that there was some discussion of the implications. Indeed it is also possible that the Queen's Council members may have considered that the royal physicians were never going to endorse Delahoyde and Lucett whom they would have regarded as competitors. After all the generalists had done all they could to keep out the specialists. The record at Lambeth Palace is silent on the point. Perhaps more surprising is the apparent poor communications between the Queen's Council and the Committee. Both groups were made up of people who were members of the Georgian social, political and economic elite and would have moved in the same rather restricted circles. There is no record at Lambeth of the Archbishop of Canterbury telling the Committee or individual members that the views of the physicians had been canvassed and that the responses had been broadly critical. There is also no indication that the clear pointers to several of the doctors knowing more than they were prepared to commit to paper were followed up. Manners-Sutton had been appointed Archbishop by the king when he had been Dean at Windsor. He would have been a familiar figure to the royal family and should have been able to gain immediate access to Kent either on a personal basis or in an official capacity.

The energetic pursuit of the Committee activities by the Queen's Council continued immediately after the physicians had been consulted. On 4th July the Archbishop of Canterbury wrote to Lord Melville asking about the trial of the Delahoyde and Lucett process and specifically for a progress report on the case of John Moon.[23] As First Lord of the Admiralty, Lord Melville was perhaps a reasonable contact point for the Archbishop given that Delahoyde and Lucett were treating naval patients. However, the Duke of Kent was the more obvious choice as chairman of the Committee and correspondence might efficiently have been carried out through the secretary Richard Troward to cover all aspects of the trial. In his letter Manners-Sutton made no reference to the questioning of the royal doctors and therefore did not raise the subject of the integrity of Delahoyde and Lucett. It is not clear why Manners-Sutton was so reticent. He may have felt some sensitivity over Melville's position as a Committee member but equally he may simply have decided that he would let the trial run its course.

By this time Moon was on the point of being discharged from the navy. He had been due to be examined by the Committee in mid-June to determine whether he was well enough to justify a formal request for his release from the navy. On the appointed day Moon appeared flushed and rather incoherent. Earl Fitzwilliam who had seen Moon the previous day was astonished by the sudden deterioration in his condition. It was decided that the assessment should be put off until the next meeting on 28th June. At this session Moon was asked to explain his condition at the previous meeting. Moon was evasive but on being pressed he admitted to having had too much beer. He admitted to 6 or 8 glasses and when further pressed answered that 'he believed a little gin in some of them'! So all this, including Moon's unconscious attempt at sabotage, went to the Archbishop of Canterbury as well as an initial report on the progress of the first four patients under the formal auspices of the Committee.[24]

The first of the four patients identified and placed under the care of Delahoyde and Lucett at Sion Vale was transferred from Hoxton on 27th June. Dr Harness visited on that day and noted that the patient John Braily was very violent. He had previously described Braily as 'a most enraged maniac'. In fact he had been transferred from Hoxton in chains because of his violence. The intention had been to begin treatment immediately but Braily's condition made this impossible. Three quarters of an hour after arrival at Sion Vale Braily had 'become so violent as to break asunder the apparatus prepared by Mr Delahoyde for his confinement during the operation'. This resulted in a delay until the 29th when Harness was again on hand to monitor the impact of the treatment directly. He took the patient's pulse before the treatment and recorded it at 108 beats per minute. Ten minutes after the treatment Harness noted that Braily was considerably calmed as he was put to bed, but his pulse, while softer was still as rapid. Three quarters of an hour later Harness checked the patient again with Delahoyde and found his manner 'in every respect more calm and his pulse reduced to seventy-six'. Braily commented to Harness that 'he had undergone a severe operation'.[25]

This account from Harness in his letter to Lord Melville on 6th July provides an extraordinary picture of the immediate impact of the curative process; not least because the patient is able to contribute his own rational, almost detached perspective. Harness added to the sense that he had just witnessed something extraordinary when he wrote to Lord Melville. On 4th July Dr Harness was again at Sion Vale and had chatted to Braily for a quarter of an hour in the garden where he had been working. Braily was entirely rational and expressed his gratitude for the treatment he had received. Having set out the account of the events for Melville, Harness summarised the Braily case up to that point in terms of complete perplexity. 'I am really at a loss to account for the sudden effects induced by the means employed, neither can I form any idea of the probability of permanency to the relief, which they evidently afford.' Time would tell as Harness added in conclusion.[26]

Dr Harness' commentary for Lord Melville was important on several levels. He had clearly not expected the almost miraculous change brought about in Braily's condition. He does not actually state that he was present when Braily was treated, but he was certainly present immediately before and immediately after the 'operation'. He had also seen the equipment used as he had witnessed the destructive impact of Braily's mania on it. The essential point is that Harness considered that he knew the 'means employed' at the start of the therapeutic process so that his assessment that it had an immediate positive impact was apparently an informed conclusion. The fact that he could not logically account for the power of the impact simply emphasises that he thought he knew what the treatment involved. This is important as Lucett was to claim exclusive knowledge of the process throughout the rest of his working life yet there are a series of clear indications that the exclusivity was not complete and that the claim to exclusivity was simply an important element in his promotional efforts.

Harness wrote up a report regarding the start of the therapeutic trial for the Committee and sent it to the Duke of Kent on 30th June. The copy of the report which went to Earl Fitzwilliam on 1st July survives and the covering letter by Dr Harness includes the concern that Mr Delahoyde 'had begun to fill the house with private patients'. Harness was critical of this diversion from the fundamental business of evaluating the claims made for the 'process' and considered that at the very least the trial was going to take longer as a result. Harness considered that Delahoyde had been wrong to do this in view of the 'uncommon handsome and zealous manner their Royal Highnesses and the Committee have taken it up'. Indeed Harness states that taking in private patients had been against the wishes of the Committee and goes on to give his view that the publicity the Committee had generated about the experiment had enabled Delahoyde to exploit the opportunity to take in private patients.[27]

Lucett is not mentioned in Harness' letter to Lord Melville or in his visit report for the Committee. This was almost certainly a reflection that Delahoyde, as the qualified doctor, had been placed in charge of the patients when the Committee was set up. In 1815 Lucett would claim that Delahoyde had been involved in profiteering and at the expense of the experiment and even at the expense of Lucett himself. No evidence survives to suggest that Harness' concerns at the beginning of July 1813 were followed up by the Committee as a whole or by any senior members. Indeed the Resolutions for the foundation of the Committee and the trial do not in fact state that the receiving house should be used exclusively for the ten patients who were expected to be placed with the practitioners. It may be that Delahoyde and Lucett were guilty of ignoring more of the spirit than the letter of the agreement, but Harness' report does suggest that the practitioners were trying to exploit the relationship with the Committee right from the start.

Meanwhile Lord Melville had responded to the enquiry from the Archbishop of Canterbury by tasking Dr Harness for information particularly on Moon. Harness in turn secured a report from Richard Troward the secretary of the Committee. This report, entitled 'A narrative of the facts relative to John Moon'[28] which was forwarded by Melville to Lambeth Palace, gave an account of Moon's case right back to his release from Bethlem on 21st December 1812 at the behest of the Duke of Kent. The letter from Captain Boyle referred to above[29] which recommended that Moon should be discharged from the navy was also included. All these papers were forwarded to Lambeth under a covering letter on 7th July. Melville's reply is in reported speech which was a normal device in business letters of the time but does make the reply seem almost disrespectful to a modern reader. This business-like response was nevertheless in contrast to the letter written by the Archbishop himself and is another indicator of the urgency with which the Queen's Council viewed the Delahoyde and Lucett experiment. The process by which the Queen's Council linked in to the activities of the Committee worked, but it was a curiously roundabout way of doing things. As the exchanges immediately above demonstrate Manners-Sutton's enquiries had eventually been passed to the secretary of the Committee. The Committee had shown its enthusiasm for informing as wide an audience as possible of its activities and would surely not have had any objection to allowing the Queen's Council to have direct access to developments through the Committee secretary? As mentioned above Manners-Sutton would have known many of those involved in the Committee and could have approached the Duke of Kent direct.

On 13th July the Archbishop of Canterbury wrote again to Lord Melville.[30] The tone of the letter was firm and it is clear that the archbishop wanted to leave no doubt that he was writing on behalf of the Queen's Council and very much in an official capacity. Whether he considered that Lord Melville should have written with a greater personal commitment is not clear, but the archbishop clearly intended to engage Melville on the detail of the experiment. Manners-Sutton wanted not only detail of Moon subsequent to his discharge, but also details about the Braily case. He had also picked up on a reference Troward had made to 'other naval patients'. The archbishop noted that Harness had given a progress report only on Braily and concluded his letter, 'If there be more [patients] it is important to know what has been the effect of Mr Delahoyde's process upon those of whom we have no records.' There can be little doubt that possible application of the 'cure' to George III was central to the archbishop's thinking. It was equally clear that Manners-Sutton had not been daunted by the critical response of the physicians treating the king when asked about Delahoyde and Lucett. In his enthusiasm to explore the potential of the 'cure' Manners-Sutton may have given implicit expression to his desperation to find some new approach to the treatment of his charge which implied that the responsibility for the king was not completely open ended. Melville's position judged by this early exchange was not one of personal involvement. He was detached and ready to await the outcome of events. For the archbishop an enforced period of waiting would follow as Melville did not reply to the letter of 13th July until 17th September and only then after the archbishop had sent a further letter of enquiry. Again this delay in a response raises the question of why the archbishop did not approach the Duke of Kent or another senior member of the Committee in the interim.

If the archbishop had come to see that the 'Delahoyde' process as a potential solution to the problem of the king's illness, there can be little doubt that this had been in the minds of the Dukes of Kent and Sussex from the start. The Duke of Sussex visited Sion Vale twice in July in order to monitor Braily's condition, while the Duke of Kent visited Braily once during that month. The Duke of Sussex had witnessed Braily's aggressive violence at Hoxton and had suggested that he should be a candidate for the trial. The duke's interest in the impact of the therapy on Braily had obviously continued as Harness mentions the Duke of Sussex visiting Sion Vale immediately after he was first treated.[31] It is confirmation that the dukes' involvement in the trial was personal and that it was not enough for them to rely on formal accounts from Harness or Delahoyde.

At the end of July Melville received information which would have given the Archbishop of Canterbury great expectations. Dr Harness reported to him in a letter dated 31st July that there had apparently been real progress in the case of John Braily. Harness had visited Sion Vale every few days during July and his letter tracked the progress of this patient. This was no instant cure although there had been an almost instant initial improvement in the patient's condition. Harness noted that Braily had felt weak early in the month immediately following his treatment and he subsequently showed signs of shaking hands and limbs and of sweating. What is clear is that Harness had unfettered access to Braily and that there was no attempt by Delahoyde or Lucett to monitor what passed in their conversations. Harness reported that Braily was working in the garden at Sion Vale and that exercise, occupation and fresh air were considered an important part of the curative process or at least a useful adjunct. Harness clearly discussed the case with Delahoyde as he noted in the letter to Melville that Delahoyde had ordered a cold bath daily for the patient.[32] This apparent openness extended beyond Dr Harness as he commented in the letter that he was aware that three of the Committee members had also visited in order to monitor progress of the patients. Formally, however, this openness did not extend to details of the initial treatment itself.

This is one of the central curiosities of the whole experiment; the contrast between the secrecy over the initial part of the treatment which was apparently carried out behind closed doors and the complete openness over what followed. What was visible was that there was no resort to restraint, even with patients like Braily who had been so violent that he had been transferred in chains to Sion Vale. It was also clear that the kind of engagement of the patient which Heberden had advocated for the king was a part of the Delahoyde and Lucett approach. Dr Harness' visits demonstrate that occupying the patient's mind and steady physical activity were considered important. Calm, after the initial treatment seems to have been the aim and would have been a complete contrast with the patients' existence in Hoxton or Bedlam or the navy for that matter.

Newspaper articles tracking the work of Delahoyde and Lucett were perhaps a further manifestation of the openness of the activities at Sion Vale, but it is also likely that this publicity reflected efforts by the practitioners to exploit progress for ultimate financial advantage. It is also interesting that the publicity at the time gave sole credit to Delahoyde and while this is understandable in view of the fact that he was the qualified doctor it may also reflect the beginning of some separation between him and Lucett. The *Caledonian Mercury* for 29th July carried a report that Mr Delahoyde had performed one of 'his miraculous cures' during 'the last three weeks under the inspection of the Duke of Sussex and several noblemen'. On the 31st July the *Ipswich Post* printed its own variation of the same story and this wording was repeated in the *Royal Cornwall Gazette* of 14th August. While the patient was not identified, it is highly likely that it was Braily. The oddity is the reference to the Duke of Sussex. The Duke of Kent was the motive force behind the

Committee and while Sussex supported him he was clearly the subsidiary character. The publicity could have been inspired by the Committee as a way of attracting additional sponsorship, but if that had been the case it seems likely that a formal statement by the Committee in the name of the chairman, the Duke of Kent, would have been issued. The flurry of publicity looks as if it reflected briefing by Delahoyde.

A more significant account of the curative process became available in a medical journal at this time. This was not picked up by the popular press even though it gave a detailed account of the process itself and provided a complete rebuttal of the *Examiner's* assault on Lucett over the supposedly failed case of Mr Morgan of Somers Town. Dated 20th July 1813 the account appeared in the *Medical and Physical Journal* under the title, 'Treatment of Insanity by Messrs Tardy and Lucett communicated by Mr Tardy, Surgeon, of Marchmont Street, to Dr Fothergill' and gave a detailed history of the Morgan case. [Dr Fothergill was the editor of the *Medical and Physical Journal*.] Tardy was entirely straightforward about the timing of his intervention as the opening of his account demonstrates, 'Sir, the new method of curing insanity so laudibly countenanced by His R. H. the Duke of Kent, and a committee of noblemen and gentlemen, having created considerable interest, I have been induced to transmit to your Journal a detailed report of the first case in which it was tried, conjointly by myself and Mr Lucett, the gentleman who communicated to me this particular plan of treatment.'

Tardy continues with a disclaimer. He refers to a number of advertisements which had appeared in 1811 which related to the Morgan case. Tardy states that these adverts had appeared without his knowledge and it is implicit that he did not approve of Lucett's initiative. It is not clear which adverts Tardy was referring to, but the most obvious ones were the open letters to the queen of August and September 1811. The *Examiner's* dismissal of Lucett based on the Morgan case had come in early 1812. If Dr Tardy had been aware of the *Examiner's* version of the Morgan case he gives no indication in his communication with Fothergill. Dr Tardy then sets out the text of the letter which was sent to the Prime Minister, Spencer Perceval, about the curative process in 1811 under his and Lucett's joint signatures. Tardy says nothing about a response. Finally Tardy focuses on the Morgan case.

In contrast to the 'case histories' which Lucett was to use in promoting his curative process later, Tardy was clearly writing for a professional audience. He sets the background to the case with an account of Morgan's age and physical and mental history. He also clearly identifies the patient as 'The Editor of the *Dublin Correspondent* newspaper'. Tardy and Lucett treated Morgan between 23rd September 1811 and the 1st and 2nd October by which time Morgan was able to sleep and behave 'with decorum'. The treatment was never finished however. Morgan had suffered from haemorrhoids for the previous nine or ten years and during the treatment he suffered serious bleeding. Tardy said that he had at first hoped that this might actually aid the treatment, but this was not the case and the Lucett treatment had to be terminated because of the severe blood loss of the patient. 'This discharge was the more to be regretted, as unequivocal symptoms of amendment had shown themselves from the moderate application' of the Lucett treatment. 'The treatment employed by Mr Lucett and myself upon this gentleman; were immersion and warm affusions on the head conducted in such a manner, by a considerable column of water, as to produce a slight concussion upon the shaven vertex. The bath was at first at 93 degrees, and subsequently increased to 107 and 108. He was kept in the bath about four minutes in the first trial, and afterwards from thirty to fourty [sic] minutes.' Tardy went on to say that the treatment had continued for a short time after the letter was sent to Mr Perceval but due to 'an incautious and sudden increase of the temperature of the bath' Morgan's haemorrhoids burst and he lost about 10 ounces of blood per day.

The Morgan case had not therefore been a failure of the Lucett process. Instead the intervention of a pre-existing condition which threatened the life of the patient had led to the treatment for insanity to be stopped. Frustratingly Dr Tardy supplies no information on how he had come to be involved with Lucett in the treatment of Morgan or why they had apparently co-operated only in the single case. Interestingly Tardy does not criticise Lucett, his methods or refer to his being unqualified. Indeed Dr Tardy did not accept that the Morgan case itself was finished. On the contrary he comments to the editor of the *Medical and Physical Journal*, 'In an establishment in which I am about to engage for the reception of insane persons, I propose to try this process with some variations on this gentleman again; and the results upon him, as well as some others, I will transmit to you for publication'. Essentially Tardy's view was that there was not enough evidence to formally endorse the Lucett process as a treatment for the insane, but it was certainly worth serious investigation.[33]

Dr Tardy's views are valuable as he was clearly a professional with a dispassionate view of Lucett and his process. He was not looking for the kind of publicity which would have accompanied an approach to the popular press. Instead he approached the professional journal of his calling and set out the incomplete, but promising experience he had had. He was clearly aware that Lucett did not have a medical background, but Tardy did not assume that Lucett was therefore a charlatan or quack. His balanced perspective perhaps demonstrates that the involvement of the royal dukes and the other important people in the formation of the Committee to investigate the Lucett process was reasonable in the light of medical and scientific knowledge of the time.

Chapter Twelve

The Trial Continues

'Why should we be ashamed to think, or to have it known, that we have a brother or a sister afflicted with insanity? It is neither so loathsome as the small-pox, nor so dangerous as a typhus fever … nor is seclusion half so requisite for the madman as for the fever patient.'[1]
General View of the present state of Lunatics and Lunatic asylums
in Great Britain and Ireland and some other kingdoms.
Sir Andrew Halliday, London 1828.

The correspondence generated by the Committee has not survived as a coherent, comprehensive whole. However, it is possible to piece together a reasonable picture from what has survived. On 3rd August 1813, Delahoyde wrote to Earl Fitzwilliam[2] with what was essentially a side copy of the report he had sent to the Committee the previous day. In the report he gave an account of the five patients he was treating under the auspices of the Committee experiment. The report was positive and it is notable that the treatment seemed to have a significantly tranquilising effect. All the patients had high pulse rates during their deranged or manic state. In all cases Delahoyde reported very significant reductions of pulse rate as well as a marked improvement in behaviour.

A letter from Dr Harness to Earl Fitzwilliam on 6th August[3] may be representative of a more comprehensive correspondence which was generated by the therapeutic trial. Again the balance of what Harness reported was very positive, but progress was not uniform. Interestingly Harness reported that one of the patients, Thomas Reilly, seemed better physically since his arrival at Sion Vale, but that his mental condition did not seem much improved. A version of this account went to the Committee as a formal report and was discussed during the third meeting of the Committee on 7th August.

Harness' letter of 6th August also included one of the more bizarre byways of the whole trial. Harness told Fitzwilliam that John Moon had been discharged 'some days since' and that in accordance with his wishes he had been returned to the area of Trowbridge in Wiltshire where his few relatives lived. Apparently Moon had been escorted by one of Mr Delahoyde's servants who reported that Moon had been greeted triumphantly by a numerous band of criminals whom Moon had supposedly led previously. Dr Harness had been sufficiently disturbed to pass on the information to the Earl of Cork who was a Committee member and an active magistrate. The plot thickened on 11th August when Lord Dundas wrote to Fitzwilliam[4] and in a postscript pointed him to the *Morning Chronicle* of 9th August and the report that someone named Moon had killed a man near Trowbridge. The thought that a former lunatic had been released as cured and had immediately killed someone would have been the stuff of nightmares for the Committee. The newspapers of the time would have had the same kind of reaction as the popular press in the UK would do now. With royal involvement, experiments with 'cures' which ran counter to the received wisdom of the age and the backing of the great and the good, the press would have had a field day. Essentially both Harness and Dundas could have avoided raising Fitzwilliam's blood pressure as well as any other members of the Committee they spoke to in similar terms. John Moon's history was well documented as Harness knew. There was no time when he could have been absent from Bethlem or the marines to pursue a career in organised crime. In fact the *Morning Chronicle* article relates a quarrel between two blacksmiths which got out of hand and ended in a fight. The blacksmith called Moon was clearly established in the area and could not have been an alumnus of Sion Vale. A careful reading should have enabled Lord Dundas to avoid raising a scare. In hindsight though the incident was a reminder that the experiment was far from risk free and that in supporting the therapeutic trial the backers were to some extent also staking their reputations.

Lord Dundas' letter to Fitzwilliam on 11th August is important as it provides evidence of the active involvement of at least two prominent members of the Committee in its development. Dundas' letter was clearly written in response to one he had received from Fitzwilliam. Dundas says that he agrees with Fitzwilliam's view that 'the progress of Delahoyde's proceedings' should be published. He says that it might have the effect of attracting additional funds 'which I have no doubt is much wanted'. Dundas goes on to note that a published report at the time would have to make it clear that it was only a progress report towards finding a cure for insanity and that perhaps in the first instance the Committee should send a progress report to all subscribers while asking them to do all they could to find additional support. There is no full account of the discussions which took place on 7th August during the third meeting of the Committee. The progress report which was published on 27th September, however, included both Harness' and Delahoyde's reports from the beginning of August.

August 1813 proceeded with apparent calm so far as the surviving records of the Committee experiment are concerned. There was one small incident which may have been related to the experiment. Queen Charlotte had a private lunch with Sir Joseph Banks and his wife and daughter on 13th August at the Banks' home, Spring Grove. Enormous detail survives on the catering arrangements, but not a word on the conversation. It is a mark of the confidence the queen had in Banks and the intimacy of the relationship that there were no servants at the lunch. Banks himself apparently dealt with the drinks, while his wife and daughter served at table. From a letter which Queen Charlotte wrote to Lady Harcourt on the same day it is clear that the queen visited Banks in order to see some exotic plants. The timing of the encounter would, however, also fit very well with the idea that the queen was given a briefing on the progress of the Committee experiment; just as the king had been given briefings over the years by Banks on scientific developments. Sadly this idea is speculative, but the encounter took place at the time when the prospects for the Delahoyde and Lucett 'cure' seemed most hopeful. The encounter is also a reminder that the Committee was composed of people who in many cases had important direct links with the royal family. Banks had after all advised Queen Charlotte on the development of Kew Gardens.[5]

At the end of August came the first indicator of potential trouble. Dr Harness wrote again to Earl Fitzwilliam on 28th August[6] with an update on the case of John Moon. Harness had been in correspondence with the Earl of Cork who had followed up the rumour that Moon had been a bandit leader. The earl's enquiries had rapidly and predictably disposed of the idea that Moon had been a crime boss in Wiltshire. He had, however, discovered that Moon had suffered a relapse, had been arrested and was in the care of a parson living in Devizes who ran a receiving house for lunatics. In a further indicator of the very real involvement the Committee members had in the experiment, Harness reported that the Duke of Kent had sent a full account of Moon's medical history to the vicar of North Bradley which was the parish Moon had been removed to. Harness expressed his astonishment that despite the fact that Moon had suffered a relapse a month previously the Duke of Kent had 'to my astonishment not a syllable' from the vicar.[7]

Moon's relapse was a serious set-back. His case had been one of the three which had been used as evidence to justify setting up the Committee and proceeding with the experiment to assess the Lucett 'cure'. He had also been treated twice. There was other troubling news in the letter. Harness reported on the progress in the treatment of John Braily. He had visited Sion Vale on 10th August and had found Braily working in the garden. He was not, however, as calm and collected as Harness had become accustomed to.

Harness had talked quietly to Braily who had complained about his situation and particularly of being annoyed by numerous people, mainly women, who either complained to him about their troubles or complained about Braily. Although Harness did not state in the letter that this was the case it would appear that the bothersome people were imaginary. Asked if he felt better than he had at Hoxton, Braily said that he certainly did, but in a sad afterthought said that he did not know how long the improvement would continue. He said that he felt his head becoming more confused.

Here was testimony from 'inside' the process. Braily had been so violent that he had had to be transferred to Delahoyde and Lucett in chains. Yet even though his condition had deteriorated, Braily was alert enough, intelligent enough and well enough to assess his own case. He had derived some benefit from the treatment as well as escaping from Hoxton, but felt that the benefit was perhaps wearing off. Delahoyde's view was that the process should be repeated and this was done that evening. When Harness visited again on 25th August he found Braily calm and collected. Harness related that he and Braily had walked in the garden for a quarter of an hour during which time the patient 'conducted himself with great propriety, but occasionally expressed himself with more than usual rapidity'. If the similarity with George III's behaviour is noted, then for Braily it meant that he was on the verge of a relapse.

Of the other three patients Harness reported mixed progress. On Daniel O'Keefe, Harness was unable to see any sign of improvement, but on Cardiff and Matters he saw progress. Both were calm and were able, apparently, to discuss, including with each other, their former delusions. The delusions were clearly serious, or had been and included the idea that Cardiff had been confined in a whale's belly. Harness stated in the letter that any mention of their delusions let alone any challenge to their reality had originally provoked a storm in response. Following treatment the two patients were able to discuss their problems calmly. Again the similarity with the obsessive delusions of the king and his response to any challenge are clear.

This report to Fitzwilliam and the similar account which Harness gave to Lord Melville in his letter of 30th August[8] show that he was not immediately pessimistic at the relapse of John Moon. It is possible that Harness was not fully aware of the complete nature of Moon's relapse, but it is possible that Harness was realistic enough not to expect an instant, total and comprehensive cure for madness in all its manifestations. What is noticeable is that Harness highlights those aspects of the patients' behaviour which came closest to the symptoms displayed by George III. So when Braily is described as speaking with 'decorum' Harness was not only contrasting the patient's language with the probable violence and obscenity when he was fully deranged at Hoxton, but also drawing a parallel with the foul language which the king displayed under the influence of his derangement.

The next step for the Committee came with a review meeting at Sion Vale on 15th September. Apparently only the Duke of Kent, Thomas Smith and Dr Harness were present while Delahoyde and Lucett were available. The purpose of the meeting was to review the condition of the public patients and the committee members concluded that all patients had improved in varying degrees. The only account of this meeting and its conclusions on record seems to be that which subsequently appeared in the *Medical and Physical Journal*. The article in the journal is largely based on the first report of the Committee which was published in late September 1813, and gives a detailed account of the progress of the Committee. The *Medical and Physical Journal* was the professional paper which Dr Tardy had approached with an account of the first use of the Lucett treatment and had clearly taken Tardy and the formation of the Committee seriously.

'The process itself is reserved by them [Delahoyde and Lucett] from the public but having been detailed by Mr Tardy of Marchmont Stuart, (sic) in our number for August last, we consider these cases as mere exemplications (sic) of his mode of treatment, and in that point of view merit the notice of our readers.'[9] There are some important conclusions to be drawn from this episode. The first is that it provides further evidence that the Duke of Kent wanted to directly oversee the assessment process and any publications issued by the Committee as well as just how important the duke's involvement in the Committee was to him. It is also significant that the *Medical and Physical Journal*, which was a serious professional publication in its day, took the activities of the Committee seriously knowing from Dr Tardy what formed the basis at least of the Lucett process. At the time the Lucett process was not assumed to be mere chicanery or quackery, despite the cool response of most of the royal doctors when asked about Delahoyde and Lucett. Indeed Dr John Clarke the specialist in obstetrics and child medicine recommended similar treatments to those mentioned by Dr Tardy for convulsions believing that 'by diffusing the circulation generally' excess blood in the brain was diverted away.[10]

At this moment there was a reminder that Lucett and Delahoyde were not the only ones who considered that they had a potential cure for insanity to offer or that it should be considered for use on the king. Dr Charles Dunne was a qualified physician who had seen many years of service attached to the British armed forces. He had also lobbied the College of Physicians in 1810 to improve the system for inspection of private asylums in order to reduce the potential for patients to be exploited by relatives. He was also a critic of the Willises and dismissed their treatment as only temporary in effect and opposed the cruelty he considered their methods involved. His attempted intervention in the case of George III was remarkably similar to Lucett's own early attempts to engage the authorities with the offer of a treatment for the king. Dunne placed an open letter in *The News* dated 13th August 1813. In a striking parallel to Lucett, Dunne offered a treatment which had not been used on the 'Royal Sufferer' and hoped, as a loyal citizen, that his proposals would be given a fair trial by the physicians attending the king. Dunne's letter reads almost like a paraphrasing of Lucett's early ventures in open letters. Dunne's treatment he claimed was, 'founded on rational principles and successfully employed'. The clear distinction with Lucett is that Dunne was more willing to discuss his proposed treatment.[11]

Dunne clearly saw himself as a specialist in the treatment of insanity. His approach to his patients was more sympathetic than the Willis method and he deplored the use of restraint and 'lowering diets'. For the most part though he had recourse to the conventional treatments of the time such as bleeding and blisters. Where Dunne differed was in his arguments that cold on the head was very effective in dealing with mania. In this advocacy he may have been one of the practitioners who had prompted Halford's lofty comment that the use of cold was nothing new. Dunne went beyond simply placing snow or wet towels on the patient's head to include refinements in which evaporation was encouraged to heighten the effect. He even advocated cold water being dropped or dripped onto one place on the head of the patient. At this point the similarity with the Lucett treatment was complete. The irony is that at this juncture, Lucett was the 'insider' as the Committee sponsored trial was under way leaving little room for Dunne to establish himself.

Meanwhile the formal link between the activities of the Committee and the Queen's Council had remained in something of a limbo since the Archbishop of Canterbury's letter to Lord Melville of 13th July. Manners-Sutton had not had a reply so on 6th September he again wrote to Lord Melville repeating the questions he had put in his earlier letter.[12] In an attempt to increase the pressure on Melville the archbishop reminded him that a quarterly meeting of the Queen's Council was due prior to reporting to the Privy Council. The contrast between the enthusiasm of the archbishop and the detachment of Lord Melville is very marked. The archbishop clearly saw the 'cure' which the Committee was investigating as a potential solution to the problem of the king. At this point in the chronology the experiments using the so called Delahoyde process were broadly favourable so Melville would not have had failure of the trial to explain his reticence. It would be surprising if there really was no informal communication between the members of the Queen's

Council and those of the Committee on the progress of the trial. They were all people who moved in the upper ranks of Georgian society so the possibility of informal contact was real. Yet no pointer to any such informal contact appears to survive and it is clear that if the Archbishop was aware of any filtration of information from the Committee to the Queen's Council he gave no sign of it in his letter to Lord Melville.

The reply when it came in a letter dated 17th September[13] was again a formal third person response. The letter states that he enclosed the only additional information he had received 'respecting the insane Naval Patients under the care of Mr Delahoyde'. The archive at Lambeth Palace does not include an enclosure but it would presumably have been the letter from Dr Harness of 30th August. Melville's coolness is again surprising but at least he promised to let Manners-Sutton have any further information he received before the end of the month in time for the quarterly meeting of the Queen's Council.

One of the most contentious aspects of the whole Committee trial and the one which fundamentally undermined the scientific nature of the whole assessment process was Lucett and Delahoyde's secrecy over exactly what was involved in the initial stage of the patient's treatment. Dr Harness' understanding of this vital first stage of the process is of crucial importance. He was the medical assessor and had expressed his astonishment at the effect achieved by 'the means employed' when commenting on the impact of the initial treatment on John Braily. This seems to indicate, as pointed out above, that he knew what was involved in the initial treatment. However, Harness does not state then or elsewhere that he had actually witnessed the treatment being performed or been told precisely what was involved. There is also no indication that Dr Harness had questioned any of the patients to determine what the initial stage of the treatment involved. Certainly he wrote no account of the process. The surviving Committee papers give no indication that any other visitor to Sion Vale had learned what the crucial first stage of the treatment involved. Without this knowledge the credibility of the whole assessment process would be undermined and the chances of the treatment being used at Windsor or anywhere else fatally compromised. It might have been acceptable during the informal stage of Kent's contact with Lucett to monitor the effect of a process in one or two instances without knowing exactly what that process entailed. When set against the ambitions expressed in the foundation of the Committee it was simply not credible to think that those ambitions could be achieved while secrecy remained about the exact nature of the process on which everything depended. Secrecy over the curative process was unacceptable if for no other reason than that the Committee would have to be able to say with certainty that the process was safe. This is a fundamental part in the process for authorising the use of a new drug today and it is to the credit of the Committee that they addressed that issue in the early nineteenth century.

There is no record of negotiations between the Committee and Lucett or any indication that full disclosure would be required before the therapeutic trial began. Certainly there was no reference to disclosure of the nature of the curative process when the Committee was set up. The only evidence as to what may have happened comes from a letter which Harness wrote to Lord Melville on 23rd September. After informing Melville that the patients at Sion Vale all seemed to have benefited from the curative process Harness goes on to say that soon 'the World may no longer consider the nostrum confidential or dangerous in its administration' and that Messrs Delahoyde and Lucett have 'appointed this day at 1 o'clock to lay the original recipe before' the Dukes of Kent and Sussex and Dr Harness. Harness describes this development as 'a measure which will hereafter afford me the advantage of speaking to its merits or otherwise'. So far as decorum in official correspondence would allow Harness gives full expression to his pleasure at this development.[14] Harness had clearly considered that he did not know enough about the treatment to enable him to fully assess its effectiveness. His commentary also indicated that he was aware that there had been criticism of the curative process. The agreement by Lucett and Delahoyde to lay the whole process before the Dukes of Kent and Sussex as well as Dr Harness suggests that there had been some discussion between the parties and a compromise had been agreed. This was that disclosure would be made to the minimum number of Committee members necessary and to the medical assessor so that the therapeutic trial would have credibility. At the same time Lucett and Delahoyde would retain sufficient control to enable them to exploit the commercial potential of the treatment in due course.

There were three fundamental questions which had to be answered if the therapeutic trial was to achieve its aims. The first two were whether the treatment was dangerous or not and whether the trial had been carried out in full knowledge of what was involved in the therapeutic process. If the proposed disclosure to the Dukes of Kent and Sussex was properly handled then this criticism of the trial which *The Gazette* had highlighted would be neutralised. Dr Heberden had expressed the view that the Lucett process was probably hazardous when he responded to the question on Delahoyde and Lucett put by the Queen's Council. Full disclosure of the therapy by Delahoyde and Lucett would potentially go a long way to answering that concern. The third fundamental question was of course to determine whether the therapy worked or not. This increasingly became the focus of attention.

Chapter Thirteen

Things Fall Apart

'The Committee who have undertaken to make enquiry into, and ascertain the extent of the process practised by Messrs Delahoyde and Lucett for the relief of persons afflicted with insanity, and to provide the means of paying the expense of such enquiry, make this their first Report.'[1]

Dated 27th and 28th September 1813.

The publication of the report dated 27th and 28th September was of fundamental importance for the Committee sponsored evaluation of the Lucett curative process. So the whole tone of the report is formal and business-like and is written in a clear economical style.[2] The report aimed to achieve a series of objectives and to cater to several distinct audiences, but the principal objective was to underline the professionalism and integrity of the whole undertaking. Unless this was achieved there would be little prospect of the Committee achieving its longer term aims. So while the report served the function of bringing the Committee members and sponsors up to date it was essentially outward looking and was intended to address a wider audience. A balance had to be struck in which the account was scrupulously honest while presenting a picture which would attract others to subscribe and keep the experiment funded. The ambition of the Committee remained intact, but the obvious sense of enthusiasm and expectation of the foundation documents is missing. The report is absolutely neutral in its references to the curative process and is careful not to raise unreasonable expectations that a cure for insanity was either imminent or certain.

After some repetition of the foundation documents covering the structure and membership of the Committee, its members and sponsors and that a total of £796-2s had been donated the account moves on to cover the therapeutic trial itself. The greatest care, understandably, was taken in the explanation of how the patients used in the experiment were chosen and by whom. The emphasis seems to have been on making it absolutely clear that the patients were genuinely ill and that their cases were serious and of long standing.

The Report refers to the aim of putting 'the process to the severest possible test' and that the patients were selected from those at Hoxton who had been classified as 'incurable' by Dr Weir, Naval Medical Inspector, Mr Haslam, Principal Apothecary of Bethlem Hospital and Mr Sharpe, Surgeon at the Hoxton asylum. The Report sets out how the Committee had supervised the selection of the patients to be treated by Delahoyde and Lucett and how four difficult patients had been decided on.

The Report then shifts to a very detailed account of the individual patients. John Braily is the first one covered and the account goes into more detail on him than the rest of the patients. Certainly his selection was intended to provide the 'severest test' for the curative process. He is described as one, 'who appeared to the Committee to be more violent, if possible, than the rest, heavily chained and handcuffed, with an horse-cloth, by way of covering, about his waist'. Braily had been confined in Hoxton asylum in September 1809, but was shortly after transferred to Bethlem where he remained for a year of treatment. It was after that period when he was returned to Hoxton that he had been classified as 'incurable'. With his violent behaviour and long-term status as 'incurable', Braily represented a very challenging case for the experiment.

There is a quite detailed account of the impact of the treatment on Braily and the perspective of the patient himself gives the account a powerful impact without hyperbole. It emphasises the fact that the experiment was dealing with individuals rather than simply a category of beings who were labelled as insane. This mattered because it had not been so far in the past that those diagnosed as insane had been considered to have lost their humanity. In the case of Braily, Dr Harness had not witnessed an instant cure, but he was nevertheless evaluating something which produced a pretty miraculous impact on someone who had been in such a violent manic state that he had been in chains shortly before. Within ten minutes of the initial treatment, Braily was 'considerably calmed'. In just under an hour from the treatment, Dr Harness was able to sit on the patient's bed and quietly discuss how Braily felt. From a violent rage Braily had been calmed to the extent that he expressed his concern that he had given 'the gentleman' a great deal of trouble and that 'he hoped he should soon be better'. The physiological evidence Harness recorded was that Braily's pulse had dropped from 108 beats per minute to 76.

The detailed account of the impact of the process was intended to give the readership of the report the best possible understanding of its value. From a current perspective the obvious missing element is what the process involved and therefore some explanation of its effectiveness. Braily had undergone, in his own words, 'a severe operation'. What that operation involved is not explained. The report continues with shorter accounts of the other three patients: William Matters, James Cardiff and Daniel O'Keefe. The accounts essentially were intended to establish that each patient was rightly considered 'incurable' and that nevertheless the process had a significant and almost immediate positive impact on them. The limitations of Georgian diagnostics were such that the pulse and general demeanour of the patient were the only criteria which could be applied with certainty in judging the impact. Nevertheless the impact was clear. In each case the patient was calmed and the pulse reduced from over 100 beats a minute to the low seventies.

Following the accounts of the selection, background and initial treatment of the four patients the report goes on to give a short version of the accounts Harness had given to Earl Fitzwilliam of his visits to Sion Vale and included the fact that John Braily's recovery was not complete and that he had had to be treated again. There was, however, a further pointer to the rigour which was employed in assessing the impact of the process on the patients which Harness had not mentioned in his letters to Fitzwilliam during August. This was that he was accompanied on his visit to Sion Vale on 10th August by Dr Weir, Naval Medical Inspector of Hospitals. Weir had regularly seen two of the patients, Matters and Cardiff when they had been held in Hoxton and his verdict on Cardiff was that he was better than he had ever seen him. The report also mentioned that other members of the Committee had taken the opportunity to visit Sion Vale.

The Report concluded that it was too soon to make a judgement on the 'permanent effects' of the process and that the purpose of the report was simply to provide 'a narrative of the facts as they have occurred'. Nevertheless the authors did allow themselves some satisfaction in noting that the 'violence of the paroxysms being evidently mitigated'. Overall the report seems fair, reasonable and balanced. There is no question of the Committee actively promoting the Lucett cure but the commitment to the evaluation process remained. The sense that the Committee still saw its involvement with the Lucett process being long term was the additional statement seeking subscriptions. 'The enclosed report is printed and circulated … for the purpose of promulgating the information it contains and of inducing such persons as may think proper to come forward with their subscriptions, and thereby aid the laudable undertaking in which the committee are engaged.'

The format of the Report was rather odd as it consisted of two parts with different dates and a small undated piece sandwiched between. The first part was dated 27th September and covered the account of the evaluation of the Lucett process outlined above and represented the bulk of the report as a whole. The second part is a short Declaration dated 28th September which was bound, as well as the undated third piece, with the body of the report. This second part of the report may have been very short, but it resolved one important issue while creating another contentious concern for the credibility of the experiment. The Declaration by the Dukes of Kent and Sussex and Dr Harness states that Messrs Delahoyde and Lucett had communicated the nature of the process for restoring insane persons 'under a pledge upon honour of secrecy' to the signatories. This crucial step of disclosure had come about 'since printing the forgoing report' and so was literally an afterthought. It was certainly an important one. To have continued to underwrite the trial of a process which remained secret from its sponsors would have seriously undermined the credibility of the entire proceedings and yet this is precisely what the Committee was apparently contemplating when the major part of the report was signed off as of 27th September.

The Declaration includes the statement that the nature of the restorative process had been communicated 'for the purpose of enabling us to form our judgement as to the safety' of that process. This assertion seems to raise a number of questions, not the least being an explanation for such an important aspect as the safety of the whole trial being handled as an apparent afterthought. If concern for the safety of the process itself had been a priority then it should have been addressed at the start before patients were involved. It is possible that this is a case of imposing current sensibilities on the past and reaching the incorrect conclusion that the fate of the patients was not of immediate concern to the Committee members. An alternative, admittedly speculative interpretation might be that at the time of the report the effect of the treatment on the initial group of patients had been broadly positive. The Dukes of Kent and Sussex will have known of the direct interest of the Queen's Council in the proceedings and may have considered the possibility that the Archbishop of Canterbury might respond to reading the original version of the report by asking whether the curative process was really safe. It would have been clearly implicit that the process was safe judging by the effect on the patients treated, but for the archbishop this would not have been enough if the patient in view was actually George III.

The Declaration also contained a significant extra statement which represented a departure from the initial terms of the experiment. The sample size of the group of patients involved in the trial of the curative process at that point was very small and this would have made the Declaration vulnerable to criticism that there was not enough evidence to make a real assessment of whether the process was safe or not. The signatories had, however, additionally declared that they were aware of a number of patients outside the remit of the Committee who had not been harmed by the curative process. This may have been a useful mechanism to counter possible criticism of the small sample size, but it actually represented a significant erosion of the scientific control and objectivity of the experiment as these patients had not been treated under the controlled terms of the Committee experiment. It also set a precedent for using reported accounts of the impact of the curative process which were outside the experiment and therefore unverifiable. This was to return in the final report of the Committee.

For the moment though a balance had been struck between the need for scientific credibility for the whole Committee experiment, the presumed commercial interests of Lucett and Delahoyde and preparation for the possible use of the 'cure' at Windsor. This suggests that there had been some negotiation between Committee representatives and Delahoyde and Lucett and that an agreement had been reached. It is also reasonable to assume that the balance was only intended to be temporary. If the process was to be used at Windsor then more people would inevitably have had to be invested into the mysteries of the process. It was also an ironic agreement in the sense that Dr Tardy had already released considerable detail about the Lucett curative process only a month before. Clearly the early nineteenth century was not an age of instant distribution of information. Tardy's intervention had been in a medical journal. This was clearly not the popular press, but it is perhaps surprising that nobody connected with the Committee or the royal family at Windsor or even George III's physicians appears to have picked up on it.

There remains the undated section placed between the main body of the report and the Declaration. This seemingly innocuous short insert is actually hugely important in the story of the therapeutic trial. The first part is the repetition of the section from the foundation documents of the Committee in which the formation of a permanent Society was proposed in the event that the evaluation of the Lucett process proved effective in treating insanity. The rest of the section is surprising and acts to disturb the generally positive impact of the report as a whole. In a note the Committee acknowledge that they had received a letter on 27th September from Messrs Delahoyde and Lucett informing the Committee that 'finding it necessary to encrease [sic] their accommodation for patients, they had quitted Sion Vale and taken the premises at Great Ealing called Ealing House'. On one level it appeared that Dr Harness' concerns that Delahoyde was filling Sion Vale with private patients had been confirmed although it was nevertheless surprising that Delahoyde and Lucett had made a unilateral decision to move from Sion Vale which had been set up under the auspices of the Committee.

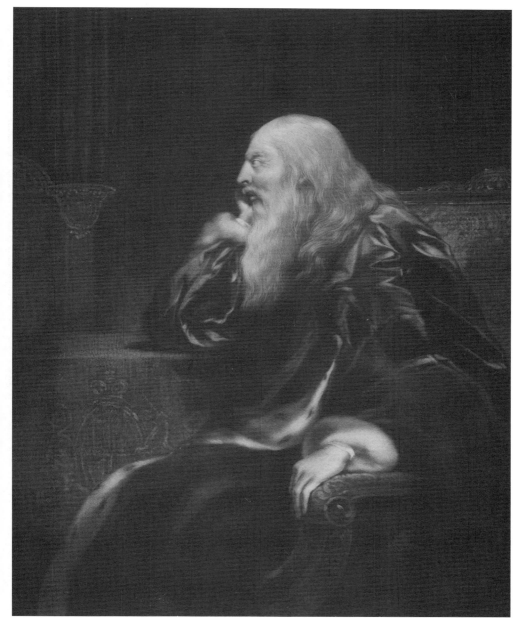

George III. Portrait in old age. Mezzotint by Samuel William Reynolds.
This image could be called 'Silent Dejection'. This was the reality of 'seclusion' which Dr Heberden had feared would break his patient's tenuous hold on reality. The portrait was made very rapidly by a visitor to Windsor and without the king being aware that his likeness was being taken. The moving portrait of George III seems to encapsulate the inner world of his imagination which had become more real than his physical existence. This is an early version of the portrait which was published later with the permission of George IV on 24th February 1820 in revised form as on the cover. (*Royal Collection Trust. Copyright Her Majesty Queen Elizabeth II, 2021/Bridgeman Images*)

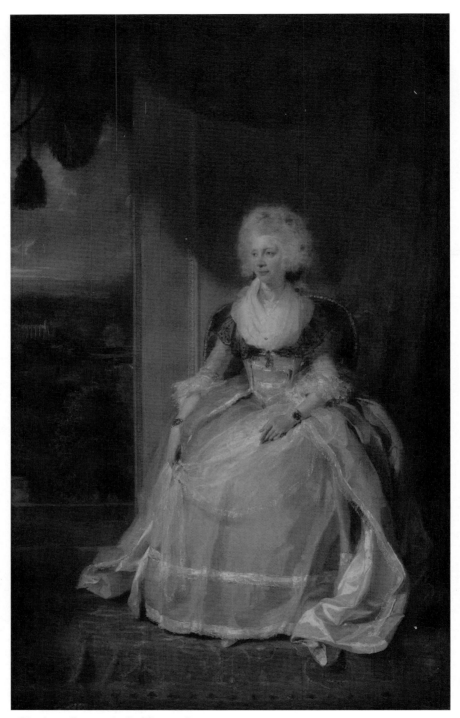

Queen Charlotte. Portrait by Sir Thomas Lawrence.
This is no 'swagger portrait' of a great lady, but a highly sensitive portrait of a preoccupied and vulnerable woman. Dated from 1789 the picture was rejected by the sitter and by George III. Perhaps neither wanted a reminder of the impact of the king's illness on the queen. (*Copyright The National Gallery, London/ Bridgeman Images*)

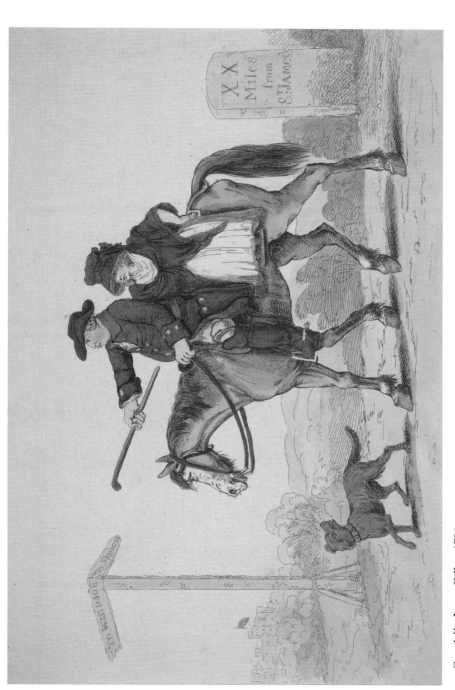

'The Constant Couple' by James Gillray 1786.

An affectionate and gentle satire of the royal couple. The emphasis on the word 'constant' is important as it highlights the closeness of the relationship between George III and Queen Charlotte before the strain of the king's illness took its toll. This cartoon marks George III's progress towards becoming the embodiment of the nation at a time when technological and political revolution seemed to threaten the natural order of society. (*Copyright The Trustees of the British Museum. All Rights Reserved*)

'Filial Piety' Thomas Rowlandson dated 25 October 1788.

Reputedly the only cartoon which depicts George III while 'mad'. The image is dated just before Dr Francis Willis was called in to treat the king. (*Copyright The Trustees of the British Museum. All Rights Reserved*)

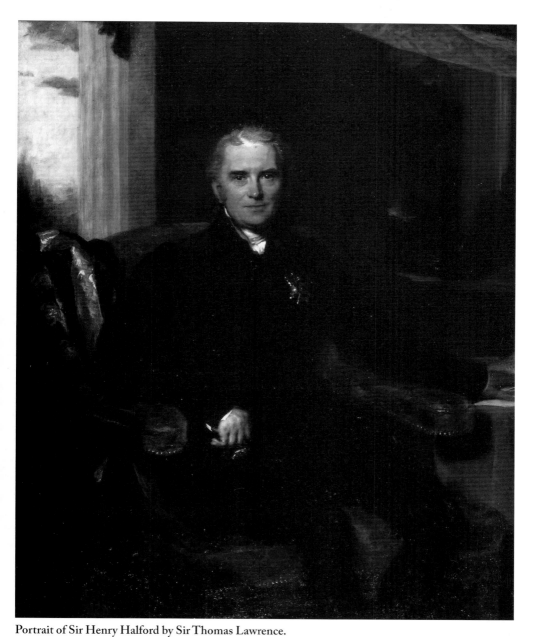

Portrait of Sir Henry Halford by Sir Thomas Lawrence.
Doyen of the medical profession, Halford looks out at the world with apparent confidence in his technical skills and his diplomatic capabilities. The pose and the fact that he was painted by the foremost portraitist of his age echo the aristocratic portraits of the age. Halford embodied the success which top medical practitioners could aspire to. (*The image is copyright Royal College of Physicians*)

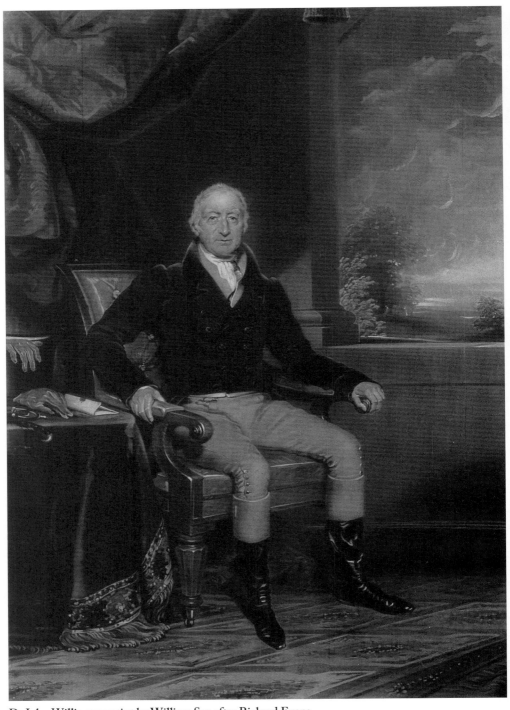

Dr John Willis mezzotint by William Say after Richard Evans.
For all the trappings of an aristocratic portrait, John Willis looks uncomfortable with the strained and exaggeratedly upright pose. It looks almost as if he is ready to spring up in response to anyone questioning his right to be sat in the great chair. (*Image courtesy of the Wellcome Trust Collection. Public Domain Mark*)

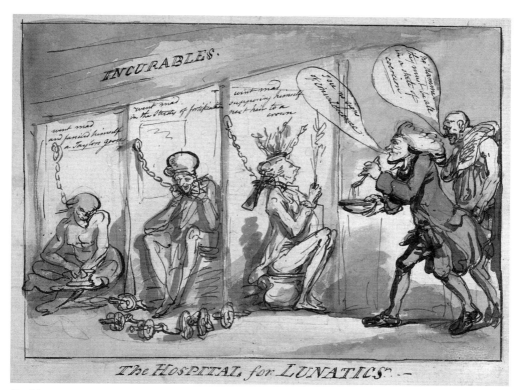

'Bethlem Hospital, London: the incurables being inspected.' Thomas Rowlandson 1789.

Although Rowlandson had a political purpose in drawing this cartoon in which eminent politicians take the place of patients at Bedlam the point is that aggressive restraint was assumed in the management of 'incurable' patients. (*Image courtesy of the Wellcome Trust Collection. Public Domain Mark*)

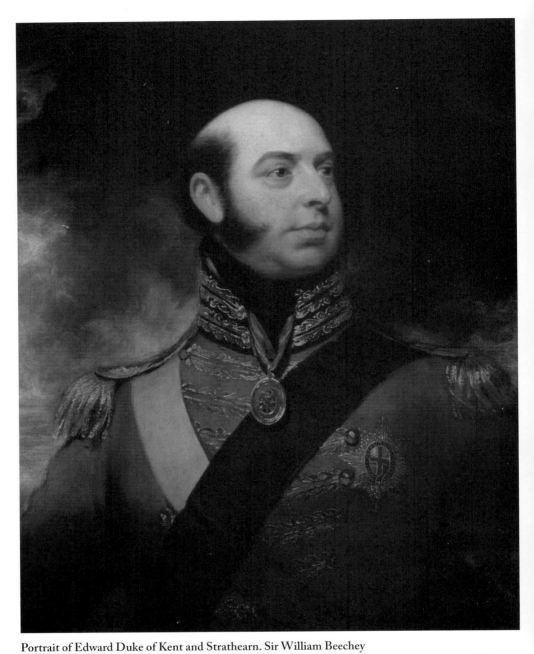

Portrait of Edward Duke of Kent and Strathearn. Sir William Beechey
The Duke of Kent's place in history is secured by his being the father of the future Queen Victoria.
His role, with his brother the Duke of Sussex, in the formation of the Committee which evaluated the
Lucett 'cure' for insanity was fundamental in making the experiment possible. It was also indicative of his
desire to explore alternative treatments which might bring relief to his father. (*Copyright National Portrait
Gallery, London*)

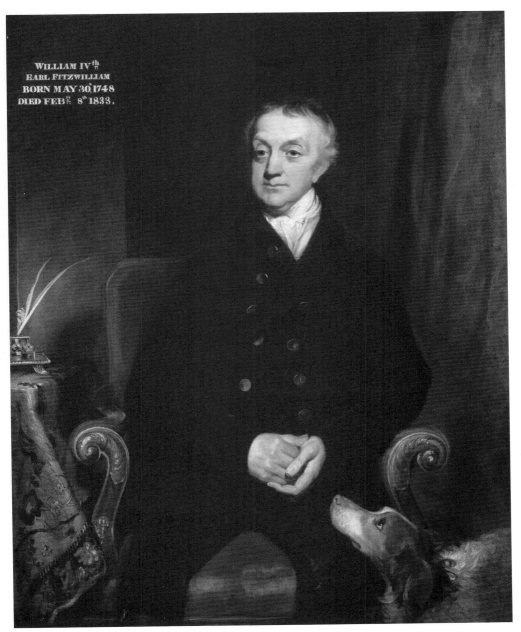

WILLIAM IVth
EARL FITZWILLIAM
BORN MAY 30, 1748
DIED FEB^{ry} 8th 1833.

Portrait of William Wentworth Fitzwilliam, 4th Earl Fitzwilliam. William Owen.
As one of the richest men in the UK Fitzwilliam was a transitional figure. He derived his wealth not simply from the traditional source of large landholdings but from mining the coal which lay on and under that land. In a literal sense he helped power the industrial revolution. (*Copyright National Portrait Gallery*)

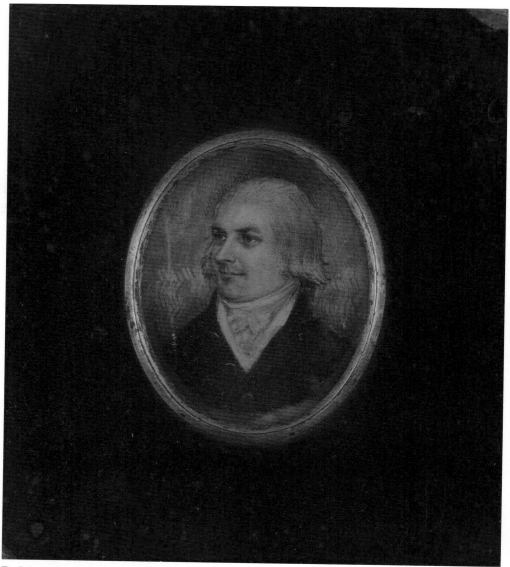

Dr John Harness. Miniature portrait.
This is no statement portrait in which the sitter faces his audience almost with disdain. Instead this is an unadorned personal likeness which must have been intended for a wife or lover as a keepsake while he was on extended voyages early in his career. (*Copyright National Maritime Museum, Greenwich, London*)

REPORT.

THE COMMITTEE, which took upon itself to investigate the Merits due to the Process, practised by MESSRS. DELAHOYDE and LUCETT, for the *Cure* of *Insane Persons*, and made its first Report on the *28th September*, 1813, has now to offer a Second and *Final* one to the Public, as the Result of its Enquiries, in the Course of which, no Pains, Labor, or Attention were spared, which it was in their Power to give to a Subject, so interesting, and so important to the Cause of Humanity.

The COMMITTEE would have wished, in Return for the Liberality of those Noblemen and Gentlemen, who, by their Subscriptions, so materially assisted the Object of the Investigation, to have been able to State, that the Result had been altogether satisfactory; but unfortunately, the Four Public Patients, whom they placed under the Care of MESSRS. DELAHOYDE and LUCETT, Viz.—*Braily, O'Keife, Cardiffe*, and *Matters;* although, at first, so essentially benefitted by the Effects of the Process, as to hold out the most flattering Prospects of ultimate Success attending the Attempt, did not retain that permanent Benefit, which had, in the first Instance, been most anxiously expected; but, at the same Time, that Candour requires this Acknowledgment with respect to the Four above-named Cases; the COMMITTEE, feels it a Duty to observe that, other Cases have also come before it, from the private Practice of MESSRS. DELAHOYDE and LUCETT, in which complete Success appeared to have attended the Effects of the Process, from which Consideration, little doubt is entertained by those who have most closely followed up the Investigation, not only that the Discovery is a most valuable one, but that it can be used with perfect safety to the Patient, when placed in the Hands of professional and scientific Men, while upon the Whole, it certainly holds out a very flattering Prospect of promoting the Recovery of those unfortunate Individuals who are afflicted with Insanity, by a Mode of Treatment, infinitely less painful to the Feelings of their Friends and Relations, than that which is frequently practised according to the old System.

EDWARD
WENTWORTH FITZWILLIAM
MILTON
DUNDAS
I. HARNESS, M. D.
R. CLARK, Chamberlain
I. DENT.

Final Report of the Committee from early 1814.
A balance is achieved and it was done publicly. The failure to produce an outright and permanent cure for insanity is set against the fact that the Lucett 'cure' did have a positive impact on mania which could contribute to the recovery of patients. The highlighting of the benign nature of the Lucett treatment compared with conventional treatment of the insane involving restraint reflects the very real revulsion at orthodox medical treatment of such patients. (*Image made available courtesy of Sheffield Libraries and Archives*)

Chertsey May the 22d 1821

Sir

The intimation given in your letter received this morning, I am not at all surprized at, I do assure you the inhabitants of Ewell need not be alarmed In respect to any person that I may think proper to receive under my care with having resided these Seven Years past adjoining the Church were I at present reside are very sufficient proofs that the Congregation nor a Single Inhabitant have never been <u>alarmed</u>, or <u>disturbed</u> and although the number of Persons at any time residing with me, I wish not to exceed four, still according to act of parliament it is necessary to have a Licence, I am inclined to think the Court who have thought proper hitherto to grant one will require more substantial evidence than surmise, and although I profess to relieve a person deranged in forty minutes, I shall never consider my residence a <u>mad</u> house or a place of <u>Confinement</u>, as never having had occasion to use those unhappy means resorted to in private and public receptacles for lunatics, and if I should be so fortunate as not to be annoyed more by the Inhabitants of Ewell than they will be by any one in my house I shall be perfectly satisfied with the result

I am
Sir
Your humble Servt
Jas Lucett

At a Vestry held this 7th Day of June 1821 the above Letter from Mr Lucett was read as the answer to the Letter directed to be sent by the last Vestry

The conclusion of James Lucett's letter to the Ewell Vestry dated 22nd May 1821.
Lucett at his best although he cannot quite resist the temptation to include some self-promotion. He nevertheless defines his views of his patients and the function of an asylum in a way which commands respect. (*Reproduced by permission of Surrey History Centre. Copyright Surrey History Centre*)

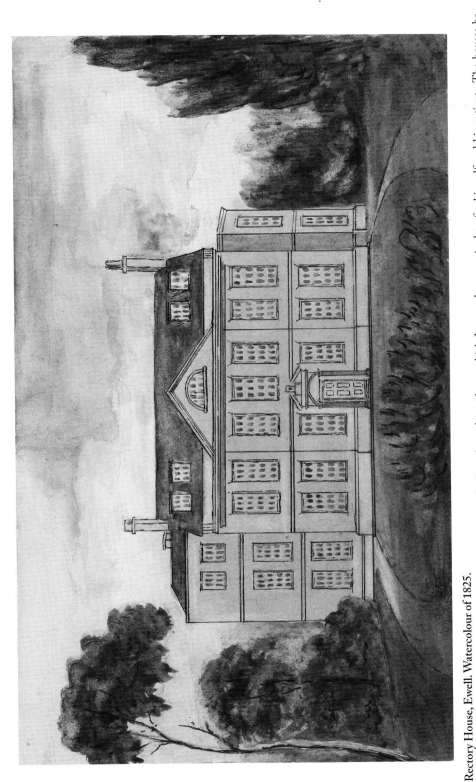

Rectory House, Ewell. Watercolour of 1825.

A naïve painting, but it nevertheless conveys clearly the kind of gentleman's residence which Lucett always aspired to for himself and his patients. The houses he occupied were intended to provide the physical manifestation of the success of his cure for insanity. (*Reproduced by permission of Surrey History Centre. Copyright Surrey History Centre*)

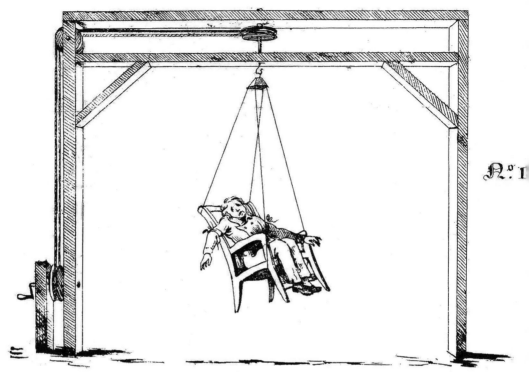

N.º 1

A picture of Dr William Hallaran's spinning chair.
It was used to treat the insane and similar equipment was suggested for use on George III. Its purpose was to disrupt manic episodes in the hope that this would aid recovery. In practice it induced violent vomiting and evacuations which had little useful therapeutic value. Picture available in Hallaran's book on *Cure for Insanity* of 1810. (*Wellcome Trust Collection. Public Domain Mark*)

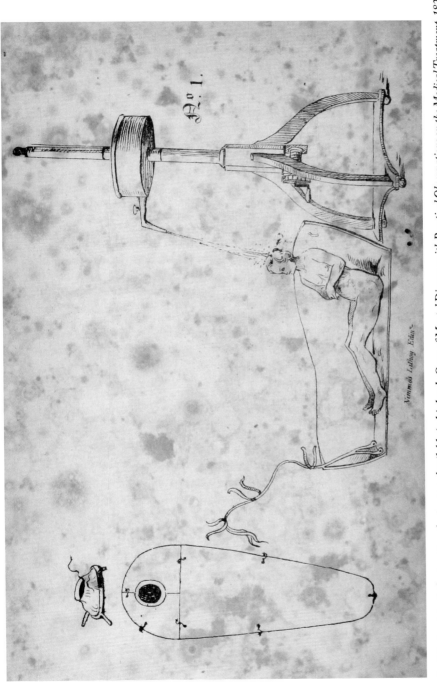

Vermmos Ludwig Edax

No. 1.

Dr Alexander Morison's bath for treating the insane. Available in his book *Cases of Mental Disease, with Practical Observations on the Medical Treatment. 1828.* Although no picture of the equipment which Lucett and Dr Tardy used to treat Mr Morgan exists this illustration matches the description given by Tardy to the *Medical and Physical Journal* in July 1813. The fact that Morison was the medical inspector of Lucett's private asylum in 1815 provides an ironic linkage as well as demonstrating that Lucett's way of treating insane patients had been taken up by one eminent and qualified practitioner 15 years later. (*Image courtesy of the Wellcome Trust Collection. Public Domain Mark*)

TO HIS MOST EXCELLENT MAJESTY *the* KING, &c.

SIRE—The humble Petition of JAMES LUCETT, Professor of a mode of treatment for the Cure of Insanity in all the various shades, by a medical treatment unknown to any other practitioner in Europe, most humbly solicits your MAJESTY's interposition to make known the same for a national benefit, by which means all mad-houses and confinement will be superseded, except in cases of malformation and organic defect, which precludes the possibility of cure. That your humble Petitioner did submit his Treatise to the inspection of his late Royal Highness the Duke of KENT, and his Royal Highness the Duke of SUSSEX, and Dr. HARNESS, to whose professional skill and judgment their Royal Highnesses appealed, and who declared the same to be a highly valuable and safe discovery, and as a mark of their approbation affixed their names and seals unto it. That your humble Petitioner did, during the late and fatal illness of his late Royal Highness the Duke of YORK, offer to submit a Treatise to the Physicians attendant for the immediate relief and ultimate restoration of his Royal Highness, to which he received his most gracious answer through Sir HERBERT TAYLOR, with thanks, requesting at the same time the communication to be laid before his professional practitioners. Your humble Petitioner did make a similar offer to submit to the Medical Counsel a Treatment, through his Grace the Duke of WELLINGTON, on the 22d of April, for the immediate relief and ultimate restoration of our late Most Gracious MAJESTY of happy memory, to which your Petitioner received answer from his Grace, that not knowing him, he declined his offer. That your humble Petitioner not wishing the discovery in his sole possession to die with him, prays your Most Gracious MAJESTY to cause an investigation of the merits of his offer to be investigated, in order that a discovery, for which your Petitioner has been awarded by Government two hundred guineas, may not be withheld any longer from the Public by the insinuations of interested persons. And your Petitioner, as in duty bound, will ever pray, &c.   JAS. LUCETT.

Mitcham, July 21, 1830.

'To His Most Excellent Majesty the *King' Morning Post* 23rd July 1830. James Lucett's response to the accession of William IV was a letter to the editor in which he not only replayed his version of the relationship with the Committee, but also effectively claimed that two of the new king's brothers – George IV and the Duke of York – had suffered from insanity. This crass promotion of his 'cure' showed Lucett at his worst.

The meeting with the royal dukes and Dr Harness on 24th September when the secrets of the Lucett process were divulged and its safety demonstrated may look like part of a comfortable progression in the trial, but it was not. The move from Sion Vale actually reflected a crisis which very nearly brought the whole therapeutic trial to an abrupt end. John Dent in his capacity as treasurer of the Committee explained nearly two years later what had really prompted the move from Sion Vale and why the revelations to the Committee about the nature of the 'cure' came when they did.[3]

Delahoyde and Lucett had joined the small meeting at the home of Mr Thomas Smith on 23rd September 1813 when it was intended to review the Committee's first report before its publication. In fact the focus of the meeting became the need to resolve the extraordinary predicament which Delahoyde and Lucett were forced to admit they were in. The practitioners admitted they were being pursued by the bailiffs in connection with debts run up at Sion Vale and that a writ had been issued against them. The pair claimed that they could not return to Sion Vale as bailiffs, were actually at the receiving house, and that without an advance of £200 they would be arrested. Dent's account of 1815 goes on to say that it was agreed that Delahoyde and Lucett would attend the dukes the following morning, 24th September 1813, in order to divulge the secrets of the 'cure'. It is not clear whether the advance of £200 was made on condition that the revelations were made although it probably was the case. The small group of Committee members were unlikely to simply hand over what was a large sum of money at the time without some guarantee of restitution. It is not clear whether Delahoyde and Lucett offered or whether Smith and Dent insisted that the revelations should be made. Dent's account certainly provides an explanation for the last minute appearance of the Declaration on the safety of the curative process in the Committee report.

The account of the practitioner's fears of immediate arrest must have spoilt their ability to appear as two professionals at their meeting with the Dukes of Kent and Sussex and Dr Harness. The revelation that Delahoyde and Lucett were in debt would have come as an unwelcome contrast to the otherwise positive assessment of the experiment. While the framework set up to monitor the patients seems to have worked satisfactorily it appears that it was not so effective in monitoring the practitioners' financial affairs. The real positive progress with the patients remained but there must have been considerable unease about the debts associated with the receiving house at Sion Vale and whether Delahoyde and Lucett were reliable partners. It is implicit that the original intention of the Committee members was that Delahoyde and Lucett would concentrate, perhaps solely, on the patients associated with the trial. After all Sion Vale appeared to have been set up by the Committee in order to make the trial possible. With Dr Harness' early notice that 'Delahoyde' was filling Sion Vale with private patients there must have been some concern over the control of the experiment, even if these private patients were used in part to provide further information about the safety of the curative process. There must also have been doubts raised over how Delahoyde and Lucett's activities had resulted in significant debts so quickly. It is also clear that the move from Sion Vale to Ealing House was the result of some settlement with the bailiffs. Although no comment seems to have survived on the change in the location of the receiving house from any of the Committee members it is likely that the whole episode caused them to feel rather let down. Earl Fitzwilliam for example was a man who valued correct behaviour and he responded to Dent's letter in 1815 by contributing to the debt which Thomas Smith had incurred in making the £200 advance to Delahoyde and Lucett for which he had not been reimbursed.

The Committee remained true to its commitment to openness about the experiment. Copies of the first report were sent to the members of both Houses of Parliament while other official bodies were informed. Richard Troward sent a copy of the report to the Chairman of the Quarter Sessions at Kingston in Surrey on 30th September for example.[4] It is not immediately obvious why this was done although in this instance the Quarter Sessions were responsible for granting licences for the establishment of private asylums in the county. It may simply be a pointer to the Committee's secretary seeking to broadcast the record of the Committee's work as widely as reasonably possible. The report was also made available for sale as the advert in the *Morning Chronicle* for 6th November demonstrates. The price of six shillings seems rather high and it would be interesting to know how many were actually sold!

After the flurry of activity around the first Report of the Committee the surviving record is quiet until the end of October when on the 30th, Richard Troward, Secretary of the Committee, wrote to Dr Harness about two of the patients: William Matters and James Cardiff. Troward's letter recorded that Delahoyde and Lucett had been in touch with the Lords Commissioners of the Admiralty and pronounced the two patients cured. The Lords Commissioners had in turn informed Troward as the representative of the Committee that they were ready to discharge the two patients from the navy if Dr Harness confirmed they were indeed cured. Harness acted.[5] In his letter to the admiralty dated 9th November 1813, Harness asked for the Lords Commissioners to be informed that he had visited the two patients and had concluded that after making 'every enquiry' about the patients that they were fit to be discharged. Harness also recommended that the two patients should also be sent to the hospital ship *Batavia* for a probationary period of a month or six weeks prior to their being returned to service or 'otherwise disposed of'. The rather alarming sounding final comment simply allowed for the patients' discharge from the navy. The probationary period before resolution of their cases was not a reflection of doubt over the effectiveness of the cure. It was a routine period of transition in the rehabilitation of naval patients when they were discharged from Hoxton or Bethlem and had applied in the case of Moon earlier in the year.[6]

More troubling was Harness' report on John Braily. Harness said that as had been recorded in the Committee Report, Braily had benefited from the curative process, but it did not amount to a complete cure. Harness said that any attempt to engage Braily on certain subjects produced incoherence and Harness concluded that he was unlikely to derive any benefit from further treatment with the process. He recommended that Braily should be returned to Hoxton. This was an important development. Harness had been briefed on the curative process by Delahoyde and Lucett so his assessment that Braily was unlikely to benefit from further treatment was reasonably informed. It was always unlikely that any curative process would be universally effective in curing the insane and it is probable that the Committee members were realistic from the outset. Nevertheless Harness' assessment of Braily was a watershed moment. It was the first documented failure of the Delahoyde and Lucett process within the context of the formal Committee experiment.

The Braily case raises the question of what the Committee was actually looking for from the Delahoyde and Lucett process. It would appear from the Braily case that this was a total cure for insanity and nothing less. Dr Harness had determined that the process had had an initial beneficial impact on Braily. This positive, though temporary, impact was put to one side entirely when Braily's relapse became complete. It is possible that Lucett's extravagant claims for a universal cure set the standard against which success or failure was to be measured. Harness was an experienced doctor though and should perhaps not have expected infallible cures in any part of medicine. He might, however, have been expected to be interested in the sedative effect of the treatment as being a potential way of breaking into the kind of manic state which the king had so alarmingly displayed. As was clear in the king's case mania could only be imperfectly controlled through physical restraint or by reducing the patient's energy level. Neither approach was desirable or humane. Alternative methods for managing mania should have been of considerable interest – even if they were only temporary.

The Braily case was also important as it began to open up a gap between Dr Harness on the one hand and Delahoyde and Lucett on the other. On 22nd November Delahoyde and Lucett wrote to the Lords Commissioners to let them know that they were ready to transfer Cardiff and Matters to the hospital ship *Batavia*. In contradiction to Harness' recommendation they said that John Braily was also ready to go to the *Batavia* as part of the process towards his ultimate release. The copy of the letter from Delahoyde and Lucett which went to Earl Fitzwilliam has a footnote written by Harness which politely expresses his consternation. 'The above remarks made by Messrs Delahoyde and Lucett I must own surprised me, as, when I saw him, in company with them and Mr Troward, upon the third of the month he really was perfectly and violently deranged.'[7]

The next development is quite mystifying on one level, but probably points to problems which otherwise appear only fleetingly in the record. On 1st December 1813 Richard Troward the secretary of the Committee wrote to Earl Fitzwilliam[8] with what purported to be a progress report on the patients under Delahoyde and Lucett's care. It begins reasonably enough with confirmation that Cardiff and Matters had been transferred to the hospital ship *Batavia* as expected. Braily had meanwhile been retained at the Delahoyde receiving house in what seems like a reasonable compromise given the doubts about his recovery expressed by Dr Harness. Troward then mentions that O'Keefe, the fourth of the patients placed at the behest of the Committee was responding well to the treatment. Thereafter the letter starts to go somewhat awry.

Troward turns his attention to 'Harrington', a musician who had been placed with Delahoyde and Lucett at the behest of the Duke of Kent. It is not clear who Harrington was, but it seems that he should not be confused with Harrison who appeared earlier in the story. As Harrington had not been mentioned before in correspondence it is likely that he was a private patient of Delahoyde and Lucett. Troward pads out his account with heart-warming demonstrations of Harrington's return to normality. This is a sales pitch rather than a formal record of a patient's progress. Troward then introduces two cases involving individuals who were clearly private patients. One was a woman from Cumberland called Fisher who could have had no connection with the armed forces. These patients were clearly people who had been placed with Delahoyde independently of the Committee and the admiralty. They may be the additional patients referred to in the Committee Report at the end of September. Troward's focus is on anecdotes to demonstrate that each of the patients had returned to normality. Each case is accompanied by an almost sentimental comment on the service to humanity which the curative process had supplied. Again the sense of a sales pitch is strong.

Troward then makes a surprising claim. This is that he had been present when the secret of the process was communicated to the Dukes of Kent and Sussex and on this basis expresses his complete confidence in the effectiveness of the cure. Troward then makes the highly significant comment that he does not know if the process 'will ever extend to Windsor' although 'if it should not, it is much to be lamented'. The reference to possible use on the king is of course significant and it is clear that Troward understood that Fitzwilliam would not be surprised by the reference. Troward had essentially confirmed that the whole Committee experiment was ultimately aimed at recovering the king. Yet Troward's introduction of Windsor comes with the suggestion that however promising the curative process might be, there was a danger that it might not be possible to deploy it. A danger, which it is implicit, was not dependent on the merits of the cure.

The reason is money. What Troward was leading up to in his letter was to point to an impending crisis. However successful the process might be proving to be, other forces were likely to bring the experiment to an end. The practitioners were in debt and Troward refers to their 'pecuniary difficulties' and to having to 'keep out of the way' which served to interrupt their ability to manage the patients as well as they would have wanted. Essentially the bailiffs were after Delahoyde and Lucett again as they had been when the advance of £200 had been made in September. Troward enters a plea of mitigation that the expenses involved in setting up the new establishment at Ealing House had been the cause of the financial difficulties. He does not go into specifics or refer to the reasons for the move from Sion Vale. It would appear that the evaluation process was coming apart as the practitioners were no longer able to carry out their duties under the terms of the Committee agreement.

This all seems to be the preparation for a bizarre change of focus. Troward was the secretary of the Committee yet he had suddenly become the advocate or apologist of Delahoyde and Lucett. Whether this role was self-appointed or the reflection of some agreement with the practitioners of the process is not clear, but the implications were extraordinary. Troward asked Earl Fitzwilliam to buy a painting, which he claimed to own, for £1,000. The money, according to Troward would be used to support the continuing activities of Delahoyde and Lucett. Troward seems to recognise that further advances by the Committee were unlikely to be granted. The proposal is backed by claims that the picture, a landscape by a painter he identifies as 'Nicholas Delabati', was the best example in the country and better than a work owned by the Marquis of Stafford. [Troward has written the name in an English form and it is probable that he was referring to the sixteenth century Italian painter Niccolo dell'Abbate.] Troward claims that he paid 1600 guineas which sum he says 'I should be glad to take again'. Perhaps more interesting is Troward's appreciation of Delahoyde and Lucett's circumstances. He argues that they were so constrained by the limitations of being involved in the experiment that they were unable to carry out their normal business. The cure worked. Of this Troward declared himself to be sure and he says that it would make money in the future. Troward then makes a fascinating reference coming after an endorsement of the cure. He says 'and now the prospect of success is flattering provided they keep their liberty – a thousand pounds would put everything with comfort'. Troward says that the practitioners have no resources they can use to solve the problem. He says 'they have no means of security beyond a personal responsibility' but says that he was ready to step forward to back the pair.

Troward's intervention was completely unprofessional and probably dishonest. He was clearly taking advantage of his status as secretary to approach one of the members over an issue which should have been a subject for consideration by the whole of the Committee. The experiment had been set up to defray the costs of the experiment and if this was not happening then it was a subject for Delahoyde and Lucett to discuss with the Committee. The records are clearly not comprehensive, but it is significant that Troward made no mention of any approach to the Committee on the issue. There is evidence that the Committee was prepared to help out in an emergency as they had done in September. Troward argues that the experiment had got in the way of the normal practice of Delahoyde and Lucett and they were losing money as a result. This is not entirely consistent as Harness had noted at the beginning of the experiment that Delahoyde seemed to be taking on too many private patients, potentially at the expense of concentrating on the experiment. From the earlier incidents in the Committee experiment it is more likely that the intervention of bailiffs was the only impediment to Delahoyde and Lucett concentrating on the experiment and that this reflected poor financial management or misuse of funds on their part. It is also noteworthy that in arguing that the 'process' was an effective cure for insanity, Troward had given examples of patients successfully cured who were not from the group sponsored by the Committee. So they were managing to continue with some of their private work according to Troward's own account.

Troward's letter has all the feel of a private initiative directed to one individual member of the committee who happened to be closely engaged in the project and extremely wealthy. What seems surprising is that Troward should have apparently considered that Fitzwilliam would accept the story unchallenged and not contact other committee members. It seems to suggest that Troward was desperate and that he was perhaps trying to rescue his own finances. If Troward's claims that he wanted to underwrite Delahoyde and Lucett had any truth in them then his intervention looks like an attempt to secure the finances to underwrite an entirely commercial interest in the process. Troward was not a medical man so his opinion of the effectiveness of the process was not a professionally informed one. It looks as if Troward thought he had spotted an opportunity in the market and wanted to exploit it and invest in it. His claimed motivation of only wanting to support Delahoyde and Lucett does not seem very convincing. It would be fascinating to know what Fitzwilliam's reaction was and how he interpreted the intervention. There is no copy of a direct reply to Troward and there is no annotation on the letter which Earl Fitzwilliam received except that it had been received on 2nd December and that reports were included with the letter. Troward's intervention may have been misplaced. Fitzwilliam had shown himself to be a man who expected precision in legal matters and it is likely that even if he did not write immediately to Troward he would have written to other senior Committee members about the incident.

Certainly Troward's apparent desire to take a direct interest in the curative process was to be replayed six months later in a letter to Fitzwilliam by Lucett's wife and in a version published by James Lucett, although by then it had taken on a rather ugly format with Lucett claiming that Troward was attempting to deprive him of the curative process. Ironically Troward may have chosen the peak of the market to make his intervention as times seem to have been getting desperate for Delahoyde and Lucett in their new receiving house in Ealing. Essentially the experiment was losing momentum. Moon, whose case had been used as part of the justification for setting up the experiment, had had to be treated again but on release had quickly relapsed. James Cardiff and William Matters had been sent to the *Batavia* hospital ship where they were showing signs of relapse. Braily had also been treated again, but was making slow progress. O'Keefe was still at the receiving house and was due to be discharged. Significantly there had been no additional transfers of patients to make up the original target of ten patients. The sense that the experiment was coming to an end is strong. Frustratingly no correspondence between members of the Committee seems to have survived so there is no clear insight, at this point, into their thinking. The most positive explanation for Troward's letter to Fitzwilliam would be that he was attempting to stimulate renewed impetus in the experiment.

There is evidence that Fitzwilliam wrote to Dr Harness in response to Troward's initiative on 6th December. Harness responded with one of his own on 14th December.[9] This letter has survived. Harness makes no mention of Troward's attempts to raise money for Delahoyde and Lucett, but does refer to Fitzwilliam's statement that he had received optimistic reports on the state of the four official patients. Harness says that the best way he can give Fitzwilliam 'a more correct statement of their cases' is by 'transcribing the official correspondence between Messrs Delahoyde and Lucett and the Lords Commissioners of the Admiralty'. It is clear that Harness wanted to correct the optimistic accounts which Troward had given Fitzwilliam of continuing progress by the official patients. The most significant element of the exchange is that it demonstrates that one of the prominent members of the Committee at least was sceptical about the reports he was getting on the progress of the experiment and that in fact there was a growing gap between Delahoyde and Lucett's perspective of the curative process and reality. It is unlikely that the perception of doubt about the effectiveness of the 'cure' was confined to Fitzwilliam and Dr Harness. Meanwhile a bombshell was about to explode.

On 26th December 1813 the *Examiner* carried an open letter addressed 'To their Royal Highnesses the Dukes of Kent and Sussex' under the title 'INSANITY – LUCETT and De La HOYD's PRACTICE'. The author was James Birch Sharpe the surgeon at Hoxton Asylum who would have been aware of the Committee activities from the start; not least because he had had a hand in selecting some of the patients for the Committee experiment. He was also one of the most experienced 'mad-doctors' of the time. The letter itself is long and from a modern perspective, verbose with an unattractive sycophantic attitude to the royal dukes. Once the stylistic characteristics of the age are stripped away the letter emerges as a brutal attack on Lucett and Delahoyde as imposters who have exploited the credulity and good nature of the public and the dukes. In making the attack Sharpe dismissed the individual cases where a cure was supposed to have taken place and criticises the rest of the medical establishment for not speaking out clearly against the imposters.

Sharpe begins by setting out his own experience of mad doctoring as a basis for the criticism to follow. His aim is clearly stated as 'my humble efforts towards unmasking that which appears to me the most daring imposition till this day never attempted to be imposed upon an enlightened, humane, and generous public'. Sharpe goes on to state that he wishes 'to assist in drawing aside that veil which seems so artfully to have been suspended between your Royal Highnesses and the truth.' The attack on Lucett and Delahoyde is delayed while Sharpe criticises the medical establishment: 'I cannot refrain from expressing to your Royal Highnesses my surprise and my astonishment at the profound silence of those, whose names are so familiar to the public, and who, in my humble opinion at least, should long ago have stepped forward to have undeceived both your Royal Highnesses and the public.' This was an extraordinary break in the professional ranks of medicine. It is not certain who the targets actually were, but given the royal audience Sharpe was addressing it is probable that he meant the physicians attending the king at Windsor. These august figures were indeed household names and they had been directly asked for their views on the Delahoyde and Lucett experiment.

After further hyperbole and further tributes to the goodness of the Duke of Kent, Sharpe really gets down to business. He had clearly read the first report of the Committee and the background to its formation. Sharpe directly contradicts the claim that Mrs Lancaster had been cured and assumes that the dukes had been unaware of the fact. These comments echo Mr David Dundas' statement to the Queen's Council on 3rd July that Mrs Lancaster had not been successfully cured. Sharpe then focuses on the case of someone called Harris. This individual does not appear elsewhere in the record. Given the seriousness of Sharpe's claims Delahoyde and Lucett could have been expected to highlight an instance of a patient being sent to participate in the trial who was not fit to undergo treatment. Nevertheless Sharpe claims that this person was sent from Hoxton to the receiving house of Delahoyde and Lucett on 29th June 1813 only to be returned to Hoxton on 1st July. According to Sharpe the patient called Harris was returned because he was said by Lucett and Delahoyde to have a fractured skull. Sharpe was unable to find evidence of a fracture but significantly did find two large 'scars' on the shoulders of 'poor Harris' which he attributed to the severity of the treatment he had received. It seems likely that 'scars' was used loosely to convey the idea that Harris had been harmed and marked by the treatment. Sharpe then turns to the case of Moon and gives an outline of his case with the inevitable and true conclusion that he had had a relapse and was held in an asylum in Devizes.

Sharpe was by this point well into his theme and the criticisms become more direct. Sharpe states that he had been approached to contribute towards the costs of the experiment and had refused. His knowledge of the failures of the treatment was his justification for not having supported the Duke of Kent and his associates. With his claimed knowledge that Mrs Lancaster had not been cured this might have been an opportunity to bring it to the attention of the Dukes and the committee. Sharpe appears not to have taken the opportunity. Having dismissed Lucett and Delahoyde for 'the consummate quackery of this wonderous plan' he moves on to attack them for venality. He claims that the pair charged enormous sums when a patient was taken on and with the potential for inconsistency Sharpe claims a further enormous sum on their recovery. He dismisses the claims to cure insanity as 'vain boasts' and that Lucett and Delahoyde are beneath the notice of the Dukes of Kent and Sussex.

Sharpe's credentials were ostensibly impeccable. He described himself as a 'Member of the Royal College of Surgeons and Student in the Royal College of Arts' on the title page of his *Elements of Anatomy; designed for the use of Students in the Fine Arts* which he published in 1818. He was also responsible for gathering the proceedings of the 1815 House of Commons Select Committee Investigation of Insane Asylums and making it available to the public in bound form. The Commons had arranged only a very limited print run of their deliberations and without Sharpe's initiative their work might well have been lost very quickly. There was a less creditable and very important association in his career, however. He was the surgeon at the Hoxton Asylum which was notorious for never turning away any patient and where the conditions were quite awful even by the standards of the time. The priority for the Hoxton asylum was to make money for the owner Sir Jonathan Miles.

Looking at the record of the Commons enquiry it becomes immediately obvious how important Dr John Weir, the naval physician who accompanied Dr Harness on visits to Delahoyde and Lucett's establishment, was as a witness. He demolished any pretence that Hoxton was an appropriate place to send the insane. He even indicated that he thought there was some understanding between Sir Jonathan Miles and Mr John Haslam [apothecary at Bethlem] to limit the number of patients who were released from Hoxton. Weir also drew attention to the presents which had been sent to him when he first began to inspect Hoxton on behalf of the navy and how he had insisted that this should stop. At Hoxton there was no attempt to treat the patients who were confined in extreme squalor and overcrowding in a regime which was underpinned by corruption.[10] Sharpe was part of this corrupt regime.

It is intriguing to note that Sharpe always gives precedence to Lucett in the *Examiner* which runs counter to the express intention of the Committee in putting Delahoyde forward as the principal in the partnership because he was medically qualified. Whether Sharpe intended simply to highlight that an unqualified person was involved in the experiment is not clear. Certainly he made no attempt to focus on Lucett's career with the Bank of England in order to demonstrate his unsuitability as a medical practitioner. The spelling of Delahoyde's name in a consciously French way seems eccentric given that there is evidence, even in mundane documentation such as insurance policies that the man himself did not use a French form for his name.[11] Perhaps Sharpe intended to suggest that not only was one party unqualified, but the other was foreign! There can be no doubt, however, that Sharpe's intervention must have been very damaging. He was actually in a good position to comment – particularly in 1813. As surgeon at Hoxton asylum he would have known about the process for selecting the patients for the trial and would also have known that some had already been returned to the asylum after a relapse. The emphasis on Delahoyde and Lucett's high charges will not have been seen as positive by members of the Committee although they may have found this rather puzzling given the pair's brushes with the bailiffs. Crucially it was the time when doubts were beginning to gather about the process and when some of the major participants in the experiment, particularly Dr Harness, knew what the process consisted of. The fact that the Inspector of Naval Hospitals, Dr Weir had written a withering report to the Admiralty in 1812 on the unsuitability of Hoxton as a place for naval lunatics and that Sharpe himself was to be criticised in 1815 for not carrying out his duties, would not have had an impact on the power of his attack on Lucett in the *Examiner*.[12]

For the moment the fortunes of Delahoyde and Lucett appeared to be prospering. The *Morning Chronicle* of 5th January 1814 carried what was actually an advertisement, but which appeared in the form of a public announcement. 'At the request of persons of distinction', Charles Delahoyde announced that 'he would spend one day a week in town for consultations on "Cases of Mental Derangement"'. The style is genteel and assumes that all would know who he was. Interestingly he makes no claims for blanket cures, but the assumption must be that his reputation preceded him. Lucett is not mentioned, which again makes Sharpe's focus on Lucett all the more surprising. Whatever Troward might have claimed in his letter to Fitzwilliam about the financial difficulties Delahoyde and Lucett were supposedly experiencing as the result of having to curtail their private practice, that practice clearly continued. Ironically at this moment of apparent triumph for Delahoyde, the end of the experiment was actually in sight.

On 21st January 1814, Dr Robertson of the hospital ship, HMS *Batavia* wrote to Dr Harness to let him know that William Matters had deteriorated and become, 'more unstable and violent'. Harness sent Fitzwilliam a letter on 3rd February[13] bringing him up to date. Lamenting that the bad weather had delayed his attempts to visit the patients Harness made the crucial judgement of the whole experiment. This was that the 'process' did not provide lasting relief. At this point Harness did not go into detail, but the message was clear. The claimed cure for insanity did not work. Harness acknowledged that the process had an immediate positive impact on the patients, but it was not a cure. Although the assessment by Harness has the feel of an immediate comment rather than a carefully weighed statement the seriousness of the situation and the inevitable impact on the whole Committee experiment was clear. In fact Harness had presented a formal report to the Committee at Mr Dent's house on 2nd February and there had been further exchanges confirming the condition of the patients.

Harness wrote again to Earl Fitzwilliam on 19th February.[14] Fitzwilliam had obviously not been able to attend the Committee meeting on 2nd February and in this crucial letter Harness gave a summary of his overall assessment of the Delahoyde and Lucett experiment. He mentioned that he had called on the Duke of Kent the previous day to deliver a copy of his final report. In discussing the experiment, Harness confined himself solely to the four patients who had actually been treated by Delahoyde and Lucett under the auspices of the Committee. His tone is careful and almost sympathetic as there is a clear note of regret in reaching the conclusion that the experiment had been a failure. Harness emphasised that he had used his open access to the patients to monitor the progress of each patient closely. 'I am persuaded that much temporary relief and mitigation of symptoms were experienced by the patients at the early application of the process.' Harness goes on to say, 'but, I lament to be under the necessity to state, that the patients received from Hoxton are at the present period relapsed, and labouring under as high a degree of derangement, as when first placed under their care.' Harness ends the letter by mentioning that he had sent a report to the Committee and that he had received communications from Weir and Robertson on the *Batavia* hospital ship confirming that the patients had suffered relapses and that Cardiff was so violent that he had been confined.

The end for the experiment had come and as before there was no attempt to hide what was now a much less positive conclusion than the interim report of 27th September 1813 had appeared to promise. The Committee published its second and final report sometime in late February or early March 1814. The copy of the report in the Sheffield Archive[15] which had belonged to Earl Fitzwilliam is undated, however, the evidence from Harness' letter suggests that it was certainly after 18th or 19th February 1814. The report is heavily influenced by the input of Dr Harness as recorded in his letter to Fitzwilliam of 19th February[16] but there is an important difference. The final report did not dismiss the Delahoyde and Lucett treatment. The report, which is of one page gives a brief account of the Committee's aims and again emphasises the importance to humanity of investigating a possible cure for insanity. It goes on to say that unfortunately the four patients, who are named, and who were placed in the care of Messrs Delahoyde and Lucett had not benefited in the long run. Although they had all shown clear immediate improvement in their condition, over time they had suffered relapses. So far the report was in accordance with the assessment expressed by Dr Harness to Fitzwilliam. The difference comes in a qualification of the failure with the public patients. 'The Committee, feels it a duty to observe that, other cases have also come before it, from the private practice of Messrs Delahoyde and Lucett, in which complete Success appears to have attended the Effects of the Process.'

It is possible that Harness' views expressed in his letter to Fitzwilliam were amplified in other correspondence which has been lost or is inaccessible. It is also clear that there was discussion amongst the Committee members during their meeting on 2nd February when the report would probably have been drafted. The final report continues, 'little doubt is entertained by those who have most closely followed up the Investigation, not only that the Discovery is a most valuable one, but that it can be used with perfect safety to the patient, when placed in the Hands of professional and Scientific Men.' This seems to represent a surprisingly positive interpretation of the assessment in Harness' letter to Fitzwilliam of 19th February given the clear statement that the patients had all suffered relapses. The conclusion of the Report reads as if it reflected lobbying by Delahoyde and Lucett. Certainly it seems to go way outside the parameters originally set for the experiment which involved making a judgement based on the rigorously controlled application of treatment to patients who had been identified and carefully assessed independently of the practitioners in the trial. To allow the claimed cure of private patients who had not been assessed independently of the practitioners to be set in the balance against controlled patients where there had been eventual failure seems to run counter to the professionalism and seriousness of the Committee.

The conclusion of the report is not accidental, however. It is carefully worded and the decision to take a wider perspective than the parameters set for the experiment is clearly intentional. The Committee members assert that the process offered, 'a very flattering Prospect of promoting the Recovery of those unfortunate Individuals who are afflicted with Insanity' and conclude, 'by a Mode of Treatment, infinitely less painful to the feelings of their Friends and Relations, than that which is frequently practiced according to the old System'. So the Committee's conclusion was that the Lucett process could contribute to the recovery of the insane even if it did not offer an outright cure. It could also do this without the distressing aspects of current treatment which affected not only the patients, but their friends and relatives. The fact that the Committee decided to take this broader view of the Lucett treatment was reasonable in some ways. For the most part the normal treatment of the insane in the late Georgian age was not a treatment at all. Patients were confined and restrained and the aspirations of the treatment went little further than their physical control – particularly in cases of mania. The House of Commons Committee enquiry of 1815 was to expose a catalogue of mistreatment of insane patients some of which touched players in the Lucett and Delahoyde story. They also touched those treating or acting as consultants in the care of the king. For friends and relations it would have been harrowing to see patients treated in the way that even George III was being treated. Many others deemed to be insane fared much worse. The Delahoyde and Lucett treatment would have seemed a model of tender care by comparison and therefore an attractive if imperfect alternative.

The administrative end came in reports by Dr Weir, the Inspector of Naval Hospitals, to Dr Harness and the Transport Office of the Admiralty and may have contributed indirectly to the final report of the Committee. On 23rd February 1814, Weir wrote, 'James Cardiff, and William Matters who have lately been returned to Hoxton, from His Majesty's hospital ship *Batavia* appear to me, to be, exactly in the same insane state they were in previous to their being placed under the care of Messrs Delahoyde and Lucett – they are both apparently in good bodily health.' On the 2nd March Weir rounded up the account of the naval patients in his report of one of his visits to Hoxton, 'I found John Brailey had been returned from Messrs Delahoyde & Co on the 23rd ultimo; his conversation was loose and unconnected, and appeared to me, to be, nearly in the same state of derangement as he has been for these several years past.'[17]

Weir's testimony on the overall impact of the Delahoyde and Lucett process is actually rather important as he provides the closest thing to an independent professional assessment of the Lucett process who was not directly involved with the Committee. He was a physician of many years' experience and was a very frequent visitor to the Hoxton asylum. Correspondence held in the National Archives indicates that he visited the naval patients at Hoxton approximately every ten days. He was not a specialist 'mad doctor' but he was very experienced for the times in judging the condition of lunatics through his oversight of the naval insane patients. The impression which is conveyed in his correspondence with the Transport Office is of a rational, pragmatic and sympathetic man who defended the interest of his patients so far as he could.

In an assessment of a seaman, John Maddox in June 1810, Weir concluded that Maddox was 'quiet and consistent – except on the subject of religion', was in the prime of life and wanted to return to the navy. Weir recommended his immediate transfer to the hospital ship *Batavia* prior to his return to service. It was clear that Weir was prepared to accept a range of behaviour which could arguably challenge 'normality'. He also took into account the wishes of the patient. In the case of a Swedish seaman who had been 'pressed' into British naval service and who had ended up confined in Hoxton, Weir simply concluded that the man was not mad and recommended his immediate discharge from the navy.

This sense of care and humanity and a willingness to accept some variation in 'normal' behaviour by both Weir and Dr Harness at the Transport Office is perhaps exemplified by the case of the naval carpenter Thomas Stokes who was confined in Hoxton as insane. In response to an enquiry from the Transport Office prompted by a petition by his wife to have him released, Weir visited Stokes and reported in his letter of 26th January 1814, 'I beg leave to acquaint you that as his complaint is extremely mild and as it is in a progressive state of amendment, I am of opinion, his recovery would be greatly accelerated, by allowing him to be returned to his family.' A marginal note dated two days later indicates that Harness had acted to have Stokes discharged and had let his wife know![18]

Weir's directness is almost shocking sometimes as the extract from a letter to officers of the Transport Office dated 3rd February 1812 shows.

'Gentlemen,
In reply to your letter of the 31st ultimo, desiring that I should report to you whether in my opinion, Lieutenant Fitzgerald is likely to be benefited by further medical treatment at Hoxton. I beg leave to acquaint you that officers of every class in the Navy, under the care of Messrs Miles and Co at Hoxton, receive no medical treatment whatever for the insane complaint. The House is merely to be considered as an Asylum for board lodging and clothing. The Seamen and Marines are sent to Bethlem for Medical Treatment according to the regulations, but like the officers receive no medical treatment during their confinement at Hoxton.'

Weir was humane, but he was scientifically still very much a man of his time. He considered that it was important to avoid irritating maniacs and he would doubtless have endorsed the 'seclusion' which was used to manage the king. He was also in favour of a reduced diet to subdue maniacs. 'To this end the diet of insane patients should, in my opinion be confined to what is termed in Naval Hospitals "Half and Low".' He went on to criticise the regime at Hoxton for over-feeding those confined there and found particular fault with the inclusion of cheese in the diet![19] Nevertheless he provides an important contemporary perspective of the trial of the Lucett process underwritten by the Committee.

Overall the conclusion of the second and final Report by the Committee was not fully consistent. A rigorous framework had been set up to test the Delahoyde and Lucett process but this had not been followed through. The plan had been to use ten patients in a trial, but only four had actually been used. It was clear that the process had some effect on the patients; even if it was short lived. From a modern perspective, and against the background of the stated desire to relieve mankind of one of its most intractable scourges, it seems strange that there was no attempt to follow up the identifiable positive effect to see if it could be improved on. Finally it must be asked why, if the trial was judged a failure on the slender evidence of four patients, the final report concluded with what reads clearly like an endorsement of the process. That endorsement was to be used in the following years by James Lucett in his efforts to promote the process and himself.

One partial explanation for the sudden end to the experiment may lie with the finances. The surviving accounts as drawn up by Mr John Dent suggest that there was an initial enthusiasm for the experiment, but that little new money flowed in in response to the positive first report by the Committee. The initial collection raised £796. 12s. This sum was augmented by a further £121 collected between 13th October 1813 and 17th November. So the total collected was £835. 12s. It is perhaps significant that in the final accounts the last disbursement was made on 2nd December 1813 which almost exactly coincides with the 'begging letter' which Richard Troward wrote to Fitzwilliam on 1st December. As all the disbursements were made to Delahoyde and Lucett through Troward, he would have been well placed to understand the reality of the finances of the experiment. Certainly on 2nd December 1813 the Committee had run out of money.

There would be an irony in a situation in which a reasonably well formulated experiment to test a process which it was claimed would cure insanity was stopped simply because the money had run out. Huge sums of money were being expended on the medical care of the king. The average expenditure for 1811 to 1819 inclusive was £33,000 per annum. Given the enthusiasm which the Queen's Council demonstrated for the work of the Committee in September 1813, it is ironic that the Council should have continued to pay 30 guineas plus expenses for every visit to Windsor by one of the medical team.[20] It is perhaps too simplistic to wonder why some diversion of funds had not been possible if the Queen's Council really was exploring all reasonable avenues for a cure.

The intervention of John Birch Sharpe through the columns of the *Examiner* would not have helped. It came at the time when the trial was unravelling and could have been a factor in the decision. Negative publicity could have caused some of the Committee members concern that they would be drawn in. In addition the criticism came from someone who represented the medical establishment at the time. There is no evidence of a direct link between the *Examiner* article and the winding up of the Committee activity, however. Shortage of money and the likelihood of difficulties in the management of Delahoyde and Lucett were the deciding factors along with the fact that the treatment did not work for the long term.

Chapter Fourteen

Lucett – A New Career

'In connecting ourselves with Lunacy we are almost compelled to share the seclusion of our patients.'[1]

William Sankey MD. Presidential Address. 1868.

After the end of the Committee experiment, the future of the therapeutic process reverted to Lucett, but things appear to have gone badly wrong immediately due to financial difficulties. On 18th May 1814 Earl Fitzwilliam received a letter from Olivia Lucett, James Lucett's wife; she had a sorry tale to tell.[2] According to Mrs Lucett her husband was confined in the King's Bench prison for debt. Mrs Lucett's account was that Delahoyde had borrowed money and, in conformity with the practice of the time, had issued bills stating that the debt would be repaid on a certain date. It was normal at the time for such bills to have a guarantor who would step in in the event that the borrower could not pay and defaulted on the debt. Olivia Lucett's claim was that Delahoyde had put Lucett's name on the bills without his knowledge and had then defaulted. Essentially Delahoyde had been involved in fraud. The impact on Lucett was that he was declared bankrupt while his heavily pregnant wife was struggling to keep herself and their other offspring going on £150 per annum which represented the salary her husband was still drawing from the Bank of England and which the Directors were about to bring to an end.[3]

The betrayal by Delahoyde did not end there. Mrs Lucett claimed that Delahoyde and Troward and 'another unprincipled character' were planning to sell the manuscript of the cure and split the money gained four ways. Mrs Lucett's outrage was clear: Delahoyde would get his debts paid off, two others who had not contributed to the experiment would gain, while Lucett the 'proprietor and injured party' would only get an equal share. The proposed purchasers of the manuscript of the cure were identified as 'the Committee of the new asylum'. There is no further detail of the asylum, but the new Bethlem hospital was being built at St George's fields and would open in 1815 so may have been the asylum Mrs Lucett was referring to. What Mrs

Lucett wanted was for Fitzwilliam to intercede with the Dukes of Kent and Sussex and the other Committee members on behalf of her husband. Mrs Lucett presumably hoped for financial support for herself and her family but there is no annotation on Mrs Lucett's letter which indicates Fitzwilliam's reaction. The letter may have been 'ghost written' by Lucett, but it has none of the self-confidence or bombast which characterised Lucett's early open letters or his later publications. The stream of consciousness style seems, even at the distance of two centuries, to be heartfelt. If the appearances are correct and this was something approaching a true account, then it was an explanation for the break-up of the partnership which Lucett was to repeat later in his own version of events.

Lucett could not have been held for long in the King's Bench as the *Morning Post* of 5th July 1814 carried a small advert in which he refers to 'continuing success attending his process'. According to the advert Lucett was at this time based in Ealing, Middlesex. The advert gives little to go on. It is not clear whether Lucett was acting alone or in concert with others, but there is no mention of Delahoyde. In hindsight this advert looks rather tentative and in a sense acts almost as a sign of life from Lucett. Whether he would bounce back after the setback of the end of the Committee trial was not clear from one small advert, but at least he had chosen, as in 1811, to use the most popular newspaper of the day to try to advance his interest. He was not alone in the market, however, and would clearly have to improve the impact of his adverts when compared with an almost exactly contemporary advert in the *Hull Advertiser* of 7th May 1814 by another practitioner caring for the insane, 'No coercion, no restraint but what is absolutely necessary to protect the attendant and to prevent self-destruction will ever be employed'. The competitor's advertisement indicated that Lucett was sensitive to the needs of the market with his emphasis on no restraint.

At this moment of crisis for Lucett the next development was one of the most bizarre in the whole Lucett story. The *Examiner* of 2nd October 1814 carried an anonymous article entitled, 'New Treatment of Lunatics'. The opening of the article was portentous, 'Strange things are spoken of the new practice of Messrs Lucett and Delahoyde, at their Lunatic Establishment near Brentford'. The article goes on to separate the two practitioners. Delahoyde is dismissed as an unknown, 'he may be a regular or an irregular practitioner', as it is Lucett who was the target of the writer. Lucett is identified as 'the founder of the practice, and lately a clerk in the Bank'. The article goes on to ridicule Lucett for claiming to have cured a Mr Morgan of Somers Town when in reality the patient had remained as deranged as ever until his eventual death. The writer congratulates Morgan for at least escaping with life from Lucett's 'hot and cold water inflictions'. 'The new practice, it seems, is first to pour almost boiling water on the heads of the afflicted and then to drench them with cold.' The writer emphasises that the practice is kept as secret as possible and says that it is no wonder. Few people would allow their friends or relatives to undergo such treatment unless they were pretty sure that a cure would result. In the case of Mr Morgan this had not occurred. The writer then explains that the Morgan case had happened three or four years previously and ends with the statement that Lucett was at that time, 'a quack and a falsifier', 'a very impudent pretender, and a very valiant teller of untruths'. The article ends with a challenge to Lucett to disprove the accusations.

There can be no surprise that Lucett should have been the focus of scepticism and criticism. He promised so much and could arguably have been said to have disappointed many eminent people with the 'failure' of the experiment. But why should a serious newspaper have attacked him at this point when the experiment under the auspices of the Committee was at an end, the partnership with Delahoyde was apparently over and Lucett himself had been in prison for debt? Lucett and Delahoyde had moved from Sion Vale to a new establishment in Ealing, but this had been under the auspices of the Committee and had been a year previous to the article being written. Surely this establishment had been broken up when the experiment came to an end? Mrs Lucett certainly referred to the break-up of the establishment in her letter to Fitzwilliam. The advert in the *Morning Post* indicated that he was operating in Ealing, however. It is also surprising that the criticism of Lucett's ability to cure the insane is based on a single case from some years previous to the experiment. There is no reference to the Committee and the experiment which seems surprising given that it was recent and had been very public. The same journal had also published Sharpe's criticisms of Delahoyde and Lucett in December 1813.

It seems likely that the apparent oversight in not mentioning the Committee experiment was intentional. Certainly to mention the Committee or any of the failed cases linked to the experiment would potentially have opened the participants, very eminent people, to ridicule for being credulous in linking themselves to Lucett. Perhaps the most significant oversight in the *Examiner* article is that the more positive account of the Morgan case sent by Dr Tardy to the *Medical and Physical Journal* is not referred to. Balance was not perhaps the aim of the *Examiner*. Certainly the focus of the article appears simply to have been to discredit Lucett. The criticism is utterly personal and characterises him as without integrity and even without education. In describing the Lucett treatment the writer compares it with the infernal and quotes Milton's *Paradise Lost* while remarking that nobody was likely to charge Lucett with a knowledge of Milton!

The anonymous writer challenged Lucett to disprove the assertions that he was a liar and a 'quack'. If the media have always thrived on controversy then the author of the attack on Lucett would have been well satisfied with the response. The following edition of the *Examiner* of 9th October indicates that Lucett had responded immediately. This edition carried a second article in which the anonymity of the correspondent is replaced by the name –'Detector'. According to this second article someone had visited the offices of the *Examiner* demanding to know the name of the author of the 'scurrilous and malignant libel upon Mr Lucett'. With smooth disingenuousness the 'Detector' went on to say that the caller, whoever he might be, had said he would spend £500 in tracking down and punishing the author. The 'Detector' claims that he has left his name at the office of the *Examiner* and after further ridicule of Lucett issues a challenge. This was that Lucett should gather a group of eminent professional gentlemen, to 'honestly lay before them his mode of practice, and procure from them a Certificate of its merits, and of his own qualifications to superintend persons afflicted with madness'.

The article ends with further criticism of Lucett for apparently blustering at a junior employee of the *Examiner* and suggests that Lucett, or his friend, should 'assume as much as possible the manners of a gentleman' if he calls again at the paper's offices. The article has the self-importance and self-satisfaction of investigative journalism in full cry. Ironically Lucett had got, with the conclusion of the second report of the Committee, something very close to the Certificate of the effectiveness and safety of the treatment process that 'Detector' challenged him to produce. The medical qualifications he was never going to produce. The mystery is that the *Examiner* or anyone else thought Lucett was worth the trouble when the Committee had come to an end and Lucett, a bankrupt, had apparently gone to jail. One thing is clear; Lucett, or a friend, was at liberty again and was no longer held in the King's Bench. What was not clear was whether Lucett had the drive to make a reality of promoting his cure for insanity or whether the failure of the therapeutic trial, bankruptcy and hostile criticism in the press would drive him back into obscurity.

The Lucett and Delahoyde trail then goes cold until the end of 1814 when Lucett, the self-publicist who had offered his services to cure the king in 1811, returned to business in what he must have intended to be a relative blaze of publicity. The *Morning Post* of 21st December 1814 carried a longer, much more confident advert than the July effort. This time Lucett noted that he was based in Datchet and goes on to state that, 'he has submitted his process to High Authority, by whom, as well as a Select Committee of Noblemen and Gentlemen, it has been sanctioned and its innocent qualities sufficiently attested'. The advert was repeated twice more in the succeeding days. This advert reads almost like a direct challenge to the 'Detector'. Lucett had clearly bounced back and decided that he was going to take on the protagonist's role and exploit his therapeutic process further. He had effectively used the conclusion of the second Committee report as the basis to promote his business. In fact the statements in the advert were a reasonably accurate reflection of his involvement with the Committee and of the final conclusion of the Committee's report. What the adverts did not do, and what Lucett would never admit, was to say that the treatment of the public patients sponsored by the Committee had failed to provide a permanent cure.

The apparently balanced conclusion of the Committee Report of early 1814 had left room for Lucett and Delahoyde to actually use it as a direct endorsement of the Lucett process. The adverts of July 1814 and more importantly, those of December 1814 had demonstrated that Lucett understood this and intended to do so. The July advert tested the water, while those of December marked a growing confidence on Lucett's part. They were nothing compared with what was to come. In late April 1815, Earl Fitzwilliam received a copy of an affidavit sworn by James Lucett before the Lord Mayor of London on 21st April at the Mansion House. The affidavit stated that Lucett was the sole possessor of the process for curing insanity which had been submitted by him to the Dukes of Kent and Sussex and Dr Harness. Lucett concluded by saying that he had never communicated the secret of the curative process to anyone else, 'in this or any other country'.[4] It would appear that Lucett had not only forgotten about Dr Tardy, but had apparently still not seen his account of the Morgan case sent to the *Medical and Physical Journal*.

There was a companion document to the affidavit sent to Fitzwilliam. This was a longhand statement in the name of Lucett in which he stated that he had 'within these four months returned patients placed under his care to their friends' although they had been certified incurable. In what may have been another riposte to the 'Detector' Lucett stated that he had certificates of the incurable status of those he had cured. He also claimed that he was able to put anyone who was interested, in touch with the relatives of the patients in order to prove they had been cured. Clearly Lucett intended to promote the 'cure' himself, but the fact that he had written to Fitzwilliam and presumably to other Committee members is significant. It would appear that Lucett was challenging them to contradict his version of events that the 'cure' worked. It was also implicit that Lucett was shifting blame for the failure to achieve a permanent cure of the public patients onto Delahoyde. Lucett clearly intended to use the final Committee report as a basis for endorsing his 'cure' and his future practice. It is not quite clear why Lucett should have decided to run the risk of prompting a hostile response from one or all of the Committee members. He may simply have been an obsessive who could not accept failure and therefore felt compelled to rewrite history. It may also have been something of a self-justification over the end of the trial and some falling out with the Committee. Any uncertainties over Lucett's aims were to be clarified by his next move.

This was the publication of a short book in mid-1815 with the long title *An Exposition of the reasons which have prevented the process for relieving and curing idiocy and lunacy and every species of insanity from having been further extended*.[5] The key word is 'prevented'. In his revised version of events Lucett wanted to show that he had a cure for insanity which forces outside his control had stopped him from developing properly. Essentially Lucett was setting out to rewrite the history of the therapeutic trial and in doing so he wanted to achieve a number of objectives. The primary one was to assert his exclusive ownership of the cure and to insist that it worked. This was relatively straightforward if he ignored the outcome of the trial. Lucett was not, however, simply looking forward to making his way as a practitioner on the fringes of medical practice and ignoring the past. He was also looking back and wanted to justify himself not just to the wider public which might have followed the promise and relative failure of the therapeutic trial but specifically to justify himself to the Dukes of Kent and Sussex and the Committee members and sponsors. In all this the events of 24th September 1813 were crucial. This was when Delahoyde and Lucett had, ostensibly, been prepared or forced to brief the Dukes of Kent and Sussex and Dr Harness on what was involved in the curative process. This briefing had been critical in giving credibility to the practitioners, the cure and the whole therapeutic trial itself.

Lucett begins *An Exposition* with the assertion that he was going to 'endevour to confine myself strictly and severely to the truth'[6]. He follows this with a denial that the briefing on the process had been complete. Lucett now claimed that he had held back the crucial information on the curative process which made its effect permanent. What had been shown in chapter twelve to have been a moment of candour was now presented as having been nothing of the sort. Lucett admits that this revelation would come as a surprise to the Dukes of Kent and Sussex and to Dr Harness. 'They will start at what I have above said, namely, that I ONLY AM in possession of the secret of the *remedy*.'[7] Lucett acknowledges the immediate implication that the briefing on the process had been a sham. He admits that 'to a certain extent they have been imposed upon' but, claims Lucett 'I was the dupe and not the author of the imposition'. So what had been understood at the time was a full and frank revelation of the curative process had become a partial explanation. 'That the process and remedy to *a certain extent*, have been communicated to their Royal Highnesses, and to Dr Harness, I do by no means deny; but I deny that the *whole* extent of the *remedy* has been communicated to them.'[8] The italics are Lucett's.

It is not immediately clear why Lucett should decide, over a year after the therapeutic trial sponsored by the Committee had come to an end, to admit that he had been guilty of bad faith if not actual deception in his dealings with his former benefactors. The fact that he made this revelation voluntarily merely adds to the puzzlement caused by his actions. Lucett expresses his profound gratitude for the support which he had received from 'their Royal Highnesses' and asks for their patience so that he can explain the reasons for his apparent bad faith. The explanation is not immediate, however. He diverts into a history of how the curative process came into his possession. This is the same story which was set out earlier so is at least consistent. He then moves on to say that although he did nothing with the remedy at first, 'certain circumstances' induced him to turn his attention to it. He claims that the 'prejudices would be very strong against me' as an unqualified practitioner and he therefore 'resolved to seek and connect [himself] with a medical man'.[9] At this point in the Lucett history he claims that the aim was simply to carry out a trial of the curative process.

Securing a qualified partner was not a straightforward business and Lucett highlights the difficulties involved in convincing a successful physician to take an interest in something entirely new and in doing so accept a relationship in which the unqualified would teach the qualified. Not surprisingly he experienced many rebuffs before he 'connected himself with Mr Delahoyde'. Further careful balancing in the narrative was required as Lucett simultaneously presented Delahoyde immediately expressing confidence in the efficacy of the curative process while claiming that he had imparted the secret of the process only 'to a certain extent'. With a medically qualified partner Lucett had a basis for taking the curative process forward. The difficulties were not at an end, however. It was essential to be able to demonstrate that the process actually worked and patients who could pay or have payment made on their behalf were not going to take a risk with an untried 'cure'. Lucett comes over as convincing in this section of his account and he makes no attempt to hide the fact that it was paying patients he was looking for. The other element Lucett highlighted was the need to demonstrate that the cure had worked on people who had really been established as insane. So, although he and Delahoyde had apparently had success with pauper patients these had suffered from the disadvantage of not being confined in institutions and they were therefore not certified as insane. So Lucett recounts that he and Delahoyde had attempted to secure patients from various hospitals and asylums without success; until they were able to count on the support of the Duke of Kent in the case of William Harrison. How this breakthrough came about Lucett does not explain, but his thesis is essentially that the Harrison case was crucial in formally establishing that the cure worked.

In Lucett's *Exposition* the importance of the Harrison case was that the patient had been 'certified as an *incurable lunatic* by Dr Munro'.[10] There could be no doubt therefore that Harrison had suffered from insanity. What Lucett does not do is to explain how the relationship with the duke had originated although it is noticeable that from what had been a personal account he suddenly uses 'we' to describe himself and Delahoyde benefiting from the duke's help. The impact of Lucett's curative process was immediate and the patient regained his reason in a matter of days and was restored to 'perfect health' in a few months. Lucett lingers over the Harrison case with a series of assertions that the former patient continued to live with his family and to work as a music teacher. The sense of the writer's discomfort over the Harrison case is increased because Lucett seems to consider it necessary to dismiss reports 'that Harrison is again confined' and rounds up his account of the case by saying that Harrison had never shown 'any symptoms of relapse' and had actually been hurt by rumours that he had suffered a relapse. This last comment is oddly emotional and in a sense Harrison seems to have become the living proof for Lucett that his cure worked.

The Harrison case was undoubtedly the pivotal point in which Lucett's assertions that he had a cure for insanity began to have real substance. He refers to it in *An Exposition* as 'one we could lay before the public in an authenticated shape with certificates of all the facts'. It was all so clear cut that 'any sceptical person could easily investigate'[11] the circumstances of the case. There had been a cost to the triumph, however, as the treatment of Harrison as well as the support of his family over several months had run up expenses which Lucett claimed he had had to cover. More importantly Lucett's triumph and the potential to take the cure forward were undermined by the fact that he had had to support the Delahoyde family as well. 'Several gentlemen now contributed considerable sums for the purpose of supporting these expences and of establishing us in such a house as would enable us to receive a different class of patients.'[12] What Lucett was describing was essentially the formation of the Committee to assess his cure, but also a base from which to treat paying patients.

His version of events avoids all detail, but the difference from the formal procedure for setting up the Committee and controlling the finances described in chapter eleven is nevertheless complete. Referring to the money donated Lucett states, 'Of these sums I received a very small part only; but being willing to believe that those in whom I put confidence were worthy of that confidence, I did not call for an account of the money so received, but assumed it would be properly applied'. The triumph of the Harrison case and Lucett's cure was effectively sabotaged by the attitude of his partner. 'Elated with the prospect of success which now opened upon him, and dazzled by the splendour of that fortune which seemed to be within his grasp, Mr Delahoyde increased his personal establishment and expences.' Lucett is presented as being a victim of his own good nature and his misplaced trust in his partner. These were no match for what he describes as a conspiracy against him.

Lucett's version of events is that it soon became clear that Delahoyde was bent on extravagance which involved milking both the Committee and private patients in order to underwrite a lifestyle of conspicuous consumption for himself and his family. In doing this Delahoyde was joined by a lawyer whom he does not name, but whom his wife had identified as Richard Troward the lawyer who had acted as secretary to the Committee. Lucett also accused Delahoyde of neglecting the patients. On the curative process itself, Lucett again claimed that it had two parts and that he had communicated only the first part of the process to Delahoyde. The second and crucial element for the long term wellbeing of patients had remained solely in Lucett's hands. Lucett had some difficulty in setting out this part of his account convincingly and his discomfort is clear. Referring to the subscriptions advanced by the Committee members and their supporters Lucett states, 'To those gentlemen I beg leave to return my most sincere thanks, and I trust they will now do me the justice to acknowledge that *I have never deceived them*[13] Lucett then proceeds to relate history as he wants it.

Having set out the background to his satisfaction Lucett returns to the crucial meeting on 24th September 1813 when he and Delahoyde had met the Dukes of Kent and Sussex and Dr Harness and set out for them the nature of the curative process. This encounter had formed the basis for the Statement dated 28th September 1813 which was attached to the first report of the Committee and which stated that the process was safe. How was Lucett now to revise the encounter which had originally seemed a moment of candour in which the two practitioners had revealed the process which was the subject of the experiment? The revised version is that Lucett had not been the protagonist during the meeting with the dukes and Dr Harness. This role had been Delahoyde's and Delahoyde's alone. Lucett essentially claims in his book that he had been an observer at the meeting.

The explanation is that Delahoyde, as the medically qualified man, had insisted on being the spokesman during the meeting. Lucett had therefore to accept his own logic that he would only secure support for an assessment of his curative process if he had a qualified medial practitioner to front for him. The problem was that he had been disappointed in the doctor he had gone into partnership with. Lucett had been too trusting and naïve in his assessment of Delahoyde. That said Lucett was apparently not so naïve as to have given Delahoyde a full picture of the cure according to his account. Delahoyde had therefore unwittingly been able to brief the dukes and Dr Harness only to the extent that Lucett had briefed him. There is some basis for the argument that Delahoyde would have assumed precedence in the discussion of the cure at the meeting with the dukes and Dr Harness. After all the Committee structure had made Delahoyde responsible for the treatment of the patients in the experiment precisely because he was a qualified physician. It was logical that this should have continued when the precise nature of the cure was to be revealed.

The first difficulty of explaining why Delahoyde had enjoyed precedence at the meeting with the dukes when Lucett was the proprietor of the process had been dealt with. The issue of what was said at the meeting had now to be addressed and again it involved a balancing act for Lucett. The meeting had been presented, at the time, as one of revelation. The dukes and Dr Harness had even signed a declaration after the meeting stating that they had been told what the treatment involved and that it was safe. In his account of 1815 Lucett presented the idea that the meeting had only been candid up to a point. That point being the limit of what Lucett claimed to have conveyed to Delahoyde. So Lucett claimed that the dukes and Dr Harness had been given the first part of the curative process with full candour. This much of the cure was beneficial and effective at least for a time. The second part which only Lucett knew was required if a cure of insanity was to be fully effective and permanent. In this way Lucett also hoped to deal with the implicit long-term failure of the process, without admitting there had been any failure, by indicating that only the first part of the process had been applied by Delahoyde to the Committee sponsored patients. Lucett was after a balance which would resolve with some kind of consistency what had happened in the past with what he wanted to happen in the future. His intention was to excuse his lack of candour with the dukes while still benefiting from royal patronage and make a sales pitch to his future clientele. There seem to have been limits even to Lucett's ability to balance conflicting ideas. The conflicting third element which Lucett could not resolve was that by claiming that he had held back on disclosing the full curative process he had undermined the value of the endorsement by the royal dukes that the process was effective and safe.

He was at least sensitive to the danger of mentioning his open letters to Queen Charlotte and addresses to the royal physicians in 1811, or to draw attention to the fact that if successful it had been intended to use the cure on George III. To draw in the fate of the king in a public document would have invited trouble. He had also implicitly addressed the issue of the failure of the experiment under the auspices of the Committee without actually admitting that there had been a failure. As he had stated previously, there was more to the process than he had revealed. These elements while effective on one level do nevertheless raise some pretty fundamental questions about whether Lucett's account is convincing. Lucett had put himself and his process forward in 1811 and had invited the royal physicians to evaluate it. Logic would therefore suggest that when he had the opportunity to have his process tested that he would have done all he could to give it the best possible chance of success – if he genuinely believed it worked. The potential rewards were almost unlimited. With success he would doubtless have been involved in treating the king and success there would have brought immediate reward while afterwards he would have been able to name his price with other patients. To hold back with the full cure was not logical, however much he mistrusted Delahoyde. Nor is deference convincing. Lucett under his own name had claimed he could cure the king in the most public way possible. Would such a confident man really have failed to find some way for his voice to be heard when meeting the dukes and Dr Harness if he had a further crucial element of the process to convey?

Lucett claims that Delahoyde was in a conspiracy with an attorney who he says saw the opportunity of repairing his 'shattered fortunes' by exploiting the process[14]. If this was Richard Troward as Mrs Lucett had claimed the year before in her letter to Fitzwilliam it could provide an alternative explanation for Troward's letter to Fitzwilliam in which he tried to raise money through the sale of the painting. Nevertheless Lucett's version of events is that the attorney was linked to Delahoyde from the first involvement of the Committee and undertook to provide the impressive sum of three thousand guineas in starting capital. The attorney also apparently promised to pay back monies advanced by the group of gentlemen in connection with the Harrison case. Perhaps unsurprisingly, Lucett claims that Troward failed in all his undertakings – despite an apparent assurance to the Duke of Kent that the gentlemen had been reimbursed. If Troward had been such a significant actual or potential investor in the curative process it is surprising that no mention of the commitments was made in the formation of the Committee. If the Lucett version of events were true then Troward would have had a conflict of interest from the start. Unfortunately Mr Troward had died before the publication of *An Exposition*.

So it was Delahoyde and Troward who took the Sion Vale establishment and it was initially very successful. Lucett claims that five thousand pounds, an enormous sum at the time, in advance payments were made on behalf of patients although he received nothing. This is to some extent consistent with Dr Harness' report that Delahoyde was taking in private patients when the focus should have been on the official patients supplied by the Committee. The money itself was largely used up through Delahoyde's extravagance according to Lucett. Curiously Lucett 'dates' the foundation of the Committee to this point in the narrative and specifically to the move from Sion Vale to a new establishment at Ealing House.[15] Allowing for Lucett's lack of precision over dates the idea that debts were mounting would fit with Dent's letter to Fitzwilliam over the need to make an advance to the practitioners in September 1813.[16]

The new establishment resulted in a further increase in the demand for treatment, but applications on behalf of potential patients were largely ignored by the attorney, while Delahoyde pursued his own dissipations. According to Lucett the creditors were closing in on Delahoyde while frustrated people who were attempting to place patients simply concluded that the whole establishment and implicitly the cure itself was a fraud. Lucett's account of the conspiracy against him was moving rapidly towards its climax. He had been the subject of false reports which were passed to the Duke of Kent. These were presumably the basis of Lucett's statement above that he had never deceived the gentlemen of the Committee. Lucett's focus now was to complete his self-justification and so he returns to the briefing on 24th September. In this final version both Delahoyde and the attorney had insisted on Lucett's silence during the briefing as part of their conspiracy to supplant him. Lucett hopes that the revelation that he had been the victim of a conspiracy would make it clear to the Dukes of Kent and Sussex that he had not 'wilfully' concealed anything from them.[17] A brief note that Lucett had managed to overcome the difficulties which had been inflicted on him by the conspirators and the news that he had a new partner in Dr Richard Smith completes the main part of *An Exposition*.

The appendix which follows is a carefully managed document. The thrust is to demonstrate the success of the process in the past and to exploit the connection with the Committee to give the cloak of respectability to Lucett's future activity treating patients. The Harrison case is used again in some detail before the focus shifts to Moon. In this instance the case history is only of the successful part of the first treatment. There is no mention of the repeat treatment of Moon, nor of his eventual relapse and confinement immediately after his release. Mrs Lancaster is used uncritically despite the public statement by Dr Sharpe that she had not been cured and the statement by Mr Dundas to the Queen's Council that when he had seen her she had not been cured.

The first report of the Committee is reprinted and presents a favourable view of the potential of the process. There is, however, no mention of the second and concluding report which was relatively unfavourable in describing the effect of the curative process as temporary. There is also no mention that all four of the public patients suffered relapses and were confined. A further example of the selectivity lies in the reprinting of the Declaration by the Dukes of Kent and Sussex with Dr Harness that the process was safe. The inescapable conclusion is that the appendix represents a cynical and disingenuous manipulation of material in order to underpin Lucett's re-launch of the curative process on the market. His use of the connection with the Committee and especially with the members of the royal family looks like blatant exploitation.

The concluding sections of the appendix of *An Exposition* are a little more nuanced. Lucett comes a little closer to an admission that there had been problems with some of his patients in a section in which he talks about convalescent patients. Entirely reasonably he talks about the need to give convalescent patients a calm and quiet environment and that badgering them with questions about their illness was calculated to cause harm. After this brief foray into reason, Lucett rapidly returns to salesmanship. He sets out the names and addresses of four people who he claims are willing to attest that the curative process works. The claim is that each is linked to a patient, who has been cured, but who, for reasons of privacy, is to remain anonymous.

An Exposition is a pretty sophisticated exercise in perception management in which the extended title is an accurate statement of what Lucett sets out to achieve and what he actually succeeds in doing. It is not a true account of the therapeutic trial. That had already been written, published and circulated by the Committee. What Lucett was doing in *An Exposition* was writing a version of the therapeutic trial which fulfilled his needs as a practitioner and businessman in launching his career in the treatment of those diagnosed as insane. He exploited the qualities which made the trial unique at the time and which made it such a potentially influential underpinning for Lucett's pretentions. It was firmly based on a scientific outlook; it was independently and expertly assessed and had remarkable and genuine backing of royalty and enormously eminent figures of the day. Lucett was not going to waste an endorsement like that.

As is clear from the examination above, Lucett's version of the therapeutic trial in *An Exposition* was highly selective but had just enough substance to make it credible. The idea that the whole trial had been sabotaged by Delahoyde's venality is not strictly true but as an explanation for why the relationship between the practitioners and the Committee did not run smoothly but was bedevilled by debts so that the planned complement of public patients was never treated it works. Dr Harness had remarked disapprovingly that Delahoyde had been filling the receiving house with private patients early in the trial while later events were to confirm Lucett's assessment that Delahoyde was a man without principles who fled to Ireland after the trial to escape his creditors. Even the idea of a conspiracy between Delahoyde and Troward acquires some credibility against the background of Troward's letter to Fitzwilliam in which he tried to sell a painting. Lucett's curative process did not provide a permanent cure for insanity, but it did have a positive therapeutic effect although of course this proved to be temporary. This vital discrepancy was removed by careful editing and it is possible that Lucett could have rationalised his lack of candour over the effectiveness of his cure with the consideration that orthodox medicine relied on an ineffective therapy which was combined with considerable mistreatment of the patients. The therapeutic trial had not gone as Lucett would have wished, but *An Exposition* was an attempt to salvage as much as possible from the wreckage of its end.

Lucett ends *An Exposition* with a little reverse self-promotion in which he even addresses the concept of the 'quack'. Not that he is one of course! Lucett says that he claims no special qualities or talents for himself. He says that he makes no claim to special knowledge or that he has invented anything. His only claim is that he happens to have in his possession a sure cure for insanity which a foreign doctor would have published in America had he lived.[18] This too is disingenuous, but there is a subtlety compared with the more obvious quackery of the inventors and sellers of miracle cures. Lucett was clearly trying to establish himself in business for the long haul. Unlike the traditional quack, Lucett was seeking ongoing relationships with his patients leading ultimately, he claimed, to a cure. The bankruptcy reported by his wife to Fitzwilliam was clearly behind him. For Lucett it is back to business using the involvement with the Committee so far as possible to bolster his efforts. The 1815 booklet is a statement of intent. Whether the Committee would really have been quite so unfortunate in the choice of their secretary is put to one side as is the unsuitability of Lucett's choice of partner. What also remained to determine was whether there really was a secret second element to Lucett's curative process or whether that had been a presentational fiction to explain failure to achieve a permanent cure.

Chapter Fifteen

'Insanity Cured Without Confinement.'

'Monsieur Moreau de Tours asserts that non-restraint is "an idea entirely Britannic, an impossibility in most cases, an illusion always, the expression itself a lie."'[1]

A concise history of the entire abolition of mechanical restraint etc.
Robert Gardiner Hill. 1857.

The *Morning Post* of 4th December 1815 carried an advertisement for Lucett and his curative process. The advert represents a significant refinement of the statement of intent set out in the short book from earlier in 1815 as it goes some way to defining his practice and distinguishing it from what was available elsewhere from 'qualified' and other practitioners. The advertisement appears under the heading, 'Insanity Cured without Confinement' and makes clear that the dominant figure is Lucett. Not only does the advert claim that the curing will be done by James Lucett, but the point of relative status is emphasised by the statement, 'with the assistance of Richard Smith, member of the Royal College of Surgeons'. There was clearly going to be no repetition of the Delahoyde episode in which Lucett was the all but invisible assistant. Perhaps even more interesting is the heading itself as this seems to play to strong fears people increasingly had over the mistreatment of the insane. The insane were not only subject to neglect in many asylums, but where actual treatment was involved, this was usually based on intimidation and the use of, or threat of, violence. Restraint involving chains and shackles was normal for most manic and certainly all violent lunatics. The king after all spent long periods in a straight waistcoat when he was deranged and a House of Commons committee had been investigating the state of insane asylums during the year. Lucett's claim to do away with such methods would have been hugely appealing to the relatives of potential patients, but it also represented a means for Lucett to claim the moral and even competence high ground. What Lucett's advert implicitly says is that he does not need primitive means of control of his patients because his methods are superior. This was a powerful message in any age and an effective form of branding for Lucett.

The advert also records a move for the Lucett establishment to Weston House in Chertsey. The choice of this building as the base for his operations is significant. It was an imposing gentleman's residence occupying a prominent position in the centre of the prosperous country town. As a base for Lucett's practice it was certainly intended to impress and to appeal to the sensibilities of the very prosperous. It was also intended to convey a sense of solidity and success for the operations carried out in it.[2] As was customary at the time for adverts involving medical treatments, Lucett's included mini case histories of patients he claimed to have successfully treated. The claim is made for complete success with all patients which seems from a modern perspective to be back in the territory of the quack. In the early nineteenth century market for medical treatment an advertisement claiming anything less than total success would have been dismissed. There is no mention of the Committee or 'Higher Authority' underwriting his activities. By the standards of the time Lucett's advert compared very favourably with the adverts for cures of all sorts of illness which were normal in newspapers of the age.

Lucett was not to enjoy an unchallenged practice, however. His area of activity was too sensitive and his claims too extraordinary for that to happen. There are pointers to controversy around Lucett in the press of the time although much of what survives originated with Lucett himself. The *Morning Post* of 31st August 1816, for example, carries an extraordinary open letter from Lucett to the editor under the title 'Mad Houses'. Essentially the letter amounts to a challenge to conventional medicine in the treatment of the insane. The letter opens in an unassuming way by referring the editor and readers back five years to his original announcement of the 'Cure of Mental Derangement'. This was of course his open letters to the queen in which he offered his cure for use with George III. There follows a brief case history which is identifiable as that of William Harrison. As might be expected from Lucett he claims that the cure of the patient was complete and that as a result the 'Lords of the Treasury did me the honour to present me with two hundred guineas'.

Lucett continues with the claim that from that time on he had given repeated proof that the cure worked, only to be opposed, with a few exceptions, by all the medical practitioners, 'more particularly those medical gentlemen who have shares in private mad–houses, whose interest it is to fill them and keep them so'. Lucett asserts that his treatment was considered a threat to their livelihoods and that being effective in curing the insane was the only offence he had committed. Lucett then claims that he is in fact only motivated by making the cure available to the nation before making an apparently extraordinary claim. This is that he had been in contact with the late Mr Perceval to ask his advice. The advice he received from the former prime minister he claims had been to offer the treatment 'without stipulation' to the physicians treating the king. This is recognisably the offer Lucett claimed to have made to the physicians attending the king in 1811. By his own account Lucett's offer was ignored by the physicians, but he cannot resist the claim that he had, with the assassination of Perceval, been 'deprived of my lamented advocate and friend'. It seems unlikely that Perceval would have actively supported an offer made by Lucett. After all he had simply passed on Dr John Willis' comments on the king's case in November 1810 to the physicians despite the fact that Willis was 'qualified' and had actually treated the king previously. Perceval had considered John Willis to have been too remote from the king's case at the time to make his views important. How much less likely he would have been to promote the views of the unknown Lucett. In a final statement of self-justification which verges on self-righteousness, Lucett claims to have offered, at the time of writing, his treatment to the nation through the House of Commons. What the reference to Perceval actually signified was that Lucett was engaged in a propaganda work in progress. He has simply put to one side the fact that the *Examiner* had already published an earlier version of the contact with Perceval in which the prime minister's reply stating that he could not support any experiment with the king's health had been included. As more time passed Lucett was to reinvent Perceval's role into that of an active supporter.

At first glance Lucett's strategy of taking on the medical establishment appears foolhardy, yet there was a certain logic to what he was doing. He was not a qualified physician and he had enough evidence that the medical profession was not going to take him seriously and would not embrace him or his cure. By presenting himself as an outsider who was opposed by the establishment Lucett created a powerful distinction between himself and them. The Report from the Committee of the House of Commons on Madhouses in England had very recently demonstrated how bad much of the conventional care of the insane was. When treatment of the insane by 'conventional medicine' ranged from the non-existent to the brutal, Lucett represented a contrast which would have seemed positive especially when combined with his irrepressible self-confidence. The Commons enquiry, which Lucett was certainly aware of, went some way to endorsing the contribution of 'unqualified' practitioners. The Tukes and their asylum The Retreat in York was presented as a model for the modern caring establishment, while Thomas Bakewell who ran a private asylum, was an important witness for the Commons enquiry and was 'unqualified'. There was even growing criticism of the brutality and unprofessional behaviour in the treatment of the insane from within the medical profession. The testimony of Dr Veitch to the Commons Committee had highlighted the corruption at Hoxton for example. Essentially being an outsider in the treatment of the insane could be good for business. After all both Dr Monro and Mr James Haslam, the qualified experts, had been dismissed from Bethlem hospital following the Commons enquiry. Incidentally Dr Edward Monro was promptly instated to replace his father in an act of defiance by the Bethlem authorities. Lucett would not of course be allowed to exploit such a line unchallenged.

Anyone publicly claiming access to secret knowledge which could bring profit or make reputations was bound to attract attention. Lucett had begun his career treating the insane with the claim that he had a secret curative process which only he knew. After all the publicity connected with the therapeutic trial under the auspices of the Duke of Kent, Lucett had sought to re-establish himself as the sole proprietor of the curative process and the only person with full knowledge of what it involved. His account in *An Exposition* in 1815 was a crucial element in backing his claims. Necessary as this might have been for Lucett to establish himself, he was also inevitably going to attract the interest of sceptics or critics who wanted to expose him as a quack or fraud. Lucett's claims would also have attracted potential rivals who would have done all they could to determine the secrets of the curative process in the hope of profiting from it. For Lucett the early part of his career was the time when he was most likely to attract attention and when, in the absence of an established track record, he would have been most vulnerable. Such unwelcome attention appeared in the *Quarterly Review* in late 1816 and was important because it included a specific, if dismissive, assertion of what the secret process involved.

Lucett's response was immediate and as was becoming almost a reflex for him it involved an open letter to the editor of the *Morning Post*. In his letter of the 23rd of November Lucett adopted a lofty tone of dismissal of the claim in the *Quarterly Review* that his cure was the mere application of hot and cold water. This claim was a 'guess' which was 'unworthy of notice' had it not been accompanied by a claim that Lucett had failed to recover a particular patient. It was a dangerous tactic to counter bad publicity when it involved repeating something discreditable, but Lucett took the risk. His response was a simple denial of any failure and as a kind of 'proof' of his confidence in his cure he offered an invitation to anyone concerned for the future of a friend or relative 'unhappily afflicted' to visit his establishment and to bring any medical practitioner they cared to with them. What Lucett does not do is to say anything about the specific nature of his treatment, but he adds a flourish which is to ask those 'who profess themselves particularly skilled in the treatment of the above disease' to 'suspend their comments on my practice' until all is revealed by the sanction of higher authority. He had at least avoided the trap of explaining his secret cure and entering into a debate on specifics. He had also used the meaningless reference to 'higher authority' preparing to endorse his cure to distract from the claims that the cure simply didn't work.

Lucett was apparently not to enjoy a period of peace in which to develop his practice. A further letter to the editor of the *Morning Post* a year later is an indication that he had been the subject of continued public criticism although no specific examples are given. Lucett indicates that 'erroneous reports have been circulated, purporting to expose my peculiar mode of treatment for the relief of Insanity'. Both irregular and regular practitioners had been involved and Lucett claims that they have 'subjected' their patients to hot and cold water treatments, the application of ice to the head, the application of the 'cold turban etc' 'on the presumption that these were my peculiar means'. Again Lucett avoids any explanation of what his 'peculiar' or personal treatment was, but he sets out a brief case history in which he claims that a medical practitioner had recently placed a young woman patient in his care whom he had been unable to recover despite using the cold turban. Lucett had succeeded over a period of four months.[3]

The 'cold turban' and the other treatments mentioned were in the forefront of contemporary qualified medical practice and were thought to be effective by reducing the circulation of blood in the head. Excess blood in the head was considered at the time to be a key element in the development of insanity; particularly in cases where mania was involved.[4] Lucett's dismissal of these treatments was not simply a re-emphasis of the exclusivity of his own treatment, but an implied statement that his practice was more advanced. Lucett had referred in his letter to regular and 'empiric' practitioners criticising him while trying to identify his curative methods. His response seems almost to welcome the interest in his work even if the conclusions were erroneous and it is just possible that the letter of December 1817 was purely an exercise in self-promotion rather than a response to specific criticism. If this was the case for an amateur propagandist and psychologist his efforts are pretty impressive.

Lucett's next effort broadens the attack on his critics and reverts to the idea that he was a victim of malicious attack. In a further letter to the editor of the *Morning Post* of 14th December 1816 Lucett again refers to earlier criticisms of him, in a neat counter-attack he suggests that the physicians running private madhouses were so opposed to him because they feared he would put them out of business by curing their client base. Essentially Lucett was increasingly confident, brazen and confrontational in his approach to conventional medicine. He also seemed to be working on the basis that even controversy was a useful form of publicity.

It should not be a surprise perhaps that Lucett's erstwhile partner made a reappearance at much the same time as Lucett was trying to establish himself and was clearly intent on exploiting the relationship with the Committee and the Dukes of Kent and Sussex just as Lucett had been doing. There is no direct evidence that Delahoyde was influenced by seeing Lucett's adverts in the press, but it seems likely that he had seen them and if anything, Delahoyde's version is the more sophisticated. The *Dublin Evening News* of 28th September 1816 and for several succeeding weeks carried adverts under the heading 'Mental derangement'. 'Mr Delahoyde, Surgeon founder of the Sion Vale Institution near London for the cure of INSANITY may now be consulted on the different species of the disease ... at Mr Heron's Apothecary No 176 North King-Street.' The advert continues with a short account of the 'success and safety' of Mr Delahoyde's system for the recovery of the insane. It refers to the appraisal and approval of the system by the two dukes and other Committee members, many of whom are referred to by name. Delahoyde even claims that he was awarded £900 by the Treasury for curing Harrison – clearly outbidding Lucett! Perhaps the only oddity about these otherwise assured claims is that Delahoyde apparently had no premises of his own. An explanation for this anomaly was not long in becoming clear.

If Delahoyde had seen the adverts as the start of a successful new career any such expectations were very soon to be destroyed by events which ironically were to be reported in the same *Dublin Evening News*. The edition of 17th December 1816 recorded the proceedings in the trial of Hinds V Middleton heard in the Court of Common Pleas in Dublin between 14th and 16th December. The case was an action of redress for the alleged assault and debauching of the plaintiff's wife and damages of six thousand pounds were sought. The plaintiff, Hinds, was an attorney in Dublin. The defendant, Middleton, was a physician and principal medical superintendent of the Hanover Park Asylum in county Carlow. The asylum was run by three doctors: Middleton, Delahoyde and Clay.

The cause seemed clear at first. Dr Middleton had taken advantage of his position to seduce a patient – Mrs Hinds. As the proceedings developed a very different story began to emerge in which a witness pointed to Delahoyde as responsible for seducing Mrs Hinds and persuading her to make accusations against Middleton. The presumption on this thesis was that Delahoyde wanted to oust Middleton from the Hanover Park Asylum. The case was to remain undecided, but Delahoyde was forced to make some very damaging admissions under pressure from several witnesses. Under cross examination he admitted that he was married and had two children and that he had abandoned them all in London. He had further to admit that he had conspired with one of the servants at the Hanover Park Asylum against Dr Middleton. Almost as an incidental point Delahoyde admitted that he had got the servant pregnant. There was still more in the sordid inventory. Delahoyde admitted that he had got Mrs Hinds drunk and persuaded her to speak out against Dr Middleton. The case against Dr Middleton was clearly collapsing, but there were yet more details of Delahoyde's licentiousness and his lack of professional standards. He admitted that he had kept a prostitute at the asylum and that he had had sexual intercourse with a patient named Alonzo.

Such a salacious story was bound to be replayed throughout the UK and additional detail appeared in some of the accounts. The *Chester Courant* for 31st December for example included the point that Dr Middleton had been in touch with Delahoyde's creditors. This may well provide a clue for why he made such a desperate attempt to discredit Middleton. After such public exposure Delahoyde would have acquired such notoriety that he would have been excluded from decent society and would have found it all but impossible to pursue a medical career. Certainly no more adverts by the founder of the Sion Vale institution were to appear. The exposure of Delahoyde is not proof that Lucett's version of the failure of the Sion Vale experiment and the conspiracy to deny him the curative process was correct. The exposure is, however, powerful circumstantial evidence that the Lucett version at least had an element of truth in it. Even Lucett's claim that he had had to support the Delahoyde family begins to look possible. The question is why Lucett exercised such apparently poor judgement and became involved with such a corrupt, unprincipled and unprofessional individual – especially given that Dr Tardy his first partner appears dully worthy on the slight evidence available.

The *Chester Courant* for 31st December replayed the *Dublin Evening News* account of the trial, but included a sensational addition concerning the Dukes of Kent and Sussex. 'Dr Delahoyde appeared a convivial pleasant fellow', the paper reported, 'and complained of injuring his finances by keeping good company. The doctor said he was the particular friend of the Duke of Kent; he and the Duke however had quarrelled but they were now reconciled, the Duke HAVING MADE HIM THE ABJECT APOLOGY. He said he knew all the Royal Dukes, they were the greatest set of .... in the world

– he had to lament his misfortune in their acquaintance – it entirely affected (sic) his ruin.' This is an extraordinary insight into Delahoyde. No part of this account will have represented an accurate statement of fact. It is not clear what the basis was for the journalists having this perspective from Delahoyde. It does not look like a formal interview. The idea that he had been 'a particular friend' of the Duke of Kent is fanciful given the nature of the relationship which had actually existed. The idea of a quarrel is more interesting and may have an element of truth in it. The end of the Committee experiment had come quite suddenly and Lucett's claim that he never 'deceived' anyone in his 1815 book leaves the sense that there had been some falling out between the senior committee members and Delahoyde and Lucett. Money seems the most likely point of contention with the mention of ruin and the earlier contact between Dr Middleton and Delahoyde's creditors. Another surprising element of this account of his supposed ruin is the absence of any reference to Lucett. This would have been a logical moment to denigrate Lucett – especially after the publication of his 1815 book, *An Exposition*, with its criticism of Delahoyde. It is probable that Delahoyde's career was at an end following the court case and after this moment of brief notoriety he disappeared from the scene.

The picture of Lucett which was emerging from the claims and counter-claims in the newspapers, however, was one of a consistently polemical individual who projected the image of a crusader on behalf of himself and the insane. Ranged against him was the entrenched establishment of medical orthodoxy which was intent on restraining and dosing patients while milking them financially and having little real thought of a cure. What was the reality behind this? For the next several years Lucett continued to advertise regularly in the press. After a while the adverts began to present Lucett as clearly the sole proprietor and sole practitioner of the 'cure' and Dr Richard Smith was no longer mentioned. For the most part the adverts were short although he continued the practice of referring to individual patients through a brief case-study. A kind of stability, even routine had apparently been established in his life. A pointer to this is that he gave the same address of Weston House, Chertsey in his adverts from 1815 to 1820. Lucett gave every impression that he was an established practitioner in a prosperous market town. This was not the itinerant practice associated with quacks. The years that he was based at Weston House in Chertsey suggest that there was considerable stability in Lucett's life behind all the controversy he stirred up in the press. He was a married man with three children to provide for. No detail of that family life survives, but other insights into the man and his practice do survive. The process of official inspection of madhouses, which had been instituted as a first step in the development of protection of the insane, in fact presents a view of Lucett the practitioner from an independent official perspective.

Starting with the 1768 Act for Regulating Madhouses and the 1774 Act for the Regulation of Private Madhouses [in England and Wales], private madhouses had been made subject of official control. This included a process of licensing and inspection. Within a radius of seven miles of London this regulation was the responsibility of the Commissioners in Lunacy who were elected by the College of Physicians. Outside London the task of licensing and inspection fell to the local courts and magistrates. The reports represented an element of protection for the patients by ensuring some outside supervision, but it was the bare minimum. Dr Charles Dunne was right to lobby the College of Physicians to do more in the way of inspection. The system included one crucial condition which was specifically intended to provide a safeguard for patients. This was that a madhouse keeper could only accept a patient with a certificate of insanity signed by a medical practitioner. This provision did something to limit the scope for unscrupulous relatives to put away individuals they hoped to confine because they were inconvenient in some way or whose wealth could be exploited. The visitations did some good. An example is that in a report dated 21st March 1815 the visiting magistrates of Surrey pulled up the proprietor of Great Foster House asylum. It appeared that the proprietor himself and other directly interested parties had been signing some of the certificates of committal of the patients. The magistrates ordered that this should stop and that disinterested medical practitioners only should sign the certificates.[5]

This system of licencing and inspection provides a methodical record of who the licensee was for each asylum and whether they were qualified medically or not. The guarantors were also recorded as well as the sum they were guaranteeing. There is considerable detail in the reports as the names of the patients were often recorded as well as who they had been committed by and when. The reports also set out which patients had left the asylums and whether they had been discharged as cured or whether they had been transferred to another establishment. There is a surprising amount of actual individual colour with comments about people being reclaimed by close family members. When transfers were made there is no detail on why the new establishment was thought preferable, however. The reports themselves concentrate on the cleanliness of the establishments and on issues such as the location and the suitability of the facilities. There was some commentary on the treatment of the patients and in the case of the reports for Surrey there are examples where the absence of restraint is recorded. Actual detail on the medical treatment is not included so for Lucett's history there is no detail of his having a special process or any reference to the Committee or the royal connection. Whether the asylum owner knew in advance when a visit was to take place is not clear. Lucett was for example not present when one visit took place and so his wife had to answer the questions of the visitors.

The record of the 'Visits of Magistrates to Lunatic Asylums' for Surrey survives and this record allows the career of James Lucett the practitioner to be tracked during the immediate years after the end of the Committee experiment. It is not a comprehensive account, but it does provide a perspective of Lucett which is in some ways surprising. Under the heading 'Middlesex Session 11th July 1815' the entry includes the following statement, 'James Lucett of Chertsey, Surgeon. Licenced to keep a house called Weston House at Chertsey for the reception of lunatics not exceeding ten in number for one year.'[6] The Licence had been applied for with Lucett himself and 'Richard Smith of Chertsey, Surgeon' providing surety of £100 each. As was standard practice in Surrey, a team of three 'visitors' or inspectors, which included two JPs and a doctor, was appointed.

The first inspection took place on 9th February 1816 when two patients were recorded at Weston House. Lucett himself was absent during the inspection so Mrs Lucett had dealt with the visitors. The inspectors recorded that they had been unable to see the record book with the certificates under which the patients had been received, but did not comment further on this fact. They did, however, comment on Weston House itself. 'We further report that we are of opinion the House is well calculated for the reception of Lunatics, as it is commodious in itself and in a retired and airy Situation.' Interestingly the inspectors clearly talked to the patients and their views of the establishment were recorded. 'The Patients stated themselves to be well satisfied with their treatment and they appeared to be under no restraint.'[7] This last point was important not only because it demonstrated that Lucett was in the vanguard of those running asylums for the insane who dispensed with the use of restraint, but in the identity of one of the inspectors. Dr Alexander Morison was later to become eminent as the author of *Outlines of lectures on mental diseases*.[8] He was to become an academic encouraging the inclusion of mental illness in the training of medical students. He even tried to become the first professor of mental diseases at Edinburgh University. He failed in this, but Macalpine and Hunter commented that Morison had no direct experience of treating the insane apart from accompanying the Surrey Magistrates on their tours of inspection.[9] It would appear that Lucett provided him with a good example of management of the insane without resorting to restraint and it is ironic that Lucett was later to describe himself as 'Professor' at about the time when Morison was failing to obtain a chair at Edinburgh University. Lucett of course was self-appointed!

This is a wonderful insight into Lucett the practitioner by a critical and well-informed audience. Their good opinion could not be assumed. Robert Stracey Irish, a prominent second generation asylum keeper near Guildford was sharply and repeatedly criticised by the same inspectors. Indeed the inspectors finally recommended his licence should not be renewed in May 1823. The premises of some asylums were criticised as being in unsuitable locations, while the crowding of patients as well as a lack of cleanliness in both patients and asylum was a repeated concern of the inspectors. Yet in Lucett's case the inspectors not only approved of the asylum itself but even recounted the views of the patients on their treatment. The reference to the lack of restraint is also important. Although the inspectors do not state specifically that the other asylums used restraint it is clearly implicit that Lucett was unusual for not doing so.

Over the course of the next year two further inspections were made. These showed that there had been a quite rapid turnover of patients, but that three patients seemed to be the normal complement of the asylum. Lucett had been present at both inspections and had produced the correct certificates for the patients. He also had to admit that one of his former patients had been returned to his care after suffering a relapse. The inspectors made no comment on the fact and this was probably because it was a normal occurrence in madhouses of the time. Perhaps more important is that the inspections seem to demonstrate that Lucett was not running a 'receptacle' for the insane where people were dumped for the long term. It would appear that the rapid turnover of patients reflected that they were discharged after a relatively short period of time.

During the next two years until mid-1819 the inspections continued with a little less frequency. The reports were favourable with no irregularities in the paperwork. The maximum number of patients recorded at any one time was five. They seemed to have been drawn from a wider radius than central London. Patients from Birmingham and East Anglia were on record as well as several transfers in of patients from Bethlem and other major asylums. Lucett himself was referred to as 'gentleman' in the later reports in place of 'surgeon' as he was described in the original licence. There is no reference to the change in the reports so the assumption is that the inspectors did not consider it significant. One unexpected omission in the inspection reports was that Dr Richard Smith was not referred to at any point. The inspection team operated on the basis that the Lucett and his wife were solely responsible for the asylum.

Things did not run entirely smoothly at Weston House, however, as the inspection report of 19th July 1819 noted. Sarah Wyer had been admitted on the previous 5th November, but the inspectors recorded that she 'died on the 9th of the same month "by strangulation during the momentary absence of the attendant"'.[10] The obvious assumption is that Wyer was killed by another patient, but there is no further explanation by the inspectors and no suggestion even that one might be expected. There was an inquest on the 14th November presided over by the coroner Charles Jennett, but the actual inquest report has not survived.[11] The record is simply the bald fact that an inquest took place with no indication whether Lucett had given evidence. Indeed the entry in the inspection report for Weston House reads almost as if it was a repetition of the conclusion of the inquest. Certainly the inspectors do not dwell on the incident which is a pity as the death of Sarah Wyer encapsulates a key separation between those who, like Lucett, advocated a regime which dispensed with restraint and those who considered restraint to be unavoidable. John Connolly was to write about the absolute need for a high ratio of attendants to patients and the need for those attendants to be of high quality and to be active participants in the treatment regime.[12] It would be interesting to know whether Lucett was questioned by the coroner on the safety of the non-restraint method and his response. Meanwhile Sarah Wyer was buried on 17th November in Camden.[13]

The advertisements which Lucett placed regularly in the press appear to be the public face of a business carried out on a commercial basis and could be assumed to be aimed at maximising profit. The picture of Lucett the asylum keeper which emerges from the official inspection reports for Weston House point to something rather different. Although he was licensed to receive up to ten patients, the maximum on record was five and that number was cared-for for only a short time. The norm was for there to be three or four patients at Weston House. Other asylums in Surrey had much higher occupancy levels and the inspectors criticised every aspect from cleanliness to cramped accommodation. Lucett's establishment escaped these criticisms and attracted only positive comments. The lack of restraint was highlighted from the start by the inspectors so Lucett really seems to have lived up to the claim in his adverts that he did not need to manacle his patients or use straitjackets. There was also the sense that Lucett was not trying to maximise his profits. The occupancy levels were so consistently low and the fluctuations within such narrow bounds that it seems reasonable to conclude that he cared for very small numbers of patients by choice. They paid, or at least the bills were paid on their behalf, but there is no evidence that he was treating only very wealthy patients. The patients were not titled and there was nothing to suggest that they were drawn from anything more elevated than just a solvent part of society. The inspection reports also record a regular change of patients confirming that individuals were not kept indefinitely simply to provide income. They also came from other parts of the country as well as from London and Surrey itself. This suggests that his newspaper advertisements were effective or perhaps that his reputation was spreading.

If adverts were a valuable resource for James Lucett in the promotion of his business, controversy, particularly when it offered the opportunity to promote himself as the victim of attacks from competitors or simply the entrenched medical establishment, was even more valuable. The *Morning Post* of 17th October 1818 carried a Letter to the Editor claiming that Lucett had received an anonymous letter. This letter threatened to expose Lucett for wrongly having claimed, in an advertisement in the paper of 29th September, to have successfully cured the daughter of a qualified physician. Having forwarded the anonymous letter to the Editor, Lucett challenged the writer to identify himself to the newspaper and he, Lucett, would provide proof of the recovery of the former patient with the permission of her father. Lucett also asked the editor to replay the original advertisement three times more. With the preliminaries over Lucett sets about the fundamental message he wants to promote. This is to remind readers of his 'indefatigable' 'exertions' to 'restore the insane to health' and to set out an additional difficult case where he had been able to achieve a cure. It may all be true, but the weight of self-promotion gives more than the suggestion of a put up job.

In 1820 Lucett moved from Weston House to Rectory House in Ewell and in doing so prompted a wonderful moment of domestic controversy. The parishioners of Ewell did not want a lunatic asylum located in the house next to their church and said so. A special Vestry meeting was held on 20th May 1821 and the decision taken to order the Churchwarden, Mr James Andrew, to write to Lucett. The letter tried to impress on Lucett the majesty of the Ewell parish and warned him that if it was his intention to use the house previously occupied by Lady Glyn to 'receive insane persons' then the parish would formally oppose the grant of a licence. The tone of the letter has the confidence of complacency and seems to assume that the act of pen being put to paper would be enough to ensure that Lucett would think again about his plans to invade the sanctity, or at least the sanctimoniousness of Ewell.[14] Setting aside a modern perspective of the reaction of the Ewell vestry there was a serious underlying concern. The vestry was, in the early nineteenth century, responsible for many of the local services which are now the responsibility of borough councils. Crucially the vestry was responsible for raising funds for and administering the Poor Law. It is quite likely therefore that the hostility to Lucett's proposal to open an asylum was in part based on a fear that some of the patients could ultimately become the financial responsibility of the Ewell parishioners.

Lucett's habitual response was always to meet a challenge head on. Perhaps more significantly it provided him with the opportunity to set out his perception of his own practice to a hostile audience. His response was sent by return and began with the statement that he was not surprised to receive the letter from Ewell and that the parishioners need not be 'alarmed'. Emphasising that he had had no local problems during the seven years he had practiced in Chertsey, Lucett stated that although he had no intention of exceeding four patients at any time he was still required by Act of Parliament to secure a licence. In a show of bravado Lucett managed to make this apparent vulnerability a point of strength in his response. 'I am inclined to think the Court who have thought proper hitherto to grant one, will require more substantial evidence than summarised …' commented Lucett in response to the threat of opposition to the granting of a licence. In his conclusion Lucett expressed himself so confidently that he became dismissive of even the Ewell Vestry.

'I shall never consider my residence a <u>mad</u> house or a place of Confinement, as never having occasion to use these unhappy means resorted to in public and private receptacles for lunatics and if I should be so fortunate as not to be more annoyed by the inhabitants of Ewell than they will be by anyone in my house I shall be perfectly satisfied with the results.' There is no hint of a concession to the good folk of Ewell, but more important is the bold statement of the philosophy behind his practice. It is uncompromisingly patient-centred and sympathetic. It is also in the vanguard of the more sensitive and caring approach to the treatment of the insane exemplified in The Retreat at York or Spring Vale, the asylum in Staffordshire of Thomas Bakewell who emphasised the need to focus on the cure of the insane rather than just their confinement. Lucett meanwhile can perhaps be forgiven the very brief foray into self-promotion with his comment that 'I profess to relieve a deranged person in forty minutes.' Over all the exchanges with Ewell vestry may provide the nearest thing to the authentic voice of James Lucett.[15] If that is the case then it is an attractive picture which he creates. He is in business, but he is not out to make as much money as he possibly can. The self-imposed limit on the number of patients would have limited profitability. He sees his charges more as house guests than as patients although he makes it clear he expects them not to be with him long. For the solvent with a relative needing help, the Lucett philosophy of no use of restraint and the small scale of practice would have been hugely attractive.

The special Vestry meeting of 2nd June conceded defeat and in a delightful insight into Lucett's mentality it emerged during the meeting that he may have already been issued with a new licence to practice in Ewell when he wrote to the vestry! It is not clear why Lucett should have made the move as the practice at Weston House had drawn only positive comment by the inspectors. Lucett had almost certainly been renting Weston House and it is possible that the lease had come to an end. Whatever the reason the move was made by 5th July 1821 when the new premises were the subject of an inspection. Judged by the report the inspectors wrote this was a more detailed inspection than previous ones and in an echo of the first report of Lucett's asylum in Chertsey, Lucett was not at home when it took place.[16]

The opening of the report was basically favourable. The house was as comfortable and well-chosen as Weston House had been, but 'not so clean or in such good order and condition as might be wished'. In fairness the inspectors went on to comment that these failings were doubtless due to the fact that Lucett had just moved. They were perhaps reassured by Mrs Lucett's assurances that the whole house was due for a major refurbishment and that work had already begun. The conclusion of the inspectors was that the patients, including one who seemed to have become rather long-term, 'appeared to be under proper care and treatment and free from all coercion'. The inspectors did, however, note administrative irregularities which were to turn into a major crisis in Lucett's practice a year later. The inspectors noted that one of the patients did not have a proper certificate of committal as this 'had not yet been received'. It also emerged that a former patient had been transferred to another asylum without a new certificate being issued. This was a requirement which the inspectors commented had been notified to keepers two years previously. There was no direct criticism made of either Lucett or the irregularities, but they were noted. The slight sense that all was not quite right is not helped by Lucett's absence at this critical moment.

The slightly sour note of the July 1821 inspection was increased when the inspectors called again on 11th January 1822. It is not clear whether Lucett's standards were slipping or whether the inspections were becoming more rigorous. The general comment on the asylum was favourable and the inspectors, 'found the same cleaner and in much better order than our last visit'. There was an irregularity in the paperwork, however. A patient had been returned home in the previous November only to be re-admitted five days later, but without a new certificate of insanity. The lapse was noted, but on two other issues there was direct criticism. The inspectors expressed their concern over the lack of cleanliness of the long-term patient Mr Mackinnon who 'was very much neglected'.

The inspectors continued, 'and we have to make it a matter of positive complaint that care is not taken to confine the patients within the walls of the establishment for the gate of the courtyard being left unlocked throughout the day the patients are at liberty to go out and actually do go out unattended into the public road'.[17] The fears of the Ewell Vestry were apparently being realised if patients were being allowed to wander in the village. The inspectors clearly saw the 'liberty' which the patients had to go out as a kind of dereliction of a custodial duty. Lucett may well have seen things rather differently. At The Retreat in York it had been the custom to allow patients to leave the asylum to visit the city. They did so as part of the development of rational behaviour and self-discipline.[18] The gates at Ewell were clearly left unlocked because custody was not the purpose of the establishment. While the inspectors may not have reacted positively it is possible that the lack of containment was intentional and was part of Lucett's regime for rehabilitation. Nevertheless the inspectors' criticism of security combined with the concerns over the neglect of Mackinnon give the impression that Lucett was perhaps lowering his standards or was being caught out more effectively. There is no indication in the report of Lucett's reaction to the criticisms. Worse was to come, but the return of controversy did not for the time being come directly from his practice as a private asylum keeper.

Lucett's reaction to the end of the Committee experiment in 1814 had been to reinvent himself as a sole practitioner in the care, or cure as he would put it, of the insane. In doing so he had given his version of the events of the Committee experiment in his book of 1815. This had not simply been a process in which he set the record straight in his terms, but was an exercise in self-promotion in which he presented himself as the potential benefactor of mankind. On 1st March 1820, following the deaths of George III and the Duke of Kent, Lucett wrote to Lord Liverpool the Prime Minister seeking his permission to offer his cure to the nation through Parliament. In doing so Lucett again set out his version of the formation of the Committee and his involvement with the royal family.[19]

Essentially the story is the one he had given before, but there are some significant detailed additions. Lucett makes it clear that he approached Spencer Perceval. It was Perceval apparently who suggested that Lucett should contact the physicians attending His Late Majesty. The implication is clear; Perceval had immediately seen the potential application of the cure to George III. Lucett claims that he took Perceval's advice and wrote to Dr Willis. From the approximate timing this would have been Dr Robert Willis. Lucett claims that Willis had responded and said that he would inform the other doctors of Lucett's offer. This version of events places the involvement with the former prime minister rather earlier and expands Perceval's role. Lucett claims that Perceval assured him that he would take an interest in the offer. Lucett also claims that he still held several letters from Perceval assuring him of his continued interest although he heard nothing more from the physicians attending the king. Unfortunately no evidence to confirm the existence of this claimed correspondence between Lucett and Perceval seems to have survived. As Dr Tardy had recounted there had been an exchange of letters with Perceval, but this had simply prompted the comment that the Prime Minister could not support any experiment with the king's health. Most of this latest version of Lucett's contact with Perceval was almost certainly fabrication. Despite Lucett's claim that with Perceval's death he had lost a 'friend and advocate' his revised account was simply intended to bolster his place in the market. It is likely that the death of the Duke of Kent would have removed someone who could have responded and countered Lucett's claims.

Lucett's account is abbreviated from here on. The late Duke of Kent commanded that William Harrison should be placed under Lucett's care. Naturally he was cured within three months and Lucett repeats the claim that he was awarded two hundred pounds by the treasury. The Committee is mentioned briefly, but the focus of Lucett's attention, as it had been in his 1815 pamphlet, was on the meeting with the dukes and Dr Harness. This meeting, as rendered for Lord Liverpool, involved Lucett showing the manuscript setting out the cure which was endorsed as 'a most important and valuable discovery'. There is an apparent sleight of hand in Lucett's account. The brief reference to the meeting with the dukes refers only to the manuscript, but when addressing Lord Liverpool on making the cure available to the nation through Parliament he refers to offering the 'manuscript with the medical treatment'.

Lucett then makes a surprising claim. This is that he had already tried in 1819 to offer the cure in the form of a petition to Parliament made on his behalf by the MP George Holme Sumner. This petition had apparently been rejected by Lord Sidmouth and Mr Vansittart out of what Lucett presumes was 'delicacy to his late Majesty's situation'. Lucett's assumption that the apparent rejection was out of concern for the then king's situation is not convincing. The king had been diagnosed as insane nine years previously and had effectively been replaced by his eldest son. Lucett nevertheless advances a question. This is to ask whether it would cause any offence to His Majesty's Ministers to publish a pamphlet setting out his offer of the cure to the government through Mr Sumner. With studied disingenuousness Lucett claims that he does not want to deprive the public of the benefits of the cure any longer. Perhaps forgetting that he had been regularly advertising his cure in the press? There was a potential risk to Lucett in advancing this account. Sumner was a Surrey MP and was in his prime at the time. He was a man who had already shown an interest in the plight of the insane as he had visited Bethlem in 1814 following the discovery of the notorious case of James Norris who had been discovered chained to a wall for nine years. Vansittart and Lord Sidmouth were also alive and available to contradict Lucett if this was appropriate. Indeed they had been Chancellor and Home Secretary in Liverpool's administration formed in 1812. Lucett could not have known whether Liverpool would consult any or all these people to give the lie to his claims.

A brief exchange of minuting followed and on 8th March Lucett had his answer.[20] This was that Lord Liverpool saw no objection to Lucett publishing an account of 'the plan which you state you have discovered for the relief and care of mental derangement'. It is not clear what Lucett's intentions were in initiating the correspondence with the Prime Minister but it is certain that the reply on Liverpool's behalf was not intended to be used as it was. Lucett went ahead with the publication of a pamphlet in 1822 entitled, *Address to a Candid and Impartial Public* which is dedicated to Lord Liverpool.[21] The linkage to the Prime Minister is increased with the opening of the address itself which attempts to imply that Liverpool endorsed the Lucett cure. 'Under the sanction of the Right Honourable the Earl of Liverpool, Mr Lucett is induced to offer to his countrymen, and to the world in general, the benefits resulting from his excellent mode of treating and curing insanity.' Compared with the 1815 book, this pamphlet is a model of concision although the content is familiar.

Out has gone the history of the cure. Instead there is a short clear and very convincing sounding account of his contact with Spencer Perceval and the then Prime Minister's desire to arrange that Lucett should see the king with the implication that he should treat the royal patient. Of course this is implicitly what Lucett claimed for the Perceval link in the letter to Liverpool. It is just that this time the claim is effectively explicit. Careful editing of the story removes all mention of the Committee, but produces a flow in which the untimely death of Perceval appears to have left the Dukes of Kent and Sussex no option but to ask to see Lucett and to subsequently endorse his cure for the mentally deranged. What is still recognisably the Harrison case follows, but this is simply the opportunity to set out again the claim that the payment of 200 guineas was made by the Treasury to Lucett for effecting the cure. Lucett must have considered that sufficient time had elapsed to make it unlikely that anyone would recall that he had himself quoted the response from Perceval in the *Examiner* of 26th January 1812, 'Mr Perceval desires me to observe to you, in reply to your letter, that he cannot venture to recommend His Majesty's physicians, to permit any experiment to be made with regard to His Majesty's health which they do not themselves approve of.'

Lucett's strategy is clear. It is to demonstrate that his cure is officially sanctioned. He adds to the impression already given by a case-history in which he claims that at the request of two named MPs he had visited Bedlam to see a patient who had an extremely bad case of mania. Lucett claims to have cured the individual in four months. There follow a further sixteen case histories where there is a further innovation. Lucett names the doctors in some instances who had failed to cure the patients whom he subsequently took on. As Lucett himself remarks in his concluding comments all the cases were 'attended with that uniform and astonishing success, which has constantly accompanied his unremitting exertions'. The whole feel of the pamphlet is of a prospectus in which Lucett was re-launching his career after ten years. It is a document of considerable disingenuousness. There is no mention of patients suffering relapses and certainly no mention of the conclusions of Dr Harness that his 'cure' offered temporary relief at best. It was perhaps a convenience that both the Duke of Kent and Spencer Perceval were dead and unable to question Lucett's account.

Lord Liverpool can have had no idea how the bland official statement that the Prime Minister had no objection to Lucett publishing the success and value of his cure for insanity could be turned into a personal endorsement for it. Lucett's advert in the *Morning Post* for 25th January 1823 was a bravura performance in self-promotion. 'Under the Patronage of the Rt Hon the Earl of Liverpool, – INSANITY CURED.' It was almost as if the Prime Minster himself was about to engage in curing the insane. Lucett was aiming for the literate and wealthy urban elite as his customer base. It may seem a little odd that such efforts of publicity were considered necessary for a patient base which was maintained at less than a handful for the most part.

Perhaps the best way of examining Lucett's efforts is to see them simply in terms of marketing. He was operating in a competitive market where there was an underlying fear of the practitioners of the time. Through association with the royal family and with the apparent endorsement of two Prime Ministers, Lucett was attempting to legitimise his position as a practitioner. He had no professional body such as the College of Surgeons to endorse his standing. It was not a static market. There were new entrants in the body of practitioners offering their services and there was a constant turnover in the potential patients bidding for their services. Lucett may have been dealing with small numbers at any one time in his own asylum, but the fact that his patients came from relatively distant locations as well as London and its environs was important. It was an indicator of the importance of having some way of validating himself at a distance. Discretion was often an important element in the concerns of patients' relatives who valued the chance to hide the stigma of insanity by dealing with a distant practitioner. Lucett was also dealing with patients by correspondence. This was a method which has always been associated with quack practitioners of cures for almost anything. In the early nineteenth century it was also an adjunct to legitimate medical practice. For those living in remote locations or for those seeking a second view of some persistent ailment correspondence could sometimes be the only way to secure advice. For the practitioner, in this case Lucett, this route presented a logical way to augment the income.

Lucett's underlying problem in promoting his treatment was his lack of a medical qualification. The concept of the 'quack' was clearly well developed at the time and although it is possible now to question the criteria which might have been applied in the early nineteenth century it was a useful term to employ with the aim of undermining any practitioner in the health industry of the time. Initially Lucett had calculated that he would do better if he worked with a qualified doctor to front the operation. The relationship with Delahoyde had ended in disaster. When that relationship ended, Lucett acquired a new partner in the shape of Richard Smith. While this relationship apparently did not end with the acrimony of the Delahoyde partnership, it was clear that by 1818 they had gone their separate ways. Thereafter the shield of a qualified partner was abandoned and Lucett had operated entirely on his own account. However, this left him vulnerable to criticism for a lack of professional competence and even potentially vulnerable to legal action. In 1823 the issue came to a head.

The first public statement came from Lucett in a letter to the editor of the *Morning Post*, dated 6th February 1823. Essentially Lucett was, as always advertising his practice through the medium of 'correspondence' in the press. There was, however, a pointer to the public controversy which was about to engulf him. Today it would be called 'grandstanding' as Lucett claimed that the owners of private madhouses opposed him because he was in danger of putting them out of business. The medical profession also came in for criticism. The edition of the *Morning Post* for 14th March carried another open letter from Lucett. In this one he seems to have been responding to criticism that the cure did not work and that he used cruelty. With oblique references to the Dukes of Kent and Sussex as well as to an entirely favourable assessment of the cure which he ascribed to Dr Harness, he tried to reassert the effectiveness of his practice. But the accusation of cruelty clearly rankled and this prompted a rebuttal from him which seems to express a genuine hurt, 'It is, I find, circulated that my means are harsh and cruel. In answer I can only say, I have ever set my face against coercion or confinement.' He goes on to say that he has none of the implements of confinement in his house and never has had. In a separate part of the letter Lucett comments that the normal treatment of mania is ineffective, 'I am enabled from experience to assert that the treatment generally known in mania is insufficient'. There can be little doubt that he was right in that.

It would be reasonable to assume that Lucett with his promotion of his 'cure' as if it was a single process saw insanity as a single illness. He did not or at least he did not see insanity as having its roots in a single cause. In the letter of 14th March he gives an inventory of several diverse reasons which could lead to derangement and insanity. In setting out the causes of insanity as he sees them, Lucett demonstrates a greater sensitivity and understanding than many contemporaries. Indeed he was clearly in the vanguard of thinking at the time on the conditions which could lead to 'insanity'. Lucett claimed that the accusations of cruelty made against him were simply attempts to discourage people from placing patients with him. The overall impression is of an apparently buoyant and confident Lucett, who was ready to pass on the benefits of his experience, but there is the sense that the underlying mood was much more defensive.

The *Morning Post* of 19th April 1823 carried an advertisement which indicates just how vulnerable Lucett had come to feel. The advert reads, 'Insanity – the Proprietor of the Discovery for the cure of Insane Persons is willing to connect himself with a gentleman qualified to engage in an establishment where the cause of the disease is removed without coercion or confinement. Letters, post-paid, to J. Lucett, Ewell, Surrey.' As always with Lucett there was more to the initiative than a sudden desire to find a qualified partner. The *Morning Post* of 6th May 1823 carried the most extraordinary advert – even by Lucett's standards. In the advert Lucett offered a thousand guineas for anyone who could prove his cure for insanity was not effective. The bravado of this advert is typical Lucett, but it almost certainly reflects public criticism which is now lost but which involved accounts of patients who had suffered a relapse or patients who had not benefited from the curative process. Lucett had suffered this before, most notably with articles in the *Examiner*. His response of an illogical, but impressive sounding challenge was combative and potentially effective. Certainly by 14th May he had returned to his more routine adverts under the heading, 'Insanity Cured without Confinement'. Calm had apparently returned, but there is no doubt that Lucett had reacted badly, perhaps overreacted, to some criticisms of him. It was also clear that he felt under pressure.

Lucett had in fact probably been rattled by a potentially serious episode which had been hanging over him and which highlighted how vulnerable he was as an unqualified practitioner if he didn't keep fully to the regulations for private asylums. *Jackson's Oxford Journal* for 2nd August 1823 and other papers carried the account of the Surrey Assizes and the case of Lawson v Lucett. Essentially Lucett was prosecuted for taking in a patient without a certificate from 'a physician, surgeon, or apothecary'. The system of requiring such a certificate was intended to provide some protection for individuals to prevent their being sectioned without any professional intervention. Lucett had an answer of course and it is one which attempted to give him the moral high ground in the face of what Lucett wanted to imply was petty bureaucratic interference. In January 1823, Lucett's receiving house had been visited by a magistrate, a 'visiting physician' and a clerk of the peace according to the portentous press reports. In fact the visitation by this apparently august body was one of the routine checks on asylums made by the Surrey Magistrates on 23rd January.[22]

When asked for a certificate for one of the two patients present at his house, Lucett admitted he did not have one and that he had not made a return to the College of Physicians. When challenged as to why he had not made the normal returns, Lucett argued that it had been out of delicacy for his patient. The gentleman was a physician himself and Lucett was concerned that such a return would prejudice his career. All this is recorded in the record of the Surrey Visiting Magistrates. During the court case a little more obvious manipulation of the defence was visible. The gentleman was certainly a physician, but was, it was claimed, staying at Lucett's home simply as a lodger who wished to benefit from country air. He had apparently suffered briefly from a fever while at Lucett's home, but had not been treated. His recovery had been rapid and while at Lucett's home he had even visited a number of his patients. Although witnesses were called to corroborate the account, the prosecution case hung on the assessment of the inspection team which contended that the gentleman had indeed shown signs of derangement and that he was in fact being treated as a patient. The verdict was against Lucett and he was fined £100.[23]

As is so often the case with Lucett, things were not quite as straightforward as they seemed in the rather cut and dried newspaper report. Under the entry for May 1824 in the financial accounts of the visiting magistrates of Surrey is the following statement: 'Mr Lucett being committed to the County Gaol and having applied for the benefit of the Insolvent consulting with the Sols

[sic] [solicitors?] to propriety of opposing his discharge.' An entry of six shillings and eight pence costs was recorded. The entry continues: 'Several applications having been made by Mr Lucett and his friends to release the debt. Visiting and conferring thereon.' A further sum of six shillings and eight pence is again entered in the account. Under December 1824 there is the following entry: 'Paid to taxed costs with Sherriff's Possesstage [sic] in an action brought for penalty incurred by Mr Lucett in harbouring a patient without certifying him to the College of Physicians in which b...[?] was insolvent.' The sum of ninety five pounds and fifteen shillings was entered as a cost at this point.[24]

What actually happened is not clear. Lucett was certainly imprisoned briefly and it would appear that this was for debt and almost certainly reflected a refusal to pay the fine imposed by the court in August 1823. The *London Gazette* for 24th June 1824 records a statement that a petition of insolvency would be dealt with at the Justice Hall of the Old Bailey in respect of, 'Lucett, James, late of Rectory House, Ewell, Surrey, Professor of a Mode of Medical Treatment for curing insanity.' What is not clear is whether Lucett was genuinely bankrupt or whether the declaration of insolvency on his part was a manoeuvre to avoid paying the fine. The magistrates' record appears to show that the fine, or most of it, was actually paid from the revenues of the licensing system. The magistrates had tried to seize and dispose of some of Lucett's possessions in order to pay the fine, but had been unable to find anything of value and even the little they did seize was not realised as the magistrates became bogged down in consultations over the legality of their actions. It is clear that Lucett was not acting alone and from the record of the Surrey asylum inspectors he seems to have mobilised effective supporters to question every aspect of the imposition of a fine and its collection. If that is the case it would represent a sort of victory for Lucett, but one which would have been at great cost to his immediate comfort and to his longer term potential to practice in Surrey.

The *London Gazette* had indicated that Lucett no longer lived in Ewell so the establishment he had there had clearly been brought to an end by the court case. The Surrey records show no indication that he applied for a licence in the county again. The only subsequent reference to him in the magistrates' inspection records is of Lucett signing an insanity certificate for a patient at an asylum which was perhaps optimistically called 'Recovery' in October 1825 when he was described as 'Professor of the Cure of Insanity'. Whatever the true details of the incident of the uncertified patient had been, Lucett was back in business at the first opportunity and with perhaps typical chutzpah he had also acquired an important sounding new title. Ironically he was also signing certificates on patients which were accepted by the authorities with which he had so recently crossed swords.[25]

Lucett's public response to the court case was not simply defiance but rather of counter-attack against the medical profession and the specialist 'mad doctors' in particular. The copy of Lucett's *Address to a candid and impartial public* of 1822 from the Hume Tracts contains an addendum which refers to the Croydon Assize of 21st July 1823. In the addendum the College of Physicians is criticised for bringing the action against Lucett, 'whereby he was fined one hundred pounds for having restored to health and liberty of one of their own members'.[26] Certainly Lucett continued to advertise for patients in August 1823 as if nothing had happened. This was even while a process for bankruptcy was pending.[27] More significant, however, was his advert of 4th August in which he referred to an investigation of Bethlem by the College of Physicians which had been very critical of the regime at the hospital. It is not clear whether Lucett was referring to a specific inspection of Bethlem of the kind carried out by Edward Wakefield in 1814, but it appears simply to be a device to focus his attack on the physicians; both as an organisation and as individuals. Lucett contrasts the inspection and criticism of the mistreatment of patients in the large asylums and his own practical interventions to cure patients. With a rhetorical swagger he refers to 'casting off the chains' of lunatics from Bethlem, St Luke's and other asylums and doubtless likens himself to Pinel. To ram the point home Lucett adds that many of the patients he had cured had previously been certified as incurable. In October 1823 Lucett took the next step in what was becoming a campaign when he started to name eminent 'mad doctors' such as Dr Monro and Dr Sutherland whose former patients he claimed to have cured when the specialists had failed. Lucett's counter-attack looks now like a populist appeal in which he highlighted the failings of a profession which was generally held in low esteem. For the time it was not an unreasonable business strategy as the speciality had not been long enough established to have achieved a positive track record, while the failure to cure George III would still have been remembered as a glaring failure.

Chapter Sixteen

Ruin and Recovery

'During the reign of George the Third ... the most immediately interesting of all arts, the alleviation of human misery by the cure of disease, has been materially improved.'[1]

Andrew Duncan MD. 1821.

The incident of Lucett's prosecution in 1823 raises a number of questions about him as a practitioner. These centre on an apparent separation between Lucett's pretentions and the reality. He claimed a unique cure for insanity and repeatedly claimed that he had put this at the disposal of mankind or that he wished to do so. Yet the reality of his operations is that they were on such a small scale that he was rarely responsible for more than three patients at any one time in his own asylum. Indeed it is possible that this was a factor in his abandonment of a search for a qualified partner. There simply wasn't enough income from so small a practice to support two practitioners. Yet Lucett was not alone in practising on an apparently small scale. Dr Francis Willis gave evidence to a Parliamentary Committee in 1789 following the king's recovery from his first crisis involving mental derangement. When asked about his experience in dealing with insane patients Willis claimed he had treated, on average, thirty patients a year for the previous twenty-eight years.[2] This would have been a nominal figure based on the throughput of his Lincolnshire asylum where he could count on sons and assistants. The number of patients he would have managed with the intensity of the king's case would have been much lower. Allowing for the fairly rapid turnover of patients which the inspections recorded while working in Chertsey and Ewell, Lucett could have come near to matching the numbers Willis personally managed. Lucett may not have been a player on a world stage as a practitioner in treating the insane, but the size of his practice may have been closer to that of Dr Francis Willis than was immediately apparent. Luck had propelled Willis to public notice when he was called in to treat the king. Willis did not have a track record of publishing scholarly works on the treatment of the insane and did not develop one after he had treated the king.

Practitioners who had positions at the asylums in operation during the eighteenth century and at the beginning of the nineteenth century were nominally responsible for large numbers of patients. In reality though institutions like Hoxton did not offer treatment for insanity, as Willis and Lucett did, but acted as holding places for the insane. Even Bethlem, which did offer treatment, did not have resident medical staff and Alexander Morison, who was the last visiting physician at the hospital, was forced to resign in 1852 after his remoteness from the patients attracted criticism. Cure, or more accurately recovery, was incidental and generally depended on spontaneous recovery rather than focused treatment in most of the asylums of the age. So institutions which did actually engage in the treatment of the insane could probably only function with a very much smaller client base than the so called 'receptacles for the insane'. They would also have had to charge well for the active involvement of the practitioner and assistants. The 1823 prosecution of Lucett nevertheless raises a question over how successful he was financially and whether there had been a separation between appearances and the reality.

The apparent inability of the bailiffs to secure anything of value to cover the debts incurred through the imposition of the fine is potentially very significant. Lucett's establishments in Chertsey and Ewell had been in imposing residences of the kind that would be occupied by a 'gentleman'. The creation of an establishment which was civilised, comfortable and exclusive would have been an essential part of the marketing of the 'cure'. It demonstrated success for the proprietor and implicitly for the cure. It seems surprising therefore that an establishment which was clearly intended to impress seemed to have had nothing of value in it. One answer is that Lucett may have anticipated being found guilty and had managed to spirit away what he owned before the bailiffs came. The Surrey assize records show that Lucett had friends who helped undermine the proceedings against him and who helped him fight the imposition of the fine at every step of the process. Lucett could have been bloody-minded enough to do all he could to thwart proceedings which he regarded as vexatious. Certainly he was a man who always pushed his perspective of events. There is another possible interpretation and it is one which succeeding events were to strengthen.

This was that Lucett may have had no alternative and that behind the genteel surface calm of Chertsey and Ewell his existence was actually very precarious. The advertisement which Lucett had placed in April expressing his willingness 'to connect himself with a gentleman qualified to engage in an establishment where the cause of the disease is removed without coercion or confinement' may well have been an attempt to gain financial and professional support before the court proceedings of 1823 against him began. It is possible that he saw that if he lost the case his whole business would be brought to an end. This would not have been because he could no longer practise, but simply because his finances were so tight that even a fine would destabilise the equilibrium to the extent that he would not be able to continue in business. It seems likely that the impressive premises which Lucett occupied in Chertsey and Ewell were rented and that even a short interruption to the income stream would be enough to bring Lucett's practice to a halt because he could not keep up payments for house and contents. The bailiffs could find nothing of value which Lucett owned because he didn't actually own the house or contents.

A final possible explanation leads into the realms of speculation, but could have a bearing on Lucett's almost destructive response to the prosecution. In March 1822 Olivia Lucett was buried in Ewell churchyard which would have adjoined the premises which Lucett had occupied with his private asylum.[3] The age given for the deceased is 32 which would make the person too old to be James Lucett's daughter, but old enough to have been his wife. The overwhelming probability is that she was Lucett's wife but unfortunately the vicar at Ewell was not in the habit of annotating the parish register as many of his colleagues did so there is no additional information to explain the death or to specifically make a link with James Lucett asylum keeper. It may of course all be a coincidence, but Olivia's illness and death could be a partial explanation for the fall off in standards noted by the inspectors in January 1822. Extending the speculation, the absence of a wife's restraining hand could also be an element in Lucett's confrontational approach towards the authorities over the uncertified patient.

It is not clear from the record when Lucett was released from debtors' prison. The *London Gazette* for 24th June 1824 records that a petition of insolvency would be dealt with at the Justice Hall of the Old Bailey. The entry refers to Lucett as 'late of Rectory House, Ewell' and as 'Professor of a Mode of Medical Treatment for curing insanity'.[4] By the end of that year Lucett was again at liberty. He did not, however, begin to advertise from a base in a new establishment of his own. Instead he joined a partnership in which he appeared to have been almost an employee rather than an actual partner. Appropriately the establishment was called 'Recovery' and was the establishment which Lucett was recorded as providing a certificate of insanity for a patient in October 1825 in the Surrey records.[5]

In early 1825 Lucett entered into an 'indenture' or legal partnership with three others in the founding of an asylum at Mitcham Green in Surrey. According to the record Lucett was not required to provide any of the capital for the enterprise. The three partners seem to have been business partners only as they were not practitioners who were involved in the treatment of the patients. Lucett was responsible for the patients under the terms of the partnership. He was expected to provide treatment for the patients based not only on his experience, but was also to make available written instructions in his possession. In other words Lucett had convinced his partners that he had a unique treatment for insanity in the form of a manuscript.[6]

An advert in *John Bull* for 17th July sets out the new arrangements and Lucett's changed status. The advert borrows from Lucett's style at the outset as it appears under the heading 'Insanity Cured' thereafter the commercial nature of the undertaking is clear. Mr W A Rocher claims credit for setting up an establishment 'replete with every comfort' and for 'having exclusively engaged Professor Lucett whose skill and experience in the mode of effecting the CURE of those who are unhappily deprived of their mental faculties'. Rocher goes on to emphasise that restraint and coercion are never used and that the intention is that patients should be 'as happy as possible'. This was doubtless all very reassuring for potential clients, but the status of Lucett is markedly different. The new title of 'Professor' which he had assumed and the respect for his expertise which Rocher emphasises, all point to Lucett's importance. Nevertheless the inescapable fact is that Lucett the gentleman has become Lucett the employee. If the loss of independence indicated by the status of employee can be traced back to the prosecution of 1823 then it would confirm that the genteel existence which he seemed to lead in Ewell and before had been financed through credit and that he was vulnerable to even minor interruptions to his cash flow. It seems entirely possible that the failure to pay the fine in 1823 was perhaps not based on a refusal based on principle but a simple lack of money.

The partnership did not last long and by the end of the year it had broken up in acrimony with Lucett's former partners pursuing a legal complaint against him. In the process the complainants revealed more about the formation of the indenture. Lucett had indeed been charged with responsibility for the medical department of the asylum and for the care and treatment of the patients. He was also to receive £500 from his partners for the 'secret process' and there is a specific reference to the papers having been sealed by the Duke of Kent, the Duke of Sussex and Dr Harness.[7] This opening salvo in the legal complaint seems to confirm that Lucett had been short of money and could only get back into business with the help of others. It is also pretty clear that

Lucett had been successful in peddling the cure which had been the basis for the Committee experiment and it was this cure which was the real focus of the partners' interest.

The complaint against Lucett rapidly descended into a series of claims and counter claims which present a sordid picture of the workings of the asylum. This was perhaps inevitable given that each side aimed at denigrating the other while justifying their own position. Nevertheless the startlingly unpleasant picture of Lucett which emerges is a surprise. His partners claimed they had 'discovered' that he had been interfering in the management of the asylum and had also indulged in, 'violent and abusive conduct towards some of the said patients and by gross and indecent conduct to some of the female patients and by incurring or threatening to incur debts in the name and style of the said establishment'. The complaints against Lucett centred on two specific areas: his financial irregularities and his inappropriate behaviour towards some of the patients. As the process advanced the complaints became more specific.[8]

Lucett was accused of issuing 'bills of exchange' or other promissory notes in the name of the asylum in order to raise money to cover his debts. These were serious charges of theft and fraud. On the personal level Lucett was accused of frequent drunkenness and abusive behaviour to other members of the staff. As the accusatory process advanced Lucett was the subject of increasingly specific offences and individual patients were named. A certain Mrs Moorat was apparently pinned down in her bed by Lucett and fondled while another patient was made so drunk by Lucett that she could not stand. Lucett's partners claimed that they had tried to settle matters amicably and to review the financial concerns, but ultimately at the beginning of December 1825 Lucett had resigned and advised his former partners to find 'a medical gentleman and his wife' to replace him. The complainants concluded that Lucett was in breach of the contract of indenture and that he had been acting with others in his removal of funds from the asylum account.

Lucett's response dated 11th January 1826 immediately focused on what, for him, was the core of the dispute. This was that the indenture contained the provision that if the other partners wound up the indenture then the 'cure' reverted to Lucett's sole use. Lucett continued his response by relating that the indenture had been drawn up by Mr Hartley [solicitor for the other partners] who had advised Lucett that the document was very long and tedious. Hartley apparently advised Lucett to take the provisions on trust and sign. Lucett claimed that he had accordingly signed without checking the document although he would never have done so if he had realised that there was any possibility that his partners would try to deprive him of the rights to the cure. In a gesture of self-importance he added that this was particularly the case as he had refused ten thousand pounds for the full rights to the cure. Lucett's behaviour seems negligent and unconvincing and there is an echo of his claimed passivity during the meeting with the royal dukes and Dr Harness to discuss the nature of the cure. His arguments that in the process of winding up the partnership the other parties had not provided the original of the contract for him but a copy seems weak. It is only in arguing that the partners had never fulfilled their financial obligations and that far from him treating the patients badly he had had to ban individual partners from contact with the patients as they had used violence against them. Lucett even names one patient who had apparently been horse-whipped by a partner.[9]

There is an unedifying catalogue of apparent abuse and exploitation on both sides, but the sincerity of both parties seems questionable throughout. Lucett was probably right to highlight the likelihood that his erstwhile partners had entered the partnership with the intention of winding it up at the first opportunity as a mechanism for claiming the rights to the cure. For his part Lucett seems to have entered the partnership as a stop gap to secure immediate access to funds and to exploit his position to reduce his debts so far as was possible. The picture of Lucett was fundamentally altered by the short time in Mitcham. Here was a man who was accused of drunkenness and misbehaviour in his treatment of patients. Nothing had pointed in this direction in the official record before. There was also the suggestion that he had been adept at managing financial transactions which were not simply illegal, but could involve a capital crime. Was this the desperate response to the financial problems brought on by the 1823 prosecution or was there more to this aspect of Lucett's behaviour?

Lucett did not give up on his efforts to re-establish himself and his practice of treating the insane although the initial effort looks tentative and clearly reflects a process of adjustment to more straightened circumstances. It was, however, more characteristic of Lucett that in less than a month after his response to his erstwhile partners he was advertising again on his own behalf. The advert in the *Morning Post* took the standard line of 'Insanity Cured' without restraint but it was now in the name of 'Professor Lucett'. Lucett may have taken an impressive-sounding new title but the decline in his fortunes was all too obvious. From the imposing address of Rectory House at Ewell to what looks like an accommodation address, 'care of Kirke's Nursery, Brompton' in February 1826.[10] He was to keep this singular address until 1828. With James Lucett nothing was ever quite straightforward. If 1826 was not proving to be a propitious year for Lucett with all the difficulties caused by the complaints brought against him by Mr Rocher and his other former partners he nevertheless chose this moment to publish a further pamphlet which demonstrated his apparent irrepressibility.

Address to the Right Honorable The Earl of Liverpool on the Cure of Insanity was a thorough-going piece of self-promotion. It was also an exercise in rewriting history which clearly entered the realms of fantasy. The use of the Prime Minister's name in the title was entirely spurious and was simply intended to attract the attention of the potential reader. In the same way Lucett's repeated claims of Lord Liverpool's '*distinguished* patronage' were complete inventions. This descent into a fantasy world is perhaps most significant in the rewriting of Lucett's contact with Spencer Perceval. From a straightforward statement that Perceval could not interfere in the treatment of the king in 1811, Lucett's revision transmogrified the then Prime Minister's role to being 'desirous of procuring permission for me to visit his late Majesty'. Only Perceval's assassination, 'prevented my having the opportunity of attending upon our late beloved Monarch'. Lucett's open letters to the Queen in 1811 and the subsequent relationship with the Duke of Kent were rendered as being about treating the king; this is just the first time he had stated this openly.[11]

The pamphlet was professionally produced and printed, but it is not clear how it was intended to be used beyond the general aim of achieving publicity for Lucett's practice. There is no price on the document and it would have been expensive to produce so was unlikely to have been a cheap 'flyer' to be handed out in large numbers. It is possible that it was used as a response to initial enquiries by the family or guardians of potential patients in which case it could have been quite effective. What it does underline is that in the early nineteenth century past records were not accessible in the way that they are now. Lucett's carefully targeted dishonesty was therefore not as dangerous as it might seem today and the chances of exposure of his lies were not very great. Even when exposure happened, as was the case of one lie in this pamphlet, the consequences were not necessarily significant. In setting out the case histories, Lucett chose in some instances to name individual physicians whom he claimed had failed to cure the patients before Lucett took them on. Sir Matthew Tierney MD of Brighton was one practitioner who was singled out as having failed to recover a patient whom Lucett claimed he successfully treated subsequently. In the context of a prosecution which took place in 1828, the discrediting of Lucett's assertions about Tierney, was part of an attempt to undermine Lucett's credibility as a witness. The choice of Tierney was an indication of Lucett's extraordinary self-assurance. At the time Lucett attempted to discredit Tierney he was Physician in Ordinary to George IV and had been one of the king's physicians since he had been Prince of Wales and while he was Prince Regent.

Despite the assurance and expense incurred in the production of the 1826 pamphlet, there is a single very clear indication that Lucett was actually experiencing serious difficulties in maintaining his practice at this time. He was obviously short of money which is not a surprise, but it appears that he was even considering giving up his practice entirely. The *Morning Post* of 25th April 1827 carried an advert under the title, 'An Eligible Situation to be Disposed Of'. The situation was, it was claimed, worth 'four to eight hundred pounds per annum' and was available 'with immediate possession'. More information was available through, 'Letters post-paid, or a personal interview with James Lucett, Professor, Old Brompton, where every information may be had'. Having tenaciously fought off his erstwhile partners from the 'Recovery' asylum in Mitcham, Lucett seems now to have been ready to sell out on what would probably have been reduced terms. It is possible that the expenses of the legal process over the Mitcham asylum exhausted his slender finances although it is possible that Lucett was attempting to attract a new financial backer. This is just a reasonable speculation, but what is sure is that this advert, which was not repeated, is the only direct evidence that Lucett had apparently considered giving up his practice of treating the insane since his first contact with the Duke of Kent.

By early 1828 'Professor' Lucett may have established the appearance of stability operating from an address at Parliament Street in central London.[12] In reality further legal proceedings were about to burst around him which were to expose the reality of his practice and pretentions. Ironically Lucett himself was not the subject of a prosecution on this occasion but was to appear as a witness in a case of forgery in which his evidence was so questionable that it prompted correspondents to contact the authorities to denounce him. The background to the case can be simply stated. The Reverend Peter Fenn was prosecuted at the Old Bailey in September 1828 for 'uttering various Bills, knowing them to be forged'.[13] This was a capital crime because Bills of Exchange were treated as cash and therefore the legislation at the time treated their fraudulent issue as being on a par with circulating forged banknotes or coins. The case was potentially further complicated by the possibility that Fenn was an assumed name and that he was almost certainly not a member of the clergy.

The trial resulted in the conviction of Fenn and he was sentenced to death. Although there can be little doubt of Fenn's guilt in the formal sense the trial raised issues which Mr Justice Gazelee drew attention to in his management of the proceedings. The case centred on whether the bills had been issued by

Fenn knowing that they would not be honoured on the date and at the bank or institution placed on the documents. Such bills also had an acceptance on them in which an individual acted as guarantor of the bill in case of failure by the bank to pay out on the bill at the end of its term. The acceptances on the bills were in the name of James Lucett and Fenn was charged with issuing the bills knowing the acceptances by Lucett were forged. Lucett gave evidence that the signatures on the bills were not his.

Although Fenn was almost certainly guilty there are pointers to his having been the subject of a conspiracy. George Vincent, the attorney who had acted on behalf of those bringing the prosecution, had written a piece for *The Times* newspaper in which he asserted Fenn's guilt and that he had confessed. Mr Justice Gazelee described 'Such publications in the newspapers ...... created great prejudices against accused parties, and might bias the minds of Juries'. Lest there was any doubt Gazelee described Vincent's actions as 'abominable'.[14] The Fenn case attracted wide public interest and anger and prompted a Criminal Petition for clemency. The series of letters and papers which formed the petition centred on Vincent's alleged conspiracy to ensure Fenn's conviction and the belief that Lucett was an untrustworthy witness. The seriousness of the petitioners is underlined by the fact that the jury members at the trial were also signatories of a petition for clemency.

The system of petitions for clemency aimed at securing consideration of a case by the Home Secretary, Robert Peel in this instance, to determine whether there were grounds for a stay of execution and a change of sentence on the basis of factors or information which were not considered at the trial. One of the most damning letters was sent by James Chapman who ironically was himself a prisoner in the Fleet Prison at the time. Lucett is the focus of Chapman's concern. 'James Lucette the principal witness against Fenn and known commonly by the name of the Mad Doctor is a man of known bad character and living on the Town for the last 20 years by the most impudent and fraudulent representations pretending his having in his possession a recipe for the effective cure of Insanity was at the time he gave his evidence under arrest and a Prisoner in the Fleet Prison and had at that time a Judge's Warrant lodged against him at the gate of the prison on an indictment with two other persons for a conspiracy for fraudulently obtaining from – – – – Bills of Exchange to a large amount for the purpose of establishing a Lunatic Asylum under the superintendence of the said James Lucette. Which Bills of Exchange they appropriated to their own use. The other parties in the Indictment were Robert Weaver of 34 Parliament Street and Simpson Fox not yet taken – Mr Harmion of Hatton Gardens is the solicitor for the prosecution.'[15]

Chapman continues his denunciation of Lucett by stating that Weaver had acted as a witness in the Fenn case in support of Lucett, but the actual witness had been Weaver's son rather than Robert Weaver who was Lucett's co-conspirator. Chapman continues by stating that Lucett and Robert Weaver [senior] had a history of issuing false bills of exchange together. Chapman continued that Lucett had used the address of the shop at 34 Parliament Street as an accommodation address for his business activities and that both James Lucett, 'the Mad Doctor', and his son of the same name were both in the habit of providing acceptances on blank bills of exchange for payment. Indeed the younger Lucett was in gaol at that time for debt. There is no doubt that Lucett had used the Parliament Street address in his business as the advert in the *Morning Post* in February 1828 had demonstrated.

Chapman had done more than pursue Lucett's involvement as a witness in the Fenn case. He had also addressed his reputation for professional honesty as a practitioner caring for the insane. The papers contained in the petition for clemency on behalf of Fenn include the short pamphlet by James Lucett of 1826 referred to earlier in this chapter. In it Lucett makes the following claim, 'I make no doubt it will be estimated by those who have thus experienced the blessing of restoration to health of Body and Mind and after every other Medical aid had proved abortive and I beg leave to make an appeal to Sir Matthew Tierney MD of Brighton relative to a Lady whose Mind and Constitution Health was considered by him past all hope of recovery.' This was clearly an example where Lucett had made a direct claim that he had cured someone whom a qualified physician had failed to help. The difference in this instance is that Chapman had sought confirmation directly from Tierney. Dr Tierney could simply have ignored the claims made by Lucett, but it is clear that Chapman had explained something of the background and his interest in determining the true nature of Lucett's medical claims. Tierney's short response is a withering dismissal of Lucett's pretentions. 'Sir, I have had your extract copied to guard against misstatements – I now add that I never saw the pamphlet from which the above is an extract and that I have no knowledge of the case referred to – Your praiseworthy intentions alone induce me to send this reply to him. Your servant, M Tierney.'[16]

This is a single example, but it is nevertheless eloquent. Tierney clearly regarded Lucett as beneath his notice and, but for the special circumstances of a legal plea for clemency on behalf of a condemned man, would have simply ignored Lucett and his claims. This is presumably the reaction which Lucett depended on professional men having when he used their names in his adverts. Tierney clearly saw Lucett as a quack and probably thought there was no point in responding to the claims of such a person. Others were moved to respond to the plea process to give their views on Lucett's bona fides. Three individuals took the trouble to make formal witnessed statements – one before the Lord Mayor of London – that Lucett and his son had been in the business of putting their names to blank bills of exchange in return for payment. They did this with no intention of underwriting the bills and indeed without the resources to do so. The statements indicated that over time bills were discounted and ultimately refused because the reputations of the 'guarantors' were so bad. What the statements make clear is that Lucett's involvement in the acceptance of bills of exchange had been going on for many years. It may have represented a significant augmentation of his income when he began, but by 1828 the returns were so small and the risks were increasing so that Lucett's continued involvement in this activity looks like desperation.

In his own appeal to Robert Peel, Fenn argued that he had not been aware at the time of his trial that Lucett had testified against him in court on a temporary release from prison where he was held for debt. Indeed Lucett had been escorted to the court by a court official. In addition Fenn pointed out that two of his accusers were the subject of legal proceedings and that his execution should be held until those proceedings had concluded and the implications for their accusations against Fenn assessed. In the event Fenn's sentence of death was commuted to transportation. Fenn had been guilty of issuing false bills of exchange, but Lucett too had been part of the process which ultimately led to the fraud. The cynicism which allowed him to testify against Fenn and to deny that a signature on the bills was his or his son's prompted a reaction amongst some of those who knew him and who considered Fenn was not the only guilty party. So far as the claims Lucett made that he was committed to the welfare of the insane they looked increasingly threadbare.[17] Lucett would never let such public criticisms of him remain unchallenged and in a letter to the editor of *The Times* dated 29th November 1828 he denied any previous contact with the other participants in the Fenn case and responded to Chapman's account, 'It may be praiseworthy in your correspondent to seek to obtain a respite for the unhappy man, but he should not do so unjustly at the expense of another individual.' The drama of the Fenn case subsided, but Lucett remained in prison. The *London Gazette* recorded that The Court for the Relief of Insolvent Debtors would consider the case of James Lucett, Professor for the Cure of Insanity on 22nd July 1829.[18]

The events of 1828 and 1829 had totally undermined Lucett's credibility as a professional healer. He had been bankrupt and had been exposed as a probable perjurer and a fraudster. His bad reputation for financial misconduct had been recorded and was a pointer to his reputation being bad with more people than had felt moved to intervene in the Fenn case. It was also clear that Lucett kept bad company as his business partners were frequently on the wrong side of the law. His former partner Antonio Rocher was moved by the Fenn case to drag up the history of the Mitcham partnership and his version of Lucett's role. He did so from the Fleet Prison where he was held and was simultaneously engaged in a legal wrangle with one of his former Mitcham associates. Yet by mid-1830 Lucett was apparently back in business with an imposing establishment in Brompton. This was an outlying part of west London which was rapidly becoming fashionable. Lucett was not ready to return to the tranquillity of life in Chertsey, however. The need or the desire for self-promotion was irresistible. It was also potentially controversial.

Chapter Seventeen

Taking on the Medical Establishment

'M Esquirol has observed that all English, French and German physicians who have devoted themselves to the study of mental diseases, recommend the confinement of the insane, and are unanimous as to the utility of this proceeding as a means of cure.'[1] *Treatise on Insanity and other Disorders of the Mind.*

James Cowles Prichard. 1837.

Lucett marked the accession of William IV with an open letter to the new monarch published in the *Morning Post* on the 23rd July 1830. As he had before, Lucett used the medium of an open letter to project his views and to attract publicity. Following his bankruptcy in 1829 it was doubtless necessary to attract some positive publicity so in familiar terms, Lucett set out his claim to sole proprietorship of a cure for insanity. There were, however, two important differences and both concerned the royal family in a direct way. The first was the claim that he had offered to submit his treatise to the physicians attending the late Duke of York with a view to bringing him relief and ultimately to restore him. This was significant because, although Lucett was a man of some presumption, this presumption had always been limited to the cure of insanity. He never claimed he could cure anything else. His claimed intervention in the case of the Duke of York was therefore effectively a statement that he considered the Duke had been deranged if not absolutely insane during his last illness.

This was not an insinuation which would have been welcomed at court and it is one which Colonel Taylor, his private secretary, gave no hint of in his record of the duke's last illness. That said, Taylor's intention was not to produce an exhaustive narrative of the duke's final illness or his medical treatment. Instead Taylor's purpose was to chronicle the Duke of York's response to the 'awful visitation of Providence' and to 'do justice to the exemplary Resolution and pious resignation with which he met and submitted to it'. If Lucett really had tried to contact York's household he might well have expected a rebuff as Sir Henry Halford was the first additional physician who was called in, while Sir Matthew Tierney was consulted when the duke briefly moved to Brighton! The Duke of York's grip on reality during his final illness seems to have been complete. Indeed he continued to work on official papers until close to his death. Only in the account of York's last day does Taylor mention the duke becoming 'delirious' although clearly his body was shutting down.[2] Zimmermann writing from Hanover would have doubtless had some understanding of Lucett's insinuations about York given his own concerns for the paroxysms the duke experienced when he was a young man in Hanover. But Zimmerman's disquiet expressed to George III about his sons would not have been available to Lucett.[3] The intervention must have been based on other evidence therefore.

The royal family and the British Government had coped with the illness and 'insanity' of George III, partly because it had not required a constitutional solution until late in his reign. The earlier crises had been of short duration but by 1810 there was an established heir and that heir had a legitimate daughter. It had also been manageable because the king was the only member of the family who had displayed the full-blown symptoms of derangement. There was a world of difference between a single unfortunate member of the family suffering from insanity and the idea that there might have been a familial vulnerability. Understandably this was not an issue which the royal family would have wanted to confront openly, as was demonstrated in chapter ten, unless there was no choice, but it was a taboo which Lucett with his irrepressible urge for self-promotion would have been insensitive to. Indeed he was intent on compounding the offence.

In the open letter Lucett also claimed to have made an offer to the Duke of Wellington to place his treatment before the Medical Council in order to provide 'immediate relief and ultimate restoration of our late Most Gracious majesty of happy memory'. He even provides the date of 22nd April. The 'Most Gracious Majesty' was George IV. In a single letter Lucett had effectively stated that the insanity which had had such a tragic impact on the last years of George III had been passed to the next generation and had affected and killed two of the sons. This should have been an incendiary assertion to say the least. Ironically the only direct response in the *Morning Post* was a letter from a Dr Hutchinson writing from Sidmouth in Devon. He asserted that Lucett was wrong in claiming sole knowledge of the cure for insanity as at his local asylum the same cure was used and had been for some years. Hutchinson even gave Lucett the credit for having made the process available to others. This response must surely rate as a splendid example of missing the wood for the trees? Ironically Dr Hutchinson's legalistic response provided an unexpected endorsement of the Lucett process as it had apparently been used for many years in Sidmouth. It was also a pointer to Lucett having had a wider practice than simply the patients who passed through his own private asylum.

The passing reference in James Chapman's letter supporting Peter Fenn, to Lucett, Weaver and Fox appropriating monies which had been falsely raised to enable them to found an asylum, does not seem to have led to further legal proceedings. Lucett was not able to keep clear of controversy for long, however, and was soon embroiled in a tragic case which ended in the suicide of the patient. The case concerned the Reverend Brackley Charles Kennett, who in 1830, was 53 years old. According to the record of the inquest reported in *The Times* of 17th December 1830, Kennett had 'laboured under insanity for about twenty years' and for most of that time had been attended by one Dr James Johnson. On Saturday, 5th December Kennett's insanity increased to such an extent that his family called in 'Professor Lucett' who lived nearby at Brompton Villa. Lucett appears to have taken Kennett to his own home and he remained with his patient until the following Wednesday when Dr Johnson visited Kennett and advised that he 'should be placed under restraint'. Lucett disagreed. He apparently asserted that he had attended many patients over the years and had never had to resort to restraint. Lucett apparently argued that soothing, calm methods were much more effective. An unseemly fracas followed in which Dr Johnson asserted a prior right of control over his patient. He saw Kennett's wife and his sister Lady Sheffield and pushed for Kennett to be removed from Lucett's home. The inquest account indicates that Kennett wished to remain with Lucett and that he threatened to commit suicide if he was forced back under the care of Johnson. The transfer was made to Kennett's house, but only after Lucett had agreed to accompany the patient.

Back in his own home Kennett briefly left Lucett who took the opportunity to leave the house although the inquest account records that he warned Lady Sheffield that there was a real danger that Kennett would commit suicide and that he should therefore be watched at all times. Tragedy followed. Kennett visited his mother who also lived in the house and took a pair of scissors she was using for needlework and stabbed himself in the neck so that he bled to death. At the inquest Lucett claimed that the evening before Kennett's death he had played whist with some flair and that it had been a mistake to remove him when he had so obviously derived benefit from his protection. The verdict was predictably one of suicide while insane, but the case was argued further in the press between the two practitioners.

The *Morning Post* of 13th December 1830 carried a letter to the editor under the title 'Melancholy Suicide'. The letter was from James Lucett. He set out essentially the account of the demise of Kennett as had been reported in the account of the inquest. The important detail which he added was that the game of whist had involved the Reverend Kennett and his wife on one side against Lucett and his wife on the other. It is a picture of domestic calm. The account presents Lucett in a good light, as might be expected, but there is no obvious evidence of manipulation in this account. There are, for example, no apparent differences in the chronology or content of Lucett's letter and the account recorded from the inquest. What is noteworthy is that Lucett styles himself, 'Medical Professor for the Cure of Insanity'. This was a piece of Lucett perception management as he was not medically qualified. Nor was he a Professor in the sense of being connected with a university faculty. In the early nineteenth century, however, there was a tendency for practitioners of particular skills to use the term 'professor' where an element of teaching was involved. Lucett would doubtless have claimed that he did carry out teaching if he had been challenged on the point, and Dr Hutchinson's letter in the press gave some credence to Lucett's assumed title. The other noteworthy element of the account was that he named Dr Johnson, Kennett's long term physician, perhaps in the belief that his name had already been published at the inquest, although there is a suggestion by Lucett that the qualified man had been unable to help his patient.

Dr Johnson's riposte was immediate and the *Morning Post* of 15th December printed it. This version is very different to the one given by Lucett, but was also different to the account from the inquest. Johnson claimed that Kennett had merely been eccentric until shortly before the crisis which began some weeks before his death. His concerns about the turbulent times had apparently pushed him over the edge and in going to Lucett's establishment he had done so to avoid a band of supposed conspirators. He soon became convinced that Lucett was in fact a member of the conspirators. When Johnson visited Kennett he found him very excited and Johnson refused to attend while he was under the influence of Lucett's system. In response Kennett was transferred to the family home, Mr Lucett accompanying. Lucett left shortly afterwards and Johnson's account is that Kennett then killed himself in his despair at Lucett's escape. Johnson claimed that Lucett had accompanied the patient during the transfer as the result of a clever stratagem by Kennett to trap him. Johnson refers his readers to the coroner and jury for the truth of his account. In some ways this account seems more worthy of Lucett and seems to contain some questionable elements in relation to the supposed conspiracy and Lucett's part in it.

Johnson's account unsurprisingly reflects well on himself as a practitioner. The problem is that nothing of Kennett's claimed obsession with conspirators or his preoccupation with unrest in the country was recorded at the inquest. Kennett was clearly from a very good family and it is possible that a mixture of deference and sensitivity towards the family could have resulted in some selectivity in the reporting. Nevertheless the obsession and preoccupations which Johnson described would actually have emphasised the tragic nature of the Reverend Kennett's decline and would have been material to the coroner's understanding of the events. The other difference is that the inquest account suggests that the insanity was of longer standing than Johnson indicated. Indeed one might ask why Kennett would have needed the long-term services of a doctor to manage mere eccentricity. What is clear is that Johnson felt his professional status had been undermined and by someone who was not a qualified medical practitioner. His attack on Lucett was direct and uncompromising. Lucett was, in Johnson's words, 'an unlicensed pretender to a secret and successful cure of insanity'.

It would have been out of character for Lucett to allow Johnson the last word, especially when it was such a damaging one. His final direct statement on the case was published on 17th December in the *Morning Post* and had the tone of outraged virtue. He says that Dr Johnson, 'may entertain an opinion that he is authorised, by virtue of his diploma, to assail the character of other men' and goes on to say that Johnson's account 'is not correct'. Lucett goes on to state that Johnson's intention was to 'prejudice me in the public estimation'. He ends what is a short intervention by his standards by asking why his note to Johnson had been answered only with a threat and why he had told Mrs Kennett that she would be prosecuted if her husband remained under the care and medical treatment of Lucett. In fact Lucett should and perhaps in reality did know that his position was vulnerable.

Dr Johnson had not finished with Lucett and his next move was another damaging one which surely reflected a closing of ranks by the medical establishment against a man who had not hesitated to denigrate them. The *Medical Gazette* for Saturday, 25th December 1830 carried a long reflective piece entitled 'Quacks and Quackery'.[4] The piece initially focused on John St John Long who was a notorious quack from the perspective of the College of Physicians but was nevertheless one of the most successful 'health practitioners' of the day. He had a wide celebrity following including members of the aristocracy and became very rich in a short time during the 1820s. He had started by treating tuberculosis but then moved on to 'treat' a range of other serious conditions including insanity. His 'treatments' were always the subject of as much secrecy as possible and patients and their families were actually sworn to secrecy before treatment began. At the time of the article in the *Medical Gazette* the College of Physicians were deliberating whether they could bring a prosecution against Long for unqualified practice.[5] While the College of Physicians were deliberating others acted and Long was prosecuted twice during 1830 for manslaughter after two of his patients died. Long was acquitted in one case and fined £250 in the other which he apparently paid in cash on the spot!

Moving from considering Long and quackery with the lofty conclusion, 'Quacks there will be as long as there are dupes to be found on whom to practice' the *Gazette* turns its attention to Lucett. 'We have received a letter, calling upon us to use our influence "in giving a death blow to quackery"' is the slightly pretentious opening of the focus on '*Professor*' Lucett and the Kennett case. The immediate target for the paper's ire is Lucett's letter to the press under the title 'Melancholy Suicide'. Not satisfied with condemning Lucett for turning a tragedy into 'a puffing advertisement' the *Gazette* draws a parallel between the manslaughter charges brought against Long and the death of Kennett which the paper attributed to his becoming 'an inmate of the Professor's asylum'. The Kennett story is replayed with the explanation for his relapse which Dr Johnson had advanced in his riposte to Lucett in the press. Finally after ridiculing Lucett and dismissing his treatment as consisting of a lack of restraint and a full diet, the *Gazette* makes its main point. Had Lucett got the requisite certificate of insanity when he took Kennett in and if he did not, 'then the Commissioners ought, without hesitation or delay, to withdraw his license'?

This was Dr Johnson's revenge and it is clear that he provided the impetus for the *Gazette* attack. It may be that Lucett was overconfident in naming Johnson and using the Kennett case to his advantage, but it was clear that Johnson had realised Lucett's vulnerability for taking in a patient without the correct documentation and warned Kennett's family accordingly. What is extraordinary is the violence of the *Gazette* attack on Lucett. To equate him with St John Long seems out of proportion given that Lucett had been called in by Kennett's family. Perhaps Lucett was lucky not to have the Fenn case replayed to his disadvantage with the indication of Lucett's involvement in financial irregularities. The charge of being a quack is based on the secrecy of Lucett's claimed cure, but this seems not to be the point of contention really. More pressing seems to be Lucett's insistence on an absence of restraint and his allowance of a full diet to patients instead of the orthodoxy of the time of restricting energy levels by a reduced diet. The *Gazette* article seems to be a counter stroke for all the disparaging comments Lucett had made about the inability of the medical profession to cure insane patients. That orthodox medicine should think he was worth the trouble is rather flattering for Lucett.

The section of the *Gazette* article dealing with Lucett concludes by indicating the responsibility of the Commissioners in Lunacy to revoke his licence if he did not have the proper certification for Kennett to be lodged in his asylum. Failure to do so, the paper pompously announced, would indicate the Commissioners 'neglected their own duty, and compromise the interests of the public'. The *Gazette* represented the interests of the medical profession so it is perhaps ironic that when the College of Physicians had been responsible for the inspection of metropolitan asylums up to 1828 their inspections had been nominal and had done nothing to improve the lot of the patient.[6]

Johnson had not been making an idle threat when he warned the Kennett family to separate themselves from Lucett. *The Times* of 19th January 1831 reported the impending prosecution of James Lucett of Brompton Villa at the insistence of the Metropolitan Commissioners in Lunacy[7] for taking in a patient without the correct certificate of insanity. In other words exactly what he had been prosecuted for in 1823 and it would seem that the Commissioners had responded to the *Gazette* article and that Dr Johnson would have his revenge. Past experience should have warned Lucett against bluster in the press, but he may have considered he had nothing to lose if Johnson had initiated proceedings against him. In that light Lucett's attempts to present himself as the victim of a jealous physician would probably have reached a wider audience than the law reports! Certainly his sense of what would play well with his market remained intact.

The Times of 25th June 1831 records in detail the report of the case of The King V Lucett in The King's Bench on 24th June 1831. As expected the prosecution case was that Lucett had taken Kennett into his asylum without the necessary certificate of insanity. The sense that a prosecution in this instance might be considered vexatious was highlighted by a statement on behalf of the authorities, 'The Commissioners did not charge the defendant with having been actuated by any improper motive in receiving Kennett without a certificate.' This seems fair enough given that Lucett had clearly been brought in at the family's request to deal with a crisis in Kennett's life. *The Times* report goes on to say that the jury could not reach a decision on whether a crime had been committed. The case hung on a fine point of law rather than any consideration of natural justice. This point was whether Kennett had been received into the defendant's exclusive care or not. In simple terms whether Lucett had taken over the case to the exclusion of Dr Johnson or not. The judge therefore directed a juryman to withdraw so that the jury could not reach a unanimous decision. That was the end of the case.[8] Lucett's adverts which followed the Kennett incident and the court judgement, such as the one in the *Morning Post* on 18th July 1831, included the addition that no patients would be forcibly taken from his care again! He had his own views on what constituted 'natural justice' and he clearly thought that he had secured it and that this would appeal to his potential clientele.

Lucett was not the only practitioner, qualified or unqualified, who experienced such problems. In the late 1820s Dr George Mann Burrows was probably the most celebrated 'mad-doctor' in the UK. His *Commentaries on Insanity* of 1828 was his defining work. He was originally a general practitioner, but from 1816 onwards he specialized in mad-doctoring. He was a strong advocate of the professionalisation of care for the insane by medically qualified professionals and wanted to improve treatment of insanity based on better scientific and physiological understanding of the disease. Burrows was to meet disaster soon after his *Commentaries* were published when he was prosecuted twice in 1829 – essentially for accepting second hand accounts from family members in assessing whether an individual was insane. In the case of Freeman Anderdon, Burrows issued a counterfeit certificate of insanity to allow two of his attendants to seize the individual. In the second case of Edward Davies, Burrows acted on family testimony to declare the individual insane and incapable of managing his financial affairs. Actually these two cases exemplified exactly why the system of professional certification of patients before they were sent to an asylum had been thought necessary. It was ironic that the advocate of scientific assessment was such an obvious transgressor. Burrows was ruined.

For Lucett the court case involving Kennett was an inconvenience rather than ruinous. He doubtless had less to loose than Burrows in terms of reputation. In terms of finances Burrows was effectively bankrupted while Lucett seems to have regarded bankruptcy as simply a question of semantics rather than practicality. As with Weston House and Rectory House, Lucett had re-established himself with some apparent style at Brompton Villa. This was a substantial property of nine bedrooms with impressive reception rooms and service facilities built around 1770 on the Day estate. This was a very prosperous area of expanding London and had already become very fashionable by the time Lucett moved there. Brompton Villa stood in two acres of ground and was secluded. It had no frontage on the busy Brompton Road, but was reached by a narrow lane off it. Only people of real substance or with access to good credit could afford the tenancy on such a property.[9]

Lucett's true financial situation is not easily accessible, however. No records or accounts of his personal or business life seem to have survived. There are, however, some pointers to how he was viewed in his own lifetime and the status he achieved. 'Gentleman' is the recurrent term used about him. At the time he lived and worked this was not an automatic and meaningless honorific. The use of the term was an indicator of his having the solvency, the education and the social standing, or the appearance of them, to justify the title. In both official documents and some newspaper reports Lucett was referred to as a 'gentleman' and there is some evidence to indicate that he fulfilled the criteria. Ironically he was also recorded as 'doctor' or 'surgeon' in many official or press references for which he did not fulfil the criteria.

Certainly the physical evidence suggests that, for the most part, Lucett enjoyed success or was able to persuade backers that the business had great potential. He lived in not just comfort, but for some periods of his life in some considerable style. The houses he occupied in pursuing his career as the keeper of a private asylum were large elegant homes which occupied secluded but convenient sites. They were properties which would have commanded considerable rents. They all had substantial service quarters and were reasonably modern. They were certainly not tumble down survivors of a previous age which were neither fashionable nor convenient and which might have been occupied cheaply. Weston House, Rectory House and Brompton Villa were all houses which were intended to make a statement of elegance and exclusivity. They would have been intended to be a physical demonstration of success implying that Lucett's practice with the mentally ill was successful and effective.

As an asylum keeper and private practitioner Lucett would have needed sufficient servants to maintain a significant establishment. Houses of the size Lucett was occupying required several servants just to keep them functioning. He would also have needed considerable direct professional support from attendants who could care for the patients and contribute to their recovery. Lucett kept patient numbers small, but without recourse to physical restraint, he would have needed attendants to engage with patients throughout their waking hours. Even the small numbers Lucett catered for would have required several attendants working in shifts to supervise the patients at all times. The Sarah Wyer case had demonstrated the dangers of even a momentary lapse in supervision. William Charles Ellis wrote in the late 1830s about the importance of large numbers of committed and intelligent attendants if restraint was to be dispensed with. Ellis considered it essential that capable attendants were well paid and had good status so they could fulfil a vital role in the recovery of patients.[10] Lucett will have had a close involvement with his patients, but it is unlikely that this would have extended to hour by hour supervision. This immediate care would have been delegated to the attendants. Such well-educated and capable people would not have been cheap. They were not mere jailers. The fact that Lucett must have been able to hire sufficient support to enable him to operate without the use of restraint should have been a pointer to a satisfactory business as well as his consistency with his stated ideals.

The period after the end of the Mitcham partnership until he established himself at Brompton Villa was not a period during which he was able to maintain the outward appearance of elegance and success. Indeed it is not clear how he would have been able to care for resident patients. During this period Lucett used accommodation addresses and there are no clues as to where his patients were housed. Kirke's Nursery does not sound like a reasonable place to accommodate insane patients while the premises at 34 Parliament Street was a shop and equally unsuitable for housing patients. Lucett continued to advertise during this period, but there is a subtle difference between the adverts which referred to his operating at a specific building and adverts which enjoined people to contact him through an accommodation address. The latter suggested a much less substantial and convincing operation. In practical terms it would seem that after Ewell at least Lucett needed someone to underwrite the operation if it was to be carried on with a properly constituted asylum.

Lucett did more than keep a private asylum, however. He travelled to visit patients housed in other accommodation and to assess potential patients. The certificate of insanity signed by him in the Surrey Magistrates records is an indicator of this activity. Certainly all the houses he occupied had quick access to major roads. So it is likely that he kept horses and it is possible that he had a carriage as well. Certainly such a vehicle would have been useful to move patients although it was possible to hire. Ironically the only part of Weston House to survive is the substantial stabling. All these aspects of the Lucett business would have added up to a substantial and expensive establishment to maintain. Again this was a pointer to the need for outside finance as well as a successful turnover of patients.

Lucett's professional career was not a straightforward success story. Eminent physicians who catered to a wealthy clientele certainly lived very well. Sir Henry Halford was admitted to the very highest levels of society for example, while Dr Battie, the author of *A treatise on Madness* and a pioneer mad-doctor or alienist of the eighteenth century lived in great style in an exquisite house on the banks of the Thames at Twickenham.[11] Lucett may have attempted to emulate such luminaries and may have succeeded to some extent, but bankruptcy was a potential reality too as has been seen.

Lucett was an educated man from a family of sufficient means and influence to be able to secure a place at the Bank of England. It would appear that his family was not of sufficient substance, however, to have endowed Lucett with the funds to enable him to live independently. His Bank salary had been sufficient to enable him to pursue the involvement with the Committee, but when the board of the Bank finally realised that Lucett had absented himself and therefore stopped his salary there was nothing to fall back on for the Lucett household as Olivia Lucett's letter of distress to Earl Fitzwilliam demonstrated. There appears to be only one perspective of life in the Lucett household which has survived. It is indirect and comes from Edward Lucett, the second son of James and Olivia Lucett, and refers to 1837 when Edward was a young adult and was on the point of leaving London as a supernumerary crew member on a ship carrying prisoners bound for Australia. Edward comments that before the voyage, 'I had experienced hitherto but little of the hardships of life.' To illustrate his knowledge of hardship he recorded, 'Once when I was at home, I thought I had been particularly ill-used, because on one occasion, during the winter, linen sheets had been spread for me instead of cotton.' After this almost laughable instance of hardship it will be no surprise that Edward Lucett was considered a gentleman and considered himself as such. He was educated at a boarding school somewhere to the west of London but there is no indication of whether he had subsequently pursued the training for any profession. So James Lucett had generated sufficient income, despite the instability in his life during the 1820s, to bring up his sons with the education and expectations of a gentleman. What is clear is that at the age of twenty-two Edward Lucett was short of money, but had the intelligence, determination and education to develop a very successful trading company in Polynesia.[12]

An explanation for Lucett's ability to set up the imposing practice at Brompton Villa was soon to appear and it came hard on the heels of the Kennett case and Lucett's prosecution. On the 2nd March 1832, James Samuel Lomax of Rose Stack Farm near Hatfield issued a Bill of Complaint against Lucett.[13] Lomax claimed that he had been persuaded by Lucett to underwrite the establishment of the asylum at Brompton Villa. He had even provided the furniture and fittings for the place. However, Lucett had quickly proved to be a drunkard and it became clear to the complainant that Lucett would not be able to make a success of the asylum. He therefore instructed a Sheriff's officer to regain possession of the furniture and effects. Lucett had apparently issued a counter claim so Lomax had resorted to a claim for debt of £1,500. This had resulted in the arrest of Lucett. Lomax argued that there had been an attempt to negotiate a settlement but Lucett had persisted in pressing his counter claim. Interestingly Lucett's counter claim, sworn in Chancery on 16th April 1833, asserted that his professional medical practice would be ruined if he was kept in jail. He therefore offered to withdraw the complaint against Lomax in return for the furniture and effects.

The echoes of the Mitcham case and that failed partnership are obvious. Even the claims that Lucett was a drunkard are familiar from the 1825 case. It may be that Lomax' move against Lucett was prompted by his prosecution for taking a patient without a medical certificate following the Kennett episode. However, it is just as likely that the relationship between the two had broken down already because Lomax had not had a return on his investment. Indeed he may have hoped to get his hands on Lucett's cure as a worthwhile speculation. Whatever the basis of this legal conflict Lucett was to appear in King V Patrick Grant and others on 30th January 1834 as a character witness. The person whose character he was commenting on was James Samuel Lomax! Lucett would doubtless have enjoyed giving his verdict that Lomax was 'a person of low extraction and character'.[14] It is ironic that Lucett should claim that his 'medical practice' would suffer if he was kept in jail. That was as close as he had officially come to claiming that he was a qualified doctor. It was also an admission that his practice was still vulnerable to any setback and that he was still financially precarious.

Lucett's days of propagandising were not over. The year 1833 saw the publication of a further slim volume in English under the title, *A Statement of Facts Relevant to the Nature and Cure of Mental Diseases.* The account is a bizarre mix. There is some rehashing of old stories and old grievances, but there is also the first sign of a transition from an inveterate self-promoter to almost a champion of the insane. He was of course self-serving, but Lucett certainly went some way to highlight the fundamental awfulness of the contemporary treatment of the mentally ill.[15] The opening of the *Statement of Facts* is a modest seeming statement in which he acknowledges the enormity of placing himself in opposition to contemporary medical thinking, but nevertheless claims he must do so. He sets out in clear terms that he was in the business of curing people of insanity while implying that the medical profession was not. Lucett then moves into a statement that he has 'a mode of treatment' which has received the approval of royalty as well as Dr John Harness the highly respected physician. He then quotes briefly from the 1814 statement that the treatment was safe. The committee and the experiments are not mentioned and the Dukes of Kent and Sussex and Dr Harness make brief appearances solely in order to endorse Lucett's cure for insanity. So far Lucett is in familiar territory rehashing his perspective. But the basic thrust is that while the medical profession as a whole had failed to make progress in the treatment of insanity, he, Lucett, had the answer.

At this point Lucett moves on to the Harrison case and although he does not actually give the name, he goes into much greater detail than he had done before. Interestingly some of what he says is even checkable. Lucett claims that Harrison would only be released by the Bethlem authorities on condition that once discharged he would not be taken back. The original correspondence relating to the conditional release does not survive in the Bethlem Hospital archive. However, the minute book on admissions and discharges for the period which does survive notes the Duke of Kent's intervention and the conditions applied. Dr Monro dismissed the idea of discharging Harrison for treatment elsewhere as folly, while Mr Haslam the apothecary, according to Lucett, said the only way to cure Harrison was to cut his head off or to hang him! Lucett claims that he was told of the conditions by the Duke of Kent and said that, after pressure from Harrison's wife and Lucett's endorsement, the Duke ordered his secretary to request the immediate discharge of the patient.

Lucett's account is not a mere chronology; it is intended as a demonstration of his perseverance against the hostility of the medical profession. With no mention of the Committee, or of his former partners he passes straight on to the first prosecution in 1823 for treating a patient without the required certificate of insanity. The hostility to him as an outsider is clear in his version of the story. The patient, a surgeon, had been treated by Dr George Mann Burrows who had also not had the correct certificate for his patient. The College of Physicians, however, prosecuted only Lucett. As is set out above, the accounts of the 1823 prosecution make no reference to another doctor having treated the patient, let alone any reference to Burrows. Lucett in his updated version of events fails to mention that he had claimed at the trial that the patient had merely been a lodger. The conspiracy, as Lucett saw it, against him continued with his contact with the promoter of a new asylum in Middlesex. Initially Lucett was encouraged to demonstrate his treatment on a very difficult patient. When he was successful, the asylum keeper wanted nothing more to do with him.

Writing in the early 1830s, Lucett's choice of Burrows and what was probably the Hanwell asylum to include in his narrative were intended to convey the idea that he was in the vanguard of developments in the treatment of the insane. George Mann Burrows had been the leading authority on insanity during the 1820s and was not simply a private clinician who had run his own asylum at The Retreat in Chelsea from 1823. His *Commentaries on the causes of insanity* of 1828 was the most comprehensive work on the identification and treatment of insanity available in the UK at the time. Despite Burrows' notoriety following prosecution for manipulating the certification process in 1829, he would still have been remembered in the early 1830s for having been an enormously successful mad-doctor. It is just possible that Lucett's claim that he had cured a patient whom Burrows had failed to recover was true. Basically Lucett's message to his audience is that he was better than the best. If Lucett had chosen to use Burrows' name because he thought he could get away with it, it was an inspired choice on another level too. For Lucett to claim that only he was prosecuted while Burrows had treated the same patient without certification of insanity in 1823 would have seemed credible in view of Burrows later history.

It is not absolutely clear which asylum Lucett was referring to in Middlesex, but The Middlesex County Asylum at Hanwell began to operate in 1831 and was to become the largest asylum in the UK. Historically it has been associated with John Connolly who was made director in 1839 and who was celebrated for his commitment to non-restraint. The Connolly connection can only have been a coincidence given the chronology of Lucett's writing and Connolly's involvement at Hanwell. Nevertheless the Hanwell asylum was built with much fanfare following the 1828 Asylums Act as the first purpose-built asylum for pauper lunatics. It reflected what would now be called cutting-edge technology and under its first superintendent, Dr William Ellis, became celebrated for its use of what was later called occupational therapy as part of the recovery process. Work, particularly, out of doors, was an integral part of the therapy at Hanwell and was exactly what Lucett had been doing at Sion Vale nearly twenty years before. So a reference to Hanwell would have been doing two things for his 1833 audience. It was saying that Lucett was so well known that the superintendents of the best asylums felt the need to consult him. The fact that ultimately the response to his ideas which was a mixture of the patronising and the dismissive simply demonstrated that a complacent medical establishment was firmly disposed against new and better practice.

Lucett moves on to consider what was going on in the asylums of the time. He argues that the certificates which had caused him such trouble were required because the asylums were places of confinement, not cure. Confinement was a life sentence and once in an asylum, patients could be abominably treated. Lucett remarks on the terrible discoveries made by the House of Commons enquiry in 1815 and highlights the dismissal of Drs Monro and Haslam from Bethlem. These were the so-called specialists and experts who personified the medical establishment Lucett argues. Lucett fails to observe that Monro had been called in in 1811 to advise on the case of George III. Interestingly Lucett claims some credit for the Commons enquiry taking place. This looks like a rush of enthusiasm on his part as he was certainly not called as a witness and there is no apparent record of any other involvement by Lucett in the enquiry.

Lucett then examines the financial incentives which operated to ensure the medical profession did not try to cure patients of insanity. This is clearly the system he saw operating with wealthy patients. The first doctor would take on a patient and treat him ineffectually and expensively for an extended period of time after which he would call in a second doctor who would go through the same process for a time. The result was that two doctors were able to certify the patient as 'incurable' and the unfortunate individual could then be confined for life. The doctors meanwhile would have profited handsomely from the process. William Belcher had described mad-houses as 'premature coffins of the mind, body and estate' and had himself been wrongly confined for seventeen years and was only released ironically due to the intervention of Dr Monro. Belcher's case was not unique, however, and he would have endorsed Lucett's analysis as he had referred to there being a 'trade in lunacy'.[16]

Lucett raises the crucial question of why these practices were not investigated and exposed. He had in a sense been at his best in addressing the issue of the injustice and exploitation of the mentally ill and for a time he had even forgotten to insert himself as a protagonist. He sets out starkly that the reason for the lack of reform was self-interest. Paraphrasing Lucett, he argues that there was too much profit to be had in charging three to five hundred pounds a year for patients whose accommodation cost fifty to sixty pounds. In the end though, Lucett's primary purpose is not actually in reform of conditions in Georgian lunatic asylums, but in promoting his treatment as the alternative to what he sees as the exploitation of the mentally ill. So, in by now familiar terms, he sets out his efforts to have his treatment examined and assessed by the House of Commons. The latest attempt he claims had been through the good offices of Sir Francis Burdett. All efforts had been frustrated, according to Lucett, but he remained positive.

The choice of Burdett as a supporter is interesting. Burdett had been a political radical during the second and third decades of the century promoting Catholic Emancipation for example, but by the time Lucett was writing in the early 1830s he had become much more conservative. In the period 1818 or 1819 when Lucett first claimed that he had tried to gain parliamentary support for his cure, Burdett had been a radical and a reformer. The plight of the insane could well have been one of his causes, but there is no apparent pointer to contact between Burdett and Lucett. Later in his career Burdett would have been a potentially damaging choice for Lucett to claim as a supporter. Burdett had appeared as a witness on behalf of John

St John Long during his trial in 1830 for the manslaughter of Catherine Cashin. Burdett had claimed that Long's treatment for tuberculosis was safe only to have his testimony and his knowledge of scientific and medical matters comprehensively dismantled by Thomas Wakley the founding editor of *The Lancet*.[17] Association with someone who had sided with a notorious quack was a connection which would probably not have done Lucett much good.

Lucett does not go any further into the claims for seeking parliamentary support for his 'cure'. Chapter and verse on the story would not be his style. He had nevertheless done sufficient to maintain the perspective that he was the outsider trying to take on the medical establishment. This was a corrupt and incompetent establishment in which profit was placed above the interest of the patient. The distinction Lucett emphasised between himself and the medical establishment was the claim that he actually cured insane patients. For the rest his attacks on the medical establishment were calculated to play to popular prejudices. It is ironic that at the time Lucett was writing his tract, John Perceval the son of the former Prime Minister Spencer Perceval, was on the point of being confined in Brislington House one of the most celebrated asylums of the day where he was to be treated abominably only to be declared sane after several years of incarceration.[18] Lucett then returns to a little melodrama and issues a challenge to all medical practitioners by suggesting that those who care for a sufferer should ask whether the practitioner can relieve the raving maniac or the sullen maniac in forty minutes. This Lucett claims he can do as he had done so many times previously to any audience that was available.

It is perhaps appropriate that Lucett the showman should end his tract with a grandiloquent flourish. 'I beg to acknowledge my sincere thanks to the illustrious personages who have patronized and supported my mode of cure, and trust my adherence to a plan that has been so universally successful in alleviating one of the most dreadful maladies the human mind can possibly be subjected to, will not only ensure me a continuance of favour and support, but gain me the approbation and respect of every philanthropist.' The final flourish is to sign himself off as the 'Public's obedient Servant'. Many of the points Lucett makes in his critical assessment of the contemporary system of care for the mentally ill were fully justified. There is a sense that after twenty years of practice in treating patients, Lucett had gained something of the dignity born out of his accumulated experience. In that light he comes over as serious and thoughtful. *A Statement of Facts* clearly demonstrates this side of his character. It is also possible that Lucett's more dignified and thoughtful persona was contrived and that it was this persona which he used with prospective patients or investors. Lucett is incorrigible, however, and simply cannot resist the need to promote himself and his treatment like a vulgar salesman.

Lucett regularly placed adverts in the newspapers throughout his career. This was entirely normal and the newspapers of the time carried multiple advertisements claiming that most of the afflictions of the human race could be cured if only the sufferers contacted the advertisers or bought their 'Universal Powders'. Many of these adverts were placed by quacks, but qualified practitioners also advertised. There was considerable variation in the frequency with which Lucett placed his adverts and this presumably was a reflection of whether he needed to drum up custom or not. Bursts of adverts over a period of a week or two were common. These were often followed by a silence for months on end. Basically the format of the adverts varied very little. He claimed exclusivity for his cure and that it worked. He dismissed the need for restraint or coercion. The variation in the adverts came in the claims he made to royal or high political patronage. Some of the claims Lucett made such as the support of Prime Ministers Spencer Perceval and later by Lord Liverpool were manifestly untrue. Yet there is no evidence that Lucett was forced to retract any of the claims and no examples appear to exist of published counter statements that he was wrong to make the claims. In the later years he was more obviously manipulative in the sense that many of the 'patrons' were already dead. This did not apply to the Dukes of Kent or Sussex, or to Dr Harness when he was advertising in the period of 1814 to 1820, however. Yet there is no evidence of a response from any of these people to Lucett's use of their names.

The advert which Lucett placed in the *Morning Post* on 7th December 1833 marks another new beginning for his practice. 'Insanity. Mr Lucett continues to receive or attend Ladies and Gentlemen DERANGED in any part of England upon the principle of CURE and not confinement. A vacancy again offers for the reception of one Lady or Gentleman in his family if the object is speedy restoration.' The immediate difference is that the address has changed to Haleston Place, Albany Road, Old Kent Road. Lucett had apparently re-established himself in south-east London in an area which at the turn of the century had been principally rural but which was developing fast. By the time Lucett moved there much of the farmland closer to the Thames had already been built over with rows of decent, but not fashionable housing. The arrival of the Surrey Canal meant that the area was mixed with considerable industrial activity amongst the housing. If Lucett lived in this area it is unlikely that he lived in the style which he had enjoyed in Brompton or before. Perhaps the rather homely style of the December advert was an appropriate reflection of a more modest but probably self-financed establishment. The advert is also noteworthy because it formally states that Lucett would still care for patients on a visiting basis – anywhere in England. It can be assumed that he had always been prepared to do this, but the relative modesty of his new home may have made this a more significant part of his practice. It is implicit from the advert that Lucett was 'reduced' to taking a single patient at a time although this is not certain. The point is that the very domesticity of the offer of a single place 'in his family' would have been a total contrast with conditions in Hoxton or any of the other large 'receptacles' for the insane. Combined with the emphasis on cure, Lucett still offered what would have been an attractive haven for many patients.

Lucett may have changed address, but the bad habits of old may have continued. The *Morning Chronicle* for 28th February 1834 carried the report of the prosecution of an individual for fraud. A false bill of exchange had been issued with Lucett's name given as the guarantor of the bill. The date of the actual trial is unclear, but Lucett is described as, 'late keeper of Brompton House Lunatic Asylum'. The way the report is written suggests that there was no question during the trial that Lucett could in any way have been complicit and that he had agreed to his name being used for a fee. There is a slightly queasy sense though that this incident could be a re-run of the Fenn case. After all the evidence advanced following the sentencing of Fenn indicates that Lucett would sign blank bills of exchange for a small fee. On past performance Lucett would always have been short of money and would have needed to augment his income as best he could.

Chapter Eighteen

Back on the Campaign Trail

'How is it possible in a hospital of nearly 300 patients, with scarcely a dozen keepers, to do justice to them?'[1]

Letter to the Governors of Bethlem Hospital
from General Palmer dated 9th October 1835.

One of the difficulties in making any assessment of James Lucett and his treatment for the insane is that independent perspectives of him are sporadic and often focus on aspects of his life, such as financial difficulties, which are tangential to his actual engagement in the care of patients. In 1834 Lucett would have been in his mid-60s given a birthdate of 1770 or 71. The previous decade had been one in which there had been some success, but also several major setbacks which had involved Lucett's incarceration in debtors' prisons and involvement in court cases, some of which indicated a serious lack of integrity on his part. It would not have been surprising therefore if he had simply faded into oblivion as a bad reputation and age began to overtake him. In fact he was soon to be engaged in an incident which attracted widespread publicity and which not only demonstrated that he was still fully engaged in treating the insane, but that he had not lost his ability to attract the support of significant members of late Georgian society. More importantly the incident and the wrangling which ensued provide an independent and generally positive perspective of Lucett and his practice.

General Charles Palmer was the MP for Bath in 1835 and had served in that role for much of the time since 1808 and had managed to combine a military career with his parliamentary role. He had the reputation for being a political radical, was an associate of Joseph Hume and was a fervent supporter of the 1832 Reform Act. Indeed his status as an MP in 1835 reflected the support of the wider franchise in Bath following the passing of the Reform Act. He had also been appointed aide de camp to the Prince Regent earlier in his career. His link with the Prince Regent was the result of his service in the 10th Hussars, the regiment which the Prince was closely associated with.

Palmer was wealthy and from a family which had long had prominence in the Bath area. A more idiosyncratic aspect of his life was his inheritance of a vineyard in France and the theatre in Bath. Over all he was solvent, moved in elevated social circles and was influential. He also to proved to be a supporter of James Lucett.[2]

In July 1835 Palmer accompanied by Lord Dudley Stuart, another reforming MP and friend, visited Bethlem hospital and saw many of the patients. One patient in particular had attracted their attention. She was Ellen Mack and had apparently been held for four months in isolation and in a straight waistcoat. Palmer and Stuart had been horrified by her extreme manic state. When Palmer visited again a week later the woman was in the same violent state. Such was Palmer's concern that he recorded, 'I resolved to bring Mr Lucett to see her'.[3] The following day with the assistance of Mr Burgess, one of the Governors of Bethlem, Palmer and Lucett visited the hospital. The low key reference to Lucett is significant because it seems to assume that calling in Lucett was the obvious thing to do in the circumstances.

The simple account of the key event of the visit was that when Lucett and Palmer visited Ellen Mack the attendant was briefly absent. During this absence Lucett tried to administer some liquid to the head of the sufferer, but was prevented from carrying out his intention by the return of the attendant. Palmer and Lucett then requested the permission of the Bethlem surgeon to allow Lucett to treat Mack. This was refused in the absence of the physicians of the hospital Drs Monro and Morison. The Morison in this case was the same Dr Alexander Morison who would have met Lucett twenty years previously when inspecting Surrey private asylums. The request that Lucett should be allowed to treat Mack was subsequently reported to Sir Peter Laurie, President of the Governors of the hospital, who vetoed any interference with the treatment by the hospital physicians.

General Palmer's response was to apply to the Court of the Aldermen in late August to have Ellen Mack transferred to Lucett so that his method of treating the patient could be tried. The court had jurisdiction over Mack's fate because she had been confined by the City of London authorities. The admission and case-note for Mack includes the comment, 'Comes from Giltspur St[reet]. Compter where she had been on a charge of being disorderly and fined 5 shillings being considered sane although eccentric. Never confined before.'[4] A 'compter' was a small prison, mainly for debtors and it appears that Mack, who had been a street vendor of fruit, had been found running wildly around the streets of Smithfield in an hysterical state. The *Examiner* of 26th April indicated that Mack had walked bare foot through the droves of cattle as a demonstration of her faith and divine protection and that this brought business to a halt in the area. The fact that she was being held in a debtors' prison suggests that she was there simply because she could not pay the fine. The transfer to Bethlem would have been a reflection that her hysterical state did not improve in prison.

The petition to the Court of the Aldermen was presented in the name of Mack's mother, but Palmer was clearly the protagonist. Indeed Mack's mother's role in the actual proceedings was nominal although she had made the long journey from Kerry to be there. Palmer was straightforward in his argument during the court proceedings. He knew nothing about Mack's mother and stated that his objective was to try the experiment *of testing the effectiveness of Lucett's treatment.* Sir Peter Laurie then gave an account of the visit by Palmer and Lucett to Bethlem to the court. Laurie also stated that he noticed the 'imbecile state' of the mother and commented that in his opinion the experiment was simply aimed at Lucett taking a convalescent patient and claiming a subsequent cure. Laurie said that he would not consent to dangerous experiments being carried out on patients and reminded the aldermen of their responsibility if the patient should die.

When Mack's mother was questioned she commented that the gentlemen, meaning Palmer, had said that her daughter would be treated like a lady and cured. The court, under the chairmanship of Sir Peter Laurie, 'unanimously' refused the petition. This was not a straightforward conclusion to the case. Sir Peter was an alderman of the City of London and had been since 1826 so he was entitled to chair the proceedings of the Court of Aldermen. He was, however, President of the Brideswell and Bethlem Hospitals so had a direct interest in the proceedings. Palmer may well have been unsuccessful because of his candour in saying that his aim was to underwrite an experiment with a patient, but Laurie's impartiality was highly questionable. There was no evidence presented that Ellen Mack was in a convalescent state, nor for the imputation that the Lucett treatment was in some way dangerous. Laurie had been involved in the politics of London and had a formal commitment to penal reform and an interest in the poor. However, it was an interest which Charles Dickens was to satirise as insincere and which led to clashes between the two.

There matters might have rested had General Palmer not felt that his integrity had been impugned or had his commitment to Lucett and Ellen Mack been less strong. Palmer was not ready to leave things as the Court of the Aldermen had concluded. On 4th September he gave notice in the House of Commons of his intention to present a petition in the Commons on 7th September 'relative to the conduct of Sir Peter Laurie and others of the Court of Aldermen of the City of London and Governors of Bethlem Hospital in the case of a female lunatic now confined there'. This statement was widely reported in the press throughout the UK as was his actual introduction of the petition on 9th September. Palmer spoke of his complaint and 'moved that a select committee of the house be set up to inquire into the nature and effect of a treatment for the cure of insanity without confinement, coercion or personal restraint'. He got no further as a Mr Baines rose stating that the attendance in the house was too low 'to discuss so important a matter' and asked for the house to be counted. This indicated that there were 31 MPs present which was less than the minimum of 40 required to transact business.[5] Palmer was not to have an opportunity to introduce his petition again as Parliament did not sit for the rest of the year.

Palmer's attempt to raise a complaint in the Commons drew a necessary statement of justification and explanation to the Sub-Committee of Bethlem Hospital on 22nd September. In outline Laurie's account was in accord with the one of Palmer and Lucett's visit to Bethlem set out above. There were some important differences of emphasis, however. In Laurie's version 'Mr Lucette (sic) selected a young female who was in a state of the greatest maniacal excitement; he surreptitiously attempted to pour a liquid on the patient's head, from a bottle which he held in his hand, unknown to the officers and servants of the establishment, and then expressed the wish to try the experiment on her which he stated would shortly quiet and cure her.' This version is probably not too far from the truth in that Lucett undoubtedly did try to begin treatment while the single attendant was dealing with another patient. Laurie's statement that Lucett acted 'unknown to the officers and servants of the establishment' has a subtle emphasis that Lucett's activities were those of an outsider and he followed this up by adding that Lucett would not be allowed to 'interfere with the practice of Drs Monro and Morison, the responsible physicians of the establishment, in whom the Governors had the greatest confidence'. Laurie set out his version of the court proceedings and concluded that he considered that the events at Bethlem had been 'nothing but an attempt to serve Mr Lucette'. General Palmer's response was not long in coming. Although Mr Burgess who had formally introduced Palmer on the day he visited with Lucett got in his comment first. Burgess was at pains to point out that he had introduced General Palmer only and not Lucett but then added in his letter to *The Times* of 25th September, 'I ought, probably, in justice to Mr Lucette, to state that I have heard of some extraordinary cures lately effected by that gentleman.'[6]

Palmer responded in the form of an open letter in the press dated 9th October addressed to the Governors of Bethlem Hospital.[7] Palmer stated that he had been asked by the Bethlem governors for a copy of his petition to the Commons about the case of Ellen Mack. It is possible that the governors knew that Palmer had been unable to carry out his intention because parliament was not sitting, but if they thought their demand might put Palmer on the defensive this is not what happened. The open letter raised the level of publicity for Palmer's complaint against the Bethlem authorities and resulted in exposure which the Governors would not have welcomed. For Lucett on the other hand it represented the best possible publicity for him and his treatment of insane patients as it was entirely favourable but was advanced by a prestigious and independent member of society. The letter began by stating that there were two possible outcomes for Ellen Mack. The first was that she should remain in Bethlem 'under close coercion and confinement' until twelve months were up when she would be discharged as 'incurable'.

The alternative was that 'the mother' of Ellen Mack 'be permitted to remove her daughter now and place her with a professional person who undertakes to remove her excitement and the necessity to use restraint. This is effectively offering a cure for the patient.' In a riposte to Sir Peter Laurie's claim, during the proceedings of the Court of the Aldermen, that to release the patient to Lucett's care would be dangerous, Palmer included the qualification that the patient could be placed with the professional person so long as she had not been injured as the result of her treatment in Bethlem! Palmer then arrives at the key issue as he sees it. This is that Laurie had rejected the petition at the court 'solely upon the question of this individual's professional character'. Palmer is careful to avoid repeating the charge made in the court that Lucett was of bad character. He asserts that he will say who and what the practitioner is.

Lucett is identified and Palmer sets out a chronology of his career. Much is familiar from the account in earlier chapters, but Palmer displays some talent in his editing; or Lucett does. The therapeutic trial is passed over and instead Lucett is said to have opened his first establishment in 1812 under the patronage of the Dukes of Kent and Sussex and other members of the nobility and gentry. Palmer emphasises that Lucett's establishment was different from all others at the time as he did not resort to restraint of the patients. Restraint was not necessary because Lucett was able to calm the most violent paroxysms and keep these paroxysms at bay until the cause of the problem had been removed. Palmer says that exceptions to Lucett's ability to effect a cure would lie with patients who suffered from some organic illness or loss of organs. Having set out the claims for Lucett's capabilities, Palmer states that it is necessary to prove what he says. Perhaps emphasising how long Lucett has been in practice Palmer gives two short accounts which are recognisably the cases of Harrison and Moon. He then makes the very important claim that Lucett's success with these two cases was the 'cause of the public inquiry that took place into the management of Bethlem Hospital, and the consequent dismissal of the whole of its medical establishment'. Palmer should have known better as the inquiry in question was the 1815 House of Commons Select Committee on Madhouses and this was not inspired by the activities of James Lucett. Palmer had been an MP at the time and should have been aware of the origins and proceedings of such an important Committee and the work of Edward Wakefield in exposing the abuses of patients at Bethlem.

Having dealt with the early career of Lucett, Palmer moves on to 1828. He refers to the case which follows as 'the next trial' and it is clear that Palmer's intention was to present this case as an officially prompted and mediated one. So he refers to Robert Gordon esq. 'of the House of Commons' as providing the impetus and as the person who chose the patient for Lucett to treat. He also emphasises that Gordon was the promotor of the asylum which was to be established at Hanwell. This was a case of 'morbid lunacy' in which the patient had lost the power of speech and the use of his limbs. He was recovered by Lucett and was able to express his gratitude to Gordon but unfortunately died some time later of heart disease. The point which Palmer wants to make is his belief that he has 'removed all doubt of Lucett's merit' but in case there is anyone yet to be convinced he had one further story to relate which involved Bethlem.

Palmer relates that 'just six weeks back' on a public visiting day, he had made a tour of the hospital in the company of the house surgeon. When the tour was at an end the two men returned to the entrance hall where they met a woman who was the wife of the landlord of a public house who had been a patient in Bethlem for six months before he was given leave of absence from Bethlem to be under the care of his wife and an attendant. Unfortunately after five months the man had become so volatile that the wife considered she could no longer cope and had returned to Bethlem for advice and assistance. 'The surgeon replied, he could do nothing for her, that the patient's time being nearly expired, and his case incurable, he could not be taken back.' Palmer intervened at this point and asked why the patient was incurable and was told by the surgeon it was because 'he had become paralytic from drinking'. 'The wife being thus dismissed I offered her the assistance of Mr Lucett which' Palmer relates 'she gratefully accepted'. Lucett was called, but while Palmer waited for his arrival he met the patient whom he found in 'a state of great excitement and delusion of mind'. The following day Palmer visited the patient and found that he had become calm and rational following treatment by Lucett. The patient was physically very weak and unwell, however, as the result of alcohol abuse and poor diet although Palmer considered that he had started to improve.

Shifting focus to the conflict with Sir Peter Laurie, Palmer explains that the publican's wife had given evidence to the Committee of Bethlem Hospital when Sir Peter had been in the chair and had said it was her view that Lucett's treatment had returned her husband to lucidity and that she was confident of her husband's full recovery. Apparently a 'noble lord' who was present at the time took an interest and helped secure the patient's formal discharge from Bethlem.

In the case of Ellen Mack, Palmer said that he resolved to bring in Lucett after two visits a week apart with Lord Dudley Stuart. On each occasion the visitors were appalled by the violence of Mack's behaviour so after the second visit Palmer returned the following day with Lucett and was signed in by Burgess one of the governors who was there by prior agreement with Palmer. When the visitors arrived at the place where Mack was 'confined' Lucett went in while Palmer explained to Burgess why he had brought Lucett and that he had a remedy which would cure her excitement. Palmer asked Burgess to call the surgeon to seek permission for Lucett to try to calm Mack. Meanwhile Lucett had been alone with the patient and had calmed her sufficiently to enable him to attempt to start treatment; however, the return of the keeper coincided with a return of Mack's paroxysms. Palmer comments 'this act of Mr Lucett being the impulse of his feeling to relieve the patient, but imprudent and unfortunate for both, as the event proved'.

The surgeon refused to sanction Lucett making any attempt to calm the patient and Palmer comments that he realised that this route to gain permission for Lucett to treat Ellen Mack would not work. The advice of Mr Burgess was to apply to the Committee of Bethlem for permission and to try to get the support of Lord Dudley Stuart who had great influence with these people. Palmer followed up on this advice and Stuart said that he would support the proposal to have Lucett treat Mack if, on making enquiries, it proved appropriate for him to do so. The result of those enquiries was a flat refusal to support Lucett's initiative. He said he had been told that Lucett was a man of bad character. Stuart told Palmer, 'he had been given so bad a character of Mr Lucett, that he was compelled to oppose my wish'. Palmer later discovered that the source of the bad report of Lucett had been the matron of Bethlem and she admitted as much to him.

With the two direct avenues for getting permission for Lucett to treat Mack blocked Palmer's only recourse was to apply for the patient's discharge. Meanwhile a further open visiting day came and Palmer had been surprised to find Ellen Mack sat up in bed chatting happily with the matron and without any restraint. A week later, when Palmer again visited Bethlem, he found Mack was back in solitude and in a straight waistcoat and as violent as ever. Palmer said his astonishment was complete when he went to the Guildhall the following morning, with the patient's mother, to find the matron in court opposing the discharge of Ellen. Palmer's words describing what came next are worth repeating. The matron 'declared the lunatic was much better and would soon be well'. On the basis of the matron's testimony and despite the pleading of the mother to have her daughter released, Sir Peter Laurie and one other alderman '*unanimously*' refused to order the release of Ellen Mack.

General Palmer's anger is manifest in his account. He describes with heavy sarcasm the claim that the decision was unanimous as being the only truth in Sir Peter's statement and that the rest of his statement was a 'misrepresentation of the fact throughout'. He then invites the governors of Bethlem to call Mary Mack and to hear from her what happened at the Guildhall and what happened between her daughter and the matron in Bethlem. 'You can judge for yourselves who is least worthy of belief and who the most *imbecile* – the President or Mary Mack.' These then were the facts of the case as Palmer put it, but he had a stinging final comment on the Ellen Mack case. He added that the surgeon at Bethlem had stated that Mack was a prostitute and this was why she had been confined in the Giltspur Street prison. In justice to her character, Palmer stated that those who knew her said she had lived an exemplary life until she was taken up mad and deranged in the street.

Palmer's assault on Bethlem had so far focused on the integrity of the President of the Governors of the hospital, but he had criticisms of the regime in the hospital which he was ready to articulate. A system of moral and medical treatment was established in the hospital, but in reality neither was actually delivered. No medicine was given to the patients with the expectation that it would cure their insanity while moral treatment was also denied. In the case of Ellen Mack it had been immediately obvious what a positive impact human contact and engagement had had on her when the matron decided for her own purposes to bestow it. Palmer asks how it is possible in a hospital with 300 patients with scarcely a dozen keepers for them to do justice to the patients? How, he asks, can the keepers be expected to deal with the pressure of so many patients with their violent mood swings and having to use restraint and isolation to control them? He ends with a further set of questions bringing the focus back to Lucett. If there was a system available Palmer asks which it is claimed would control mania and which would then lead on to the treatment of the causes of insanity would it not be right in the name of humanity to use it and spread it widely? Palmer concludes that he firmly believes that Lucett had such a remedy and that the Governors should perhaps use a positive response to Mary Mack's petition to instigate a public trial of Lucett's capabilities on Ellen Mack.

There can be no doubt of the genuine commitment which General Palmer had for Lucett and his treatment of the insane. He was a man who was not afraid of controversy. He supported Catholic Emancipation despite his links with the royal family as an aide de camp and was strongly committed to the justice of widening the popular franchise. Nevertheless his verbal assault on Sir Peter Laurie was shockingly blunt. His account of the Ellen Mack case makes it clear that Laurie and others at Bethlem had been prepared to conspire to ensure that this patient would not be treated by Lucett and to do so in the most cynical way by exploiting their ability to acknowledge or deny her humanity. There is even some internal evidence of a conspiracy to keep Mack from being treated by Lucett. During the proceedings of the Court of the Aldermen evidence was given that Ellen Mack was improving and was expected to recover. Yet when the year which Bethlem allowed patients to remain at the hospital was complete they were for the most part discharged to another asylum – one of the 'receptacles for the insane' as Lucett and others called them. When Ellen Mack completed her year in Bethlem she was discharged as 'uncured' and 'fit' for the incurable list of Bethlem on 20th May 1836. The discharge order was signed by Alexander Morison.[8] This would suggest that she was kept at Bethlem for a time as an incurable patient. Where she went in the long term is not immediately clear although she certainly did not remain at Bethlem. What is also certain is that the immediate recovery so confidently expected by the matron and Sir Peter Laurie at the Court of the Alderman was not realised.

Laurie was a former Lord Mayor of London and became the head of the Union Bank. He was a man of very considerable influence, yet Palmer was prepared to call him a liar in the most public way possible. His anger at the way the administration of Bethlem had acted was very strong and was probably inflamed by the way that even the surgeon of Bethlem had casually denigrated Ellen Mack and robbed her of her dignity by calling her a prostitute. Palmer seems to have acted out of a sense that there had been an injustice committed against a vulnerable individual. He had also highlighted the fact that the regime at Bethlem remained as appalling as it had before 1815 and that staffing levels meant there was no effective care for the patients. Lucett had clearly convinced him that there was an alternative to the malign neglect which still seemed to operate at Bethlem despite the House of Commons enquiry of 1815 and this seems to have underwritten Palmer's outrage that the Bethlem regime was fundamentally wrong. The

Sun newspaper expressed the view, in what would now be called an editorial that the Governors should inquire into the criticisms General Palmer had levelled at the hospital.[9] Lucett may well have been looking for business for himself, but he also prompted publicity for the fact that not only had Bethlem remained a place where little was done to actively encourage the recovery of the insane, but was also a place where the patients were largely powerless against the hospital authorities even when they had influential support. The quotation from General Palmer at the beginning of this chapter encapsulates the fundamental problem at Bethlem. Sufficient resources were not available to provide for an active involvement with the patients. It would take an end to the autonomy of Bethlem Hospital and its governors and the appointment of resident medical staff in the place of visiting staff like Morison and Dr Edward Monro before that could begin to be realised.

Chapter Nineteen

A Sorry End

'The effects produced were a decrease of the velocity, but an increase
of the fullness of the pulse; a quieting of disturbed and erratic mental
action, followed by calm sleep of several hours continuance.'[1]

The modern practice of physic etc. by Robert Thomas.
The 8th American edition of 1825, quoting the
impact of the Lucett treatment of mania as related by Mr Tardy.

The episode of the Ellen Mack case and Lucett's association with
General Palmer was a clear demonstration that Lucett was still very
much in business and that he was well enough known for members
of the social elite to call on his services. There were fewer advertisements
for his services although the one in the *Sun* dated 24th September 1836 is
a demonstration that he still used them even if he perhaps didn't appear to
have needed them on a regular basis. There was a further pointer from an
unexpected quarter that Lucett was very much active and had lost none of his
ambition. Indeed he appeared to be extending the range of his activities. *La
Folie* was a French version of Lucett's 1833 pamphlet which was produced in
1838.[2] It was not simply a translation of Lucett's 1833 edition, as it had been
modified to meet the French market. There is no hint of where the impetus
for the initiative came from. Lucett had dedicated some of his writing to
sponsors or patrons, real or imagined, in the past. *La Folie* does not have a
dedication which might have given a clue. Lucett had been a consistent self-
publicist, but there is no previous hint that he had done so beyond the UK,
however. To have arranged for his views on insanity and his claims to be able
to treat patients successfully to be circulated in France in French suggests
that it was not simply a whim and that he must have had significant support.

For the most part the material is familiar from the 1833 pamphlet in English
and Lucett's earlier writings but there were some interesting refinements.
It is relatively brief at fifteen pages and the style is an economical account
of uninterrupted progress in his practice. He claims to be able to cure all
forms of insanity, except those caused by a blow to the head. ['*conformation*

vicieuse du cerveau']. This was an interesting if reasonable qualification of his consistent earlier claims to universal cures for insanity. He also defined the horrors of mechanical restraint in a way that he had never done before. In his adverts and his writings for the UK market, Lucett had simply assumed that his readers would know what the implications of 'restraint' or 'compulsion' were. In *La Folie* Lucett set out a detailed description of the mechanical restraint applied in the Norris case highlighted by Wakefield's inspection of Bethlem in 1814.[3]

The basic message of *La Folie* is clear and is publicity for himself and his practice. As in his earlier work in English he claims he wants to make his cure available to humanity and that he wants to prove that his curative process works by putting it to a public test. 'This could be done,' writes Lucett, 'in an asylum which could use my curative process. Obviously I would refuse all payment if I failed. If on the other hand I was successful, I would expect payment in the form of an acknowledgement of the effectiveness of my cure.' Lucett goes on to say that he was confident that this was what would happen. There follows seven brief case studies of the sort which are familiar from Lucett's earlier output and which were common amongst contemporary health practitioners. There is then a final statement of a kind which he had never made in his writing in English. This was that if he were 'to fail to demonstrate that superiority' [of his cure] 'then the world would hear no more of his pretentions'.[4] He had never formally acknowledged the possibility that he might not be able to cure a patient of insanity. There is none of the antipathy to the medical establishment in this account and nothing of the battles he had engaged in where he had previously presented himself as the victim of the medical establishment. The salesman's bluster is muted. This is not quite Prospero signing off, but it might be a pointer to the French initiative being a new start. There are, however, no obvious indications that the Lucett process was actually tested in France or that he tried to practise there. The practicalities of how Lucett thought he could practise in France are not addressed in the pamphlet or apparently elsewhere. There is a certain symmetry in Lucett's last public statement being in France as Philippe Pinel's attack on mechanical restraint more than a generation before could almost have been an inspiration for *La Folie* and for Lucett. When Lucett published *La Folie* he would have been about 67. Although there seem to have been no adverts for his services after the one at the end of 1836 and he did not mark the accession of Queen Victoria in June 1837 with an open letter in the press, the venture into the French market suggests he was still active late in the 1830s and after a career of over a quarter of a century had not changed his basic message.

If Lucett's residence in Brompton Villa represented a high point in Lucett's career, the re-establishment of his career from an address off the Old Kent Road by 1833 did not represent a total collapse in his fortunes. It was a decent if not a fashionable area and was close to Bethlem and not far from St Luke's asylum on the other side of the Thames. It is probable that he would not have had the space at this address to take in multiple patients and to house the necessary attendants in the same way that he was able to in Brompton and during earlier incarnations. Nevertheless as the association with General Palmer and the publication of *La Folie* demonstrated he was able to maintain all the appearance of an established professional throughout the decade. This was not an obvious and inevitable slide into an irreversible loss of fortune. It is perhaps worth focusing on *La Folie* a little further as the last public initiative of James Lucett.

La Folie is a puzzle. It comes right at the end of Lucett's career yet it was a clear statement that he was attempting to enter an entirely new market. It would be possible to speculate that Lucett was in fact a first generation immigrant from France who not only spoke French, but had connections there which he could call on for support. Even allowing for the circumstantial 'evidence' that his youngest son Edward died in Papeete, Tahiti in September 1853 where he had been a merchant and the lead partner in *Lucett and Collie* the idea that James Lucett suddenly decided to exploit roots in France at the end of his career is just not convincing.[5] People may have chosen to spell his surname 'Lucette' from time to time but if he really had family connections in France which he could call on he would certainly have exploited them at the earliest opportunity in his career, not towards the end. That said the publishing of a pamphlet in France would undoubtedly have called for some support in Paris to engage and pay a printer and arrange distribution at the very least. What *La Folie* indicates is that in 1838 Lucett was still working and still looking for opportunities to exploit the 'curative process'. He had found people in the UK who were ready to underwrite his practice even if, like Mr Rocher, they might ultimately have aimed to deprive Lucett of his 'cure'. It is not impossible that he found a French backer who was impressed by Lucett and the account he would have given of the success of the 'cure'. The point surely is that *La Folie* was not the production of someone heading for the workhouse.

This raises the nature of the cure. 'Insanity Cured without Restraint' was Lucett's mantra for a quarter of a century and it would be easy to assume that his approach to his clinical practice was equally unchanging. His offer to cure insane patients and his undertaking to do so without employing the violence of physical restraint were fixed and these reflected the essential needs in the

246 George III's Illnesses and His Doctors

market he catered for. He was right to focus on the absence of restraint as this is what singled him out in the 'marketplace', but this did not mean that Lucett's treatment was the same in clinical terms from the start to the end of his career, or that it was applied in the same way to all patients. Dr Tardy had set out in detail the 'Lucett process' employed in the case of Mr Morgan in 1811, but that does not mean that the same process was necessarily being used on Lucett's patients in 1835. Indeed it is clear from the furore over Lucett's attempt to treat Ellen Mack in Bethlem that his approach to this patient was entirely different. General Palmer's testimony indicates that Lucett was applying liquid from a small bottle to Mack's head while he simultaneously engaged her attention by talking to her. In a very short space of time Lucett had calmed Mack but she returned to a manic state the moment the official keeper returned. The brief accounts from the inquest and prosecution in connection with the Kennett case again demonstrate that the 'process' described by Dr Tardy and reported on by Dr Harness during the therapeutic trial had not been used with Ellen Mack or the Reverend Kennett.

Yet Lucett referred to his curative process as if it was a single remedy. He even went in for some theatre with his reference to a sealed box containing the original manuscript of the cure which had been deposited with the Dukes of Kent and Sussex as witnesses when he was dealing with Mr Rocher in 1823. Theatre is probably the right word and Lucett employed it ruthlessly to claim exclusivity for himself as a practitioner with potential patients and their guardians and with potential financial backers for his practice. The account of a secret document which had been shared with two royal dukes under controlled conditions was a powerful way of marking Lucett out as a unique practitioner. In reality, however, Lucett was not bound to any single line of treatment determined by a document, real or imagined, which he had supposedly inherited from his father.

Dr Francis Willis did not set out his clinical practice as a single unvaried procedure – it developed through experience. Lucett probably began as an opportunist stimulated by the plight of his king, but his long-term commitment to treating patients diagnosed as suffering from insanity was real. It was his livelihood of course even though he claimed regularly in his writing up to and including *La Folie* that he simply wished to place his cure at the disposal of humanity. There can be little doubt that these grandiose claims were a more sophisticated and impressive sounding way of advertising his practice. It was certainly a way of linking himself and his practice to the appearance of endorsement at the highest level. At the end of the day though Lucett was an empiricist, perhaps in the old negative sense to begin with, but over time he left the quack behind him and made the transition to the modern sense of the word. He learned by trial and error and accumulated a wide experience from patients suffering from insanity as it was diagnosed in the early nineteenth century. It is perhaps ironic that the grandson of Dr Francis Willis who treated the king in 1788, also called Francis Willis, was in practice in Lincolnshire in the 1850s and catered for the most aristocratic segment of the market in lunacy. Perhaps it should not be a surprise that this Willis continued the methods of his grandfather with a rigid adherence to mechanical restraint for which he was censured by the Lunacy Commissioners. An additional irony is that one of his patients was a relative of Earl Fitzwilliam.

The 1841 Census is generally referred to as the first modern census in Britain as the occupants of all habitable addresses were recorded for the night of 6th June. James Lucett, with a birthdate of 1771 and recorded as a 'former clerk at the Bank', was resident at the Camberwell Workhouse in south London at the time of the 1841 census.[6] The record for Lucett remains silent for the rest of the 1840s until in January 1851 his death is recorded at the same Camberwell Workhouse. If, as seems likely in the absence of alternative options, these records do relate to the same individual there would be a final irony that the man referred to invariably as 'gentleman' as well as 'surgeon', 'doctor' and 'professor' had lived and died in the Camberwell workhouse.[7]

In the two years following the publication of *La Folie* something happened which meant that Lucett lost all independence and was placed at the mercies of the Poor Law system. For someone who had achieved some success, including on an international level as the quote at the beginning of this chapter demonstrates, and had enjoyed the title of 'gentleman' as well as a professional status the workhouse was the most terrible end to his career. It seems unlikely that the market of 'insane' patients suddenly evaporated or that Lucett was barred from practising. The growth in the number of county asylums in the middle of the nineteenth century was proof of the demand. There was also an increasing consciousness that a diagnosis of insanity could be used by the unscrupulous to neutralise or exploit vulnerable individuals and that some private asylums held patients who should not have been confined. In that context Lucett would have been an attractive practitioner who could be relied on not to engage in holding people against their interests. Lucett's emphasis on cure and a rapid turnover of patients ran counter to unjustified confinement. Even if the home he occupied off the Old Kent Road was not suitable for the reception and treatment of several resident patients, the advert from 1833 showed that he had made a virtue of taking in single patients in a family environment. Lucett had never catered for large numbers of patients at any point in his career so it should have been possible for Lucett to maintain some income even though he was getting older. He had one of the largest conurbations in the world on his doorstep and a practice which in 1833 had involved advertising for work on a visiting basis. The relationship with General Palmer demonstrated that this was a reality.

There is a unique survival from the period at the end of Lucett's practice which provides a glimpse of Lucett through the eyes of a family member. Edward Lucett was the second son of James and Olivia Lucett and, as noted above, was to become a merchant in Tahiti dealing in pearls. His book *Rovings in the Pacific* is of considerable interest as it charts Polynesia, New Zealand and Australia at the time when European settlement was beginning to have a significant impact. The introduction to *Rovings* explains the background to his decision to take the role of a crew member on a ship taking convicts to Australia. Edward does not go into details but conveys a strong sense of oppression and a powerful desire to get away from London. He had suffered from pleurisy which had been 'brought on by blighted hopes and ruined affections'. It was while recovering from illness that he decided to take a ship to Australia. His actual decision to go was made suddenly and he made a brief visit to the place where he had been at school just before he left. This is not a conventional sentimental visit as all his recollections are negative and seem to centre on floggings he received while at school. He even sees some of his former schoolmates and contrasts their apparent contentment with his own unhappiness. The tone is one of self-pity, but it is possible that his outlook reflected being in a convalescent state after a life-threatening illness and being crossed in love. How he had been making a living is not revealed; perhaps because Edward Lucett's book is not really concerned with the past.

Edward Lucett was 22 and living at home and after visiting his former school he returned there. 'On the road I met my father; the poor old gentleman reeled like a drunken man when I made the announcement that I was off; but there was no help for him or me, so I steadily pursued my purpose resolving that no unavailing weakness should overcome me. That afternoon I was at home to join the last dinner I was ever destined to partake beneath my father's roof tree.'[8] That evening he joined the ship which sailed on 28th March 1837.[9] This could be the start of a novel by Dickens with the hero stepping out into the unknown to make his fortune. He was clearly an educated and articulate man yet home life in the Lucett household or in London was clearly unbearable. It was not an easy decision to leave and he spoke with some affection of his father but there had clearly been no discussion immediately before Edward made his decision to go abroad.

After this fleeting glimpse of Lucett in relative old age, but still at liberty, he was very soon to disappear into a confinement of his own. If one word characterised Lucett throughout his career up to the end of the 1830s it was resilience. From the moment Lucett responded to George III's relapse at the end of 1810 by publicising his claim for a cure for insanity, Lucett had put aside a secure job with the Bank of England and assumed a role on the margins of respectable medical practice. It was a development fraught with risk and Lucett certainly encountered a series of set-backs. He also achieved some success, but what is clear from the available record is that his capacity to exploit and even create opportunities seemed to know no bounds. Lucett's exploitation of a banal correspondence with Lord Liverpool to create the appearance of a direct endorsement of his treatment of insane patients was a master-stroke of pure effrontery. Lucett was not cowed by prosecution, whether by the authorities or by his erstwhile partners. From every set-back and every bankruptcy Lucett had demonstrated the resilience to bounce-back – even if it involved highly risky and illegal involvement with financial instruments. Lucett was a brazen risk-taker when it came to furthering his career as a practitioner with the insane.

So entering the realms of pure speculation did illness or alcohol result in Lucett suddenly becoming disabled? A stroke or a serious heart attack could have ended his capacity to practise and his history suggests that he would have had little to fall back on financially. There is only the most skeletal background on Lucett's family. His wife Olivia made a brief foray into the consciousness of Earl Fitzwilliam in 1814 but otherwise only appears in reports of the Surrey inspectors of private asylums assisting her husband in running their private asylums. A woman of the same name died in Ewell in 1822 and was almost certainly Lucett's wife. If she was, then Lucett's obvious professional and financial problems only came after her death. It is probable that Lucett remarried in 1824 in St Mary's church Newington. The marriage certificate describes Lucett as a 'widower' so this would fit with the death of his first wife two years earlier.[10] This second wife was Elizabeth Martha Emmett and she was living in Camberwell at the Ship public house with Olivia the daughter of the marriage when the 1841 census was taken. It was normal, at that time, for family members from several generations to live together and yet, despite probably having three sons and a daughter alive from the first marriage and a daughter and second wife living close by, no one seemed willing or able to provide support for Lucett senior. There is no obvious explanation, but workhouses acted as refuges for the sick as well as the indigent so it is possible that Lucett was not simply abandoned by his surviving family members. The Camberwell Workhouse in Havil

Street had a significant hospital wing by 1840 and indeed had a section for pauper lunatics. But the records of admissions and discharges for the period of Lucett's residence have been destroyed or discarded so the explanation for Lucett's admission is lost. Whatever the explanation, Lucett lived out his last ten years of life in the Camberwell Workhouse and died there in 1851.[11]

Chapter Twenty

George III – The Last Years

'... since the time of Dr Willis the system of coercion has been the one most generally adopted. Confinement, darkness and meagre diet, have been the specifics too commonly resorted to; and the consequence of these means has been, that the affection of the mind from the weakened state of the body, has become, in the greater number of cases, more permanent.'

Letter of Dr Charles Dunne to the College of
Physicians. 31st October 1810.[1]

James Lucett may have descended into the obscurity of the institutional routine of Camberwell Workhouse, but George III was also deprived of his liberty for most of the last decade of his life. In George's case, however, the record of his enforced routine survives in considerable detail. In many ways the worst fears of the Dukes of Kent and Sussex, as well as some of their siblings, were realised after the Willis brothers were given complete control of the king from early 1812. The imposition of rigorous 'seclusion' which had been put in place initially because it was believed it would give the best chance of the patient's recovery continued unabated. The regular physicians who had been treating the king since 1810 were pushed to one side although they did not accept being marginalised without protest. In their complaint to the Queen's Council in early February 1812 Halford, Heberden and Baillie said they were required to be 'mute observers of the King's condition' unable to contribute to his health or comfort.[2]

Access to the king was granted only with the specific agreement of one of the two Willis brothers. Even the remaining physicians charged with care of the king's bodily health were not allowed to speak to their patient unless this was considered absolutely necessary and endorsed by the Willises. Indeed one of the Willis brothers was present at all visits – including by members of the king's immediate family. Dr Heberden had expressed his fears that the king would turn in on himself in the absence of new ideas and impressions exacerbated in his view by the fact that the patient was blind. The quotation above from Dr Dunne coincided with the onset of the king's relapse and if he was inspired by the renewed illness of his king, Dunne's prediction of the long-term impact of seclusion was prescient. He had mentioned 'darkness' as one of the characteristics of 'seclusion' as it was normally applied and patients were literally isolated in a darkened room. In the king's case he was blind throughout the period in which the Willis brothers had complete control of the king so his isolation would have been very intense. George did not recover under the Willis system, instead he turned in on himself and recycled people and events from the past to create an imaginary world.

Such was the intensity of the king's self-absorption that many observers have suggested that he suffered increasingly from deafness. Apparently even his medical attendants reported that they thought he might be going deaf. The possibility was investigated in 1817 and John Willis and Henry Halford reported their conclusions to the Queen's Council. 'We have now ascertained it with considerable accuracy that His Majesty's deafness has not materially increased of late. HM's thoughts are sometimes so entirely occupied and engrossed, and His distemper gives rise so frequently to a waywardness that we are not surprised that the attendants should have supposed HM to have suffered an aggravation of this infirmity.'[3] There is almost a refined cruelty in the careful assessment of a blind man's hearing when on a day-to-day basis the only world of sound he could hope to indulge was the music he played.

The delusion that he was married to Lady Pembroke was overtaken and was as nothing compared to George's renunciation of the real world. 'He considers himself no longer an inhabitant of the world', wrote Princess Elizabeth in 1814.[4] It is impossible to know whether George understood what was happening to him but there was some apparent awareness that he existed in a limbo world. He was overheard referring to a piece of music that he had been playing and saying that he had been fond of it 'when he was in the world'.[5] Whatever George thought he was aware enough to consider that the links with his former existence were increasingly tenuous. Fanny Burney [Madame d'Arblay] wrote to her father in May 1813 and included her assessment of the king's condition. 'The beloved King is in the best state possible for his present melancholy situation; that is, wholly free from real bodily suffering or imaginary mental misery, for he is persuaded that he is always conversing with angels.'[6] Fanny had been intensely loyal to Queen Charlotte during the crisis of 1788/9 and had witnessed her royal patron's struggle to master the impact of her husband's terrible illness. Burney had remained a friend of the queen and was committed to the king. Her assessment would therefore have searched for whatever good she could find in the king's condition. It was a rationalisation which she was not alone in holding to.

Princess Elizabeth, third daughter of George III and Queen Charlotte, was a thoughtful observer of the world around her and yet she too rationalised what was beyond her reach to influence. In her impotence when it came to doing anything practical about her father's situation she took much the same line as Fanny Burney had done. Writing to Lady Harcourt in October 1814 she remarked, 'tho' in a most melancholy state for us, yet a happy one for himself, for they all say he is without a care when he is not approaching a paroxysm, and that thank God, is so seldom'.[7] What is clear is that some of the heat had gone out of the king's illness and a routine and relative calm had been achieved, but it seems that the Willis brothers may have been influencing Princess Elizabeth's perception of her father's situation. In a separate letter to Lady Harcourt dated 14th October 1814, Princess Elizabeth quoted the Willis brothers' guidance.[8] 'Dr Robert Willis assures me, as well as John Willis .... that He is perfectly happy, most likely never so happy for he has no cares, enjoys his music, his company etc.' It is of course entirely possible that the Willis brothers were putting the best perspective on the king's situation as a way of comforting the Princess and it seems to have had that effect on Elizabeth. It is one thing for Fanny Burney and Princess Elizabeth to reach the consoling conclusion that the king was not suffering independently and for themselves, it is quite another for the Willis brothers to promote that view. The Willis perspective seems self-interested to say the least. To argue that George had never been so happy seems patronising when considering the patient and ironic when set against the professional confidence with which they took over the king's case. The Willis statement was undoubtedly honest in one important respect, however. They clearly did not think their patient would recover.

The reports published in the press on the king's condition became infrequent and took on the dullness of a pointless routine. The orthodoxy of the isolation of the patient was maintained and little filtered into the king's suite at Windsor from the outside world as the years passed. Dr Dunne's charge that the Willis system made patients 'imbecile' was arguably fulfilled. Queen Charlotte tried to bridge the gap between herself and her husband by visiting from time to time, but George did not recognise her. Her brief comments on her husband's condition emphasised the quiet calm. 'The King is quiet and composed', she reported at the end of 1814, while in January 1817 she commented, 'the dear King very comfortable in every sense'.[9] The queen was in a limbo of her own. She was effectively a widow yet her husband was alive. Her role as queen consort had been reduced to a shell.

In late 1817 the sudden death of her granddaughter the Princess Charlotte, apparently in childbirth, coincided with a crisis in the queen's own health. She had been suffering from a weak heart which brought on shortness of breath and other increasingly serious symptoms. As 1818 advanced Queen Charlotte's health was finally broken and she became effectively bed-ridden. Yet even at this stage she wanted to make one last visit to see her husband. It was not to be as the attempt to move the queen from London to Windsor got as far as Kew before she became so ill she could go no further. There she lingered for five months as her condition deteriorated until she died at Kew on 17th November.

The reports to the Queen's Council, renamed the Duke of York's Council following the death of Queen Charlotte, present a picture of calm, almost sterile routine. A report published by the Council reporting the impact of the death of Queen Charlotte described the king's condition as 'tranquillity undisturbed'. *The Gentleman's Magazine* commented on the report, 'We cannot conceive anything more affecting; more distressing, than this description of the tranquillity of the King during a visitation of domestic calamity which would have touched him so nearly had he possessed his reason.'[10] In January 1819 Sir Henry Halford was given permission by the Duke of York's Council, but subject to the agreement of the Willis brothers, to try to engage the king in conversation. The initiative, if that is the right word, failed. George seemed to be impressed by his senior physician, whom he had liked and trusted, suddenly speaking to him. He was noted as having raised his eyes and hands towards the ceiling, but he said nothing. What this meant is unknown, but it could have been an expression of exasperation that this gesture of humanity had come so late.

It had been possible to establish a routine at Windsor because the king was clearly not manic for most of the time. He apparently required less sleep than someone who would have been considered very old at the time and he was certainly not helpless. The daily report to the Duke of York's Council for the 15th November 1819 mentions that George had played the harpsichord that day while the entry for 10th December 1819 mentions that he had dressed himself 'as usual'. This was just over a month before he died at the age of 82. There are nevertheless recurrent references to the king's very disordered mind, but these references seem to carry less weight than the reports on the king's satisfaction with his meals. Perhaps it was right to emphasise the mealtimes as they were the high point of the day when the king, dressed in his Windsor uniform, wore his orders in a ritual which seemed to give him some pleasure. As Burney had indicated in 1813 the king may not have been suffering, but he was apparently only tangentially engaged with the real world. What is also clear is that the reports were based on detached observation of the king rather than a relationship based on engagement with the patient.[11]

George III's mania may have abated somewhat during his last years of isolation at Windsor and his paroxysms may have been rare as a result, but at the end of 1819 he suffered a series of extreme paroxysms from which he was physically unable to recover. He died on 29th January 1820. George III had not been forgotten and a very large crowd filled Windsor on the evening of 16th February when the funeral took place. The Duke of York was present when his father died although it is doubtful whether the father recognised his favourite son. The duke gave an account of the king's last moments in a letter to George IV. This account and others to be found in the Jerningham Letters and many of the biographies of George III record the gentle clarity with which he expressed his requests to be made comfortable as he was dying. The Duke of York reported to his brother 'that his last moments were free from bodily suffering and mental distress'. The absence of 'mental distress' can be taken to mean that George showed no signs of a disordered mind. The Duke of York's account included calm requests by his father that his lips should be wetted only when he opened his mouth. When the request was complied with, he graciously expressed his thanks. Sir Henry Halford and others had remarked at various points over the years that even when the patient had been delirious his underlying memory and even his reason had remained intact. This seems to have been apparent at the end.

Looking back it is difficult to understand why the Queen's Council, subsequently called the Duke of York's Council, persisted apparently unquestioningly with the Willis system without modification or relaxation long after it was clear that it was doing no good and long after the Willis brothers had themselves concluded that the king would not recover. The Willis brothers had originally been given total control over management of the king's case following his further relapse in mid-1811 when it became clear that the regime of the generalist physicians led by Sir Henry Halford had failed to recover the patient. They not only managed the 'medical' treatment of the patient, but determined the circumstances in which any visitors were to be allowed to see the king and whether they were allowed to communicate with him. The Willises failed to recover the patient in their turn and by the end of 1813 this failure was surely manifest to them and to the Council? From that point onwards the management of George III had more to do with custody than care.

Against this dismal background the experiment with Lucett and Delahoyde must have seemed like a potential way out of the sterile paralysis which had developed at Windsor. The almost desperate enthusiasm of the

Archbishop of Canterbury's interest in the trial of the Lucett process makes perfect sense against the failure of 'seclusion'. It also makes sense that any alternative to the Willis treatment would need proof that it worked if the Willis system was to be overturned. As discussed above, the Willis system represented orthodoxy and the 'proven' or at least accepted way of treating those diagnosed as suffering from insanity at the time. To go outside the established treatments for so important a patient as the king risked the credibility of the authorities. This is why the Lucett process was so important as it would seem to have been the last and only occasion when an alternative treatment for George III was under active consideration. When the Lucett process failed to deliver the certainty of a permanent cure the patient was condemned to continue a limbo existence with a therapy which had already been demonstrated to be a failure. William Munk took the view at the end of the nineteenth century that the Queen's Council had allowed the Willises 'undue' and 'injurious authority' due to their 'special and exceptional experience' in the care of the insane.[12]

One element in the explanation for George's continued treatment was who he was. During the early months of 1811 George's condition had improved enormously and the physicians debated the determinants of recovery. As has been seen they opted for an absence of 'delusions' and 'extravagances'. They were certainly applying very high standards and this was not necessarily driven by the patient's interests. The assessment process of 1811 was clearly determined by the need to demonstrate that the patient's recovery was complete in all respects. Convalescence in an ordinary patient could be a period of relative relaxation and calm with a gradual return to normality. In George III's case it seems to have been a period of tighter scrutiny during which 'a slight allusion' to a delusion would count against the determination of his recovery. It is perhaps a subjective view but in 1804 the assessment of recovery seems to have been more gradual and the patient was returned to much of his normal life as part of the convalescence. In George's case, however, normal life was a public life. There was the round of official public engagements in which his every action would be the subject of wide scrutiny. Even at Windsor the people of the town were accustomed to seeing the king promenading on the North Terrace of the castle with his suite of family members and attendants. Even this private diversion was a public occasion for many. The sense that the king had been returned to normality too soon in 1804 was strongly felt and Robert Wilson's testimony seen, in chapter three, perhaps seems extreme simply because it was written down. This background could explain the reluctance to declare the king recovered in April 1811 and to continue with treatment until recovery was complete. George was judged by higher standards than might have been applied to a private individual simply because of who he was.

It is likely, however, that there was no specific binary decision to adhere to the full Willis regime indefinitely or until the patient had recovered. It seems probable that for the early years, in the period from mid-1812 until the end of 1814, the Queen's Council was simply reluctant to make any admission of failure with such an important charge so the treatment continued. Thereafter inertia probably set in. The king was simply too mentally disordered to be allowed anything beyond a very circumscribed life while in reality the Willis regime continued because there was no viable alternative treatment. It is even possible that there was some 'group thinking' amongst the Council members which pursued the lines of the views expressed by Fanny Burney and Princess Elizabeth. They may have considered that the king was as comfortable and happy as was possible under the circumstances; even if they were unwilling to commit such views to official documents.

The corollary of the continued medical control of the king was the expense involved. This fell to the private resources of the king and queen. From 1812 until the death of their patient there was at least one of the Willis brothers at Windsor each day while the three regular physicians visited two days a week each. Mr Dundas, the Windsor apothecary, attended twice a week. Yet the day-to-day management of the king was handled by attendants while the doctors were increasingly observers except when their patient suffered occasional paroxysms. Colonel Taylor who had been the king's secretary and who continued to administer the king's private purse asked the Queen's Council to allow reductions in the attendance of the physicians. Taylor was even supported by Lord Liverpool the Prime Minister yet the Council rejected any reduction in the medical coverage. The total cost of the medical attendance for the period from 5th January 1812 to George III's death was calculated at £271,691 18s 0d based on Colonel Taylor's figures.[13] This would cover the period when the expectation of recovery had passed. During the period from November 1810 to the end of 1811 when the king was actively treated in the expectation that he would recover the cost of medical attendance ran at between £34 and 35 thousand per annum.[14]

It is ironic to say the least that Dr John Willis was to spend eight years sharing charge of George III with his brother when he considered at the time when he was first brought in that it was already too late to do anything useful. In his letter to Lord Lonsdale dated 26th January 1812 he remarked, 'He is I think worse than ever.' and 'I am in the heart of absurdity wishing myself out.' At the time when John Willis and his brother were displacing the regular physicians at Windsor John Willis was to give a candid assessment of the king's case in a letter to Lord Lonsdale dated 29th January. 'I am still without leave of absence – and cannot help feeling hardly treated – to come in when the game is over – and forced to play on without the chance of winning – I shall presently feel it a duty to myself to make a firm remonstrance --- [the king] indisputably much worse in my opinion since the last attack of paroxysm – more fixed and chronic.' Willis' tone of self-pity is deeply unattractive, but his absolute conviction that the king would not recover is left in no doubt. Whether he made any 'remonstrance' or whether he actually made any real effort to leave his responsibilities at Windsor is not clear. His actions seem to demonstrate a complete adherence to his control over the patient. Harpsichords were placed where the patient could respond but seclusion from human contact was maintained.[15]

The king's extended custody also highlighted the legal vulnerability of patients who had been diagnosed as insane. Custody is an emotive word, but it underlies the essentially unique status which patients, including George himself, acquire once they have been diagnosed as suffering from a form of insanity. Treatment is no longer optional, but becomes a legal requirement. George III's slow descent into oblivion was a tragedy, but to paraphrase Burrows, it could be argued that his illness was a case of good coming out of evil not simply on the therapeutic level but on the legal one as well. His case underlined the growing preoccupation with the possibility of people being confined without justification and the need therefore to improve and strengthen the process by which people were 'certified' as insane. The process was slowed by repeated rejection of draft legislation in the House of Lords, but the 1828 Act to Regulate the Care and Treatment of Insane Persons in England strengthened the safeguards for individuals who were subject to the certification process. Ironically this protection actually served to emphasise the fact that certification once granted was in reality legal confinement. This was in the future though. When the crowds gathered in Windsor on the evening of 16th February 1820 for George III's funeral they did so out of respect. They were not there to stigmatise the lunatic, but to express their sympathy and solidarity with the human being. In the not-so-distant past lunatics had been considered as no longer fully human. In Windsor the silent crowds were there to express their sympathy with his suffering and to reaffirm George's humanity.

Chapter Twenty-One

They Never Met

'... quackery, being a dangerous evil, should not have been taxed, but absolutely prohibited under the most severe penalties; for vice ought not to be tolerated in a good government, but rigorously surpressed.'
James Makittrick Adair. Preface to *Medical Cautions Chiefly for the Consideration of Invalids etc.* 1787.

'As to the disease itself, it may, perhaps, still be said that a great deal remains to be ascertained of its true nature; but experience has at length taught us all that is necessary for its proper treatment.'
Sir Alexander Halliday.[1] *A General View of the Present State of Lunatics and Lunatic Asylums in GB and Ireland.* 1827.

There was a clear perception of what a quack was in the late eighteenth and early nineteenth centuries. Indeed this timespan probably encompassed the heyday of quacks in the UK before the arrival of the internet! The anonymous author in 1844 of *Quacks and Quackery* defined a quack as 'A boastful pretender to arts which he does not understand'.[2] The author emphasises that the rivalry between the medical profession and quacks is more important than the rivalry between 'big enders' and their opposite numbers in *Gulliver's Travels*. It was a matter of life and death for the patient and yet he says that many physicians believed that quacks were beneath their notice. The author disagrees. He argues that the medical profession could not afford to allow the quack to exploit the credulity of the public and to engage the press, government, nobility and even royalty to support their outrageous claims. These comments could almost have been focused on James Lucett. The author says that quacks should be opposed at every turn and quackery outlawed. The author's trenchant statements are misplaced, however. Even in 1844 the subject of quackery was more complex than the anonymous author would allow; not least in the area of the treatment of insanity.

It was not just quacks who were beneath the notice of the regular physician. The Reverend Dr Francis Willis was regarded as a quack by many of the faculty,[3] while Lord Sheffield referred to him as 'not much better than a mountebank' when he was brought in to treat George III.[4] How he would have viewed the fact that his family were later to call on the services of 'Professor' James Lucett in the Kennett case is unknowable! The methods which the specialist mad-doctors used in treating their patients and the fact that these methods had been used on the king reinforced their low status. Certainly those 'qualified' physicians who chose to specialise in the treatment of the insane were regarded with disdain by many regular physicians. As late as 1868 the specialist in treating the insane Dr William Sankey would state, 'In connecting ourselves with lunacy we are almost compelled to share the seclusion of our patients.'[5] Those caring for George III in 1811 were resistant to the imposition of the specialist 'mad doctors' in large part because they did not believe the specialists had any significant expertise to contribute. There was though an inescapable element of disdain for the specialists amongst the established physicians; especially in the case of Sir Henry Halford. Therefore what were the criteria that anyone could reasonably use when looking for help for themselves or a relative or friend who was mentally ill? There were no courses for professionals treating the insane and no professional bodies which represented the specialists in treating the insane. So Francis Willis and James Lucett, had to gain knowledge through experience. And so it all came full circle because empirically based learning was seen as a characteristic of the quack in the view of much of the medical establishment at the beginning of the nineteenth century. Quack and empiric were synonymous at that time.

The concept of the 'quack' was essentially dominated by two classes of practitioner. The first and most numerous was the itinerant seller of generalised cures for a range of ailments. Most had ineffective but innocuous ingredients while a few had potentially harmful constituents. The sellers were successful precisely because they were itinerant. They had moved on before the failure of the 'cure all' became clear. The other common class of quack practitioner was again an itinerant. These were practitioners who travelled the country offering consultations and treatment for specific conditions. They were often in direct competition with regular resident practitioners but again relied on their rapid travel to avoid possible recriminations when their extravagant claims for success were shown to be wanting. There were quacks who were established in specific locations, however, and so had a regular clientele. They tended to be fringe practitioners who specialised in complaints which were not mainstream ailments although there were some quacks who practised from a fixed base and claimed to treat mainstream ailments. These were obviously in direct competition with regular qualified practitioners. Lucett was, from the perspective of established medicine, an example of the fringe category. He practised from an establishment where he took in patients and focused on a single complaint which was on the margins for respectable medicine.

The author of *Quacks and Quackery* was dismissive of the people whose 'credulity' led them to seek the services of quacks as if it was a straightforward business to determine between the qualified and the imposter and that even if a qualified practitioner was identified that this person would by definition provide a better service. People were motivated by a complex range of considerations in determining whom to trust. To paraphrase Roy Porter, the essential ingredient in making any decision across the board over who was or was not a quack was hindsight. The physicians who treated the king after his relapse in 1810 and the Willis brothers who took over treatment in 1811 when the patient's condition deteriorated further were all 'qualified' practitioners. Yet under the terms of the definition of the anonymous author of *Quacks and Quackery* they were quacks too. They pretended to a knowledge which they did not have. They applied the accepted therapies uncritically, and in the case of the king these therapies were not just ineffective but harmful as became increasingly obvious to interested observers.

George III's illness encapsulated the dilemmas involved in dealing with the insane in the early nineteenth century. Francis Willis had raised expectations in 1789 when he asserted that insanity was curable. George Mann Burrows noted the increase in cases of insanity as it lost some of its stigma and it appeared that something could be done for the sufferers. Yet chapters five and six charted the growing realisation that the physicians treating the king were actually helpless and that the full rigours of the specialist treatment were equally ineffective. It was actually worse than that because the treatment was for the most part non-specific and the remedies were used on a wide range of other unrelated complaints. This was very close to the actions of the itinerant quack selling nostrums which it was claimed would cure a wide range of distinct and very different illnesses. The remedies were also damaging or dangerous as was set out in chapter eight and would arguably have interfered with a process of natural healing which might have applied to many patients. The arguments which the author of *Quacks and Quackery* was making were self-interested. The monopoly in the treatment of the insane which he and the medical profession aspired to was neither inevitable nor necessarily justified. It might seem inevitable now in the UK or the US, but other countries have developed different systems of psychiatry where there is no assumption that the practitioner must be medically qualified.

The Dukes of Kent and Sussex would doubtless have resented the idea that they were credulous in their association with James Lucett. They would have known that he had no medical training when they first made contact with him. It probably did not matter to them. After all desperation drove people then and still drives people now to seek help almost anywhere when the qualified practitioners were deemed to have failed. The late eighteenth and early nineteenth centuries was a time of experimentation. Water treatments were very much in vogue for a wide range of illnesses and it is perhaps significant that the Dukes of Kent and Sussex appear again in that context. The *Morning Post* for 25th June 1812 reported a meeting held in the Freemason's Tavern chaired by the Duke of Kent and seconded by his brother. The radical MP Joseph Hume was present at the meeting and opened proceedings. What the group were examining was the potential to use a redundant London smallpox hospital as a sea-bathing infirmary. A publication by M L Este is linked to the project. This was the comprehensively named.[6] *On Baths, Water, Swimming, Shampooing* published in 1812. There is no indication that the proposed hospital or the benefits of water treatments were considered in this case for use on the insane. The timing, however, when the relationship between the dukes and Lucett was developing and the dedication of Este's book to the dukes 'with permission' raises the possibility that they could have been looking more widely than the Lucett process for potential treatments for their father.

Other practitioners did see the potential of water treatments in one form or other for the insane although for the most part the focus on water was a general one based on the benefits of cleanliness. Turton cautiously recommended cold baths for 'furious madness' while as we have seen Charles Dunne took water treatments seriously – including or even especially for the insane.[7] Both John Williams and William Laing drew attention to the sedative effect of warm baths with a marked slowing of the pulse.[8] But neither was a ringing endorsement of the use of warm water baths with maniacs. The uncertainty over the application of water treatments was summed up in Sir Arthur Clarke's comments in 1827 that 'in all cases of insanity whatever tends to remove blood from the head should be employed' but goes on to say 'The utility of bathing in maniacal cases, remains yet to be ascertained; it has never, I believe been exclusively used at the Retreat near York, it has been thought rather to aggravate the symptoms of mania.'[9]

There was an inescapable sense of rush in the winding up of the Committee experiment. As was clear in chapter thirteen this was probably driven to a large extent by the lack of finance to continue the experiment and some difficulty in managing the relationship with Lucett and Delahoyde. Indeed the Committee may have felt that the practitioners were increasingly exploiting the support they were receiving for their own ends. On the public level the Committee had been set up to evaluate the Lucett curative process for the benefit of humanity. Doubtless the Committee members were sincerely committed to this aim. They also had a more immediate and actually rather more manageable aim, however, as was clear in the account of the Committee experiment above. This aim was never stated publically although it was clearly agreed among the committee members and was the dominant immediate purpose of the whole experiment. This was to determine whether the curative process could safely be used on the king with a reasonable expectation that it would recover him. While the actual Committee-based experiment had lasted only a few months, the Duke of Kent and a small group of gentlemen had been engaged on the project for over a year *before* the formation of the Committee in a timescale which grew out of the failure by the regular physicians and the specialist mad-doctors to cure the king. The whole involvement with Lucett had been driven by the case of George III. By December 1813 they had clearly determined that the Lucett process was not a simple cure which could permanently resolve the very difficult cases which had probably been carefully selected to mirror the case of the king.

Dr Harness had been clear that the Lucett process did have an immediate effect on deranged and manic patients. He could not explain why this should be so, but he was in no doubt that the effect was real. Today the inexplicable is a sure basis for further enquiry and experimentation. The Committee formed by the Duke of Kent was not, however, a Georgian equivalent of the Crick Institute set up to conduct novel scientific research. It was a temporary coming together of a group of gentlemen from the social and intellectual elite of the day to determine whether a trial of a therapeutic process would deliver a reliable cure for the king. When that immediate purpose did not materialise they were not equipped or ready for the long-term commitment to explore and explain the short-term positive impact of the Lucett process; or to improve it.

Of course Lucett would have lobbied for a public statement which backed the value of his process. He was after all an effective self-promotor. The Committee were ready to do this not through a lack of integrity and a willingness to connive with Lucett, nor through a lack of professionalism in establishing basic scientific parameters for the therapeutic trial which were simply abandoned when this was convenient. The apparent inconsistency between the stated aims at the establishment of the experiment and the conclusion of the final report is in fact a resolution of the public and private elements of the whole experiment. James Lucett was not going to be let loose on the king, but he had done enough to demonstrate that his curative process did have a real, if temporary, impact on mania. In the Georgian era that was a really significant development. By underwriting Lucett in their final report the Committee was saying that the process was safe and potentially beneficial in managing manic patients. It was also an invitation for others to explore further and to try to explain and improve the therapeutic impact which Dr Harness had found so inexplicable.

Lucett had claimed a lot when he first attracted the attention of the Duke of Kent and while he had not been able to deliver fully on his claims he had done enough to justify and secure a limited endorsement by the Committee. The king's case had therefore launched the career of Lucett as a practitioner in the care of the insane and on the superficial level another member had been added to the ranks of late Georgian quacks. 'Insanity Cured Without Constraint' was the key to Lucett's practice. On the former he was only partially successful. Yet his therapy worked to the extent that it could break a manic cycle without the use of heavy metals or other poisons and narcotics. There were also pointers to the use of education and work experience as they would now be called to bolster recovery. The evidence from Surrey was that there was a rapid turnover of patients and that they were treated with dignity and given considerable freedom and were even free to talk to the asylum inspectors. Most important of all is that Lucett really did not use restraint. He committed to using no chains or straight waistcoats and he delivered. That alone would have been enough to have had an important positive impact on the Dukes of Kent and Sussex and their associates when compared with the treatment the king had actually received at the hands of the qualified doctors.

After the end of the Committee-sponsored experiment Lucett was to continue to work with patients who were diagnosed as insane for the following twenty-five years at least. He did so amidst controversy and with clear evidence later in that timespan that he was engaged in illegal financial dealings. He was accused of bad behaviour towards patients and of drunkenness yet this was by people who wanted to discredit him and gain control of Lucett's process. He was a shameless self-promotor and manipulated his contacts with senior figures to his advantage. Lucett continued to trade on his contact with the Duke of Kent long after the duke had died and certainly used the most superficial correspondence with the Prime Minister, or more accurately Prime Ministers, to bolster his credibility. Yet there were crucial and consistent elements of his career which metaphorically lifted him from the debtor's prison where he found himself from time to time. He campaigned against the use of restraint in the management of the insane and he practised what he promoted. His commitment to treating the insane with a care and humanity which was uncommon at the time fits badly with the idea that he was just a quack.

The other characteristic which separated Lucett from the conventional quack was the fact that he did not seek to maximise his profit from his patients. He had criticised asylum keepers who maximised their profit by charging £300 per year to accommodate each patient, when the true cost would have been £60, and asylum keepers who kept patients as long as possible to maintain their income. Indeed this latter practice was an element in the growing concern that sane people were being wrongly incarcerated in private asylums and was a factor in the formation of the 'Alleged Lunatics Friend Society' in 1845. Maximising numbers, regardless of the impact on patients, was another road to profitability which was common in places like Hoxton and some of the private asylums in Surrey. Lucett kept the number of patients in his asylum very low. An element in the low numbers was that Lucett took a direct role in the management of patients as part of his curative strategy although such an arrangement would have reduced the requirement for and cost of attendants. It is perhaps evidence for a modest business that when Lucett advertised his business in April 1827 he claimed an annual turnover of four to eight hundred pounds.

Lucett was not the only unqualified practitioner to push against the orthodoxy represented by the Willis clan and the vast majority of contemporary medical practitioners. The creation of the Retreat at York in 1792 represented a fundamental rejection of the callous and ineffective treatment of insane patients. The Retreat was the creation of Quakers led by William Tuke, a coffee and tea merchant, who had been outraged by the awful conditions at the local York asylum. The regime at the Retreat emphasised humane treatment and aimed to engage the patients as individuals in their own recovery. Restraint was still used but as a last resort and did not involve chains and iron manacles. Samuel Tuke wrote an account of the founding and ethos of the establishment in *Description of the Retreat near York* in which he condemned the conventional emphasis on gaining ascendency over patients through fear and confinement. He also criticised the long term use of strong emetics and purgatives as being very dangerous. Although the death of a Quaker from the York fellowship had provided the immediate impetus for the foundation of the Retreat, the suffering of the king had also been a general inspiration.[10]

Thomas Bakewell was another unqualified advocate for the insane. The proprietor of the Spring Vale asylum in Staffordshire, Bakewell was influential in promoting the need for reform in the treatment of the insane. In his evidence to the Parliamentary Select Committee in 1815 he claimed that too many insane patients were not being properly treated and that the large asylums in London were almost designed to prevent recovery. Interestingly Bakewell, claimed that his own small establishment did a better job of curing patients than even The Retreat in York, which while he thought it treated patients well, did not in his view have a fundamental commitment to curing. A major concern in Bakewell's evidence was the financial interest of private asylum keepers in keeping patients for extended periods of time and the problem of the rapacious relative exploiting the insane. Bakewell suggested that the word 'incurable' should not be used with patients as they should retain the hope of a cure and set out his thoughts for a network of national hospitals for the insane.[11]

Where the Retreat and Spring Vale coincided was in their continued employment of restraint. It was done with reluctance and as a last resort, but it was still considered a necessary option for extreme paroxysms and to protect the patient from themselves. Lucett was in the vanguard of the movement for humane treatment for the insane and he was in advance of many celebrated figures in his complete rejection of restraint. Robert Gardiner-Hill was credited with removing restraint including straight waistcoats at Lincoln Asylum when he was appointed medical superintendent in 1839. He did so, but twenty years after Lucett had begun practising without restraint.[12] Indeed the case of Lincoln was used as a contrast with the reluctance to abandon restraint at the Dundee asylum a few years later. In his book of 1841, Dr Richard Poole cited Lucett positively as showing the way in treating the insane without restraint twenty-five years before.[13]

Indeed the late 1830s was the moment when the non-restraint movement achieved momentum. In a lecture given in June 1838, Gardiner Hill advocated the 'Total abolition of Severity of every species and degree' for patients of lunatic asylums and argued that this was both desirable and practical; the key was proper supervision of patients both day and night. He quoted an attendant from the Glasgow Royal Asylum for Lunatics who referred to it 'taking a month to tame a patient'. This was not the way so far as Gardiner Hill was concerned with its implied threat of violence.[14] John Connolly is the other celebrated member of the non-restraint movement and he was able to put this into practice in 1839 when he became Resident physician at the Hanwell asylum. This mattered because Hanwell was the first large asylum where mechanical restraint was abolished. Yet these developments took place at the time when Lucett was coming to the end of his career and even then they faced strong opposition. Indeed restraint and other bad practices returned at the Lincoln asylum in 1847, while Gardiner Hill recorded the impact of the hostility his views on non-restraint attracted. 'I was shut out from other important posts because I was author of that "absurd dogma" that *restraint is never necessary.*[15]

Lucett confronted the same ills of the formal medical system responsible for the insane and he did so earlier than Gardiner Hill and Connolly. Opposing restraint while promoting more humane treatment for the insane would not have been easy for most of the first half of the nineteenth century in the UK. So Lucett would inevitably have attracted hostile attention. He attacked the corruption and exploitation in the system as well as the continued use of restraint which meant that most contemporary asylums were places of danger, degradation and even of punishment for patients. He was self-serving, of course, because he had set up in opposition to the legally authorised system and that opposition was part of his branding. His voice was, however, one in the early groundswell of voices which argued that patients diagnosed as suffering from insanity needed and deserved better treatment. It did not matter that his voice was also one of a perjurer as was seen in the Fenn case. This is not a morality play on either the individual or the general level. Lucett was not a particularly admirable individual and he was certainly not part of some inevitable march of history towards a better future or on the practical level towards the inevitable perfection of the treatment of insanity. Lucett operated at a time when the 'unqualified' were able to make a significant contribution to improved care for the insane through asylum reform and better day-to-day care of patients. Perfection was certainly not achieved and still has not, but there was improvement.

George III's case provided the stimulus for a scientific response to the problem of effective treatment for the insane. The trial of the Lucett 'curative process' reflected both the needs of the single patient but also the impulse of the age to apply scientific methods. As a scientific trial for a psychiatric therapy it was the first. As a clinical trial of a medical remedy the Committee applied many of the criteria for judging Lucett's process which were to be used increasingly during the nineteenth century and into the twentieth and the outcome was appropriate as the final report endorsed empirical evidence in stating that the process was safe and useful even though it was not an outright cure for insanity. The Duke of Kent and his associates in the Committee understood the barriers which existed against any departure from accepted treatment for the insane in the case of the king. The Prime Minister, Spencer Perceval, had warned Lucett and Tardy of this in clear terms. It has also been clear that the so called 'mad doctors' were nevertheless regarded as a marginalised group who were barely respectable. The Committee experiment confronted these barriers directly. Respectability was essential and the Committee sought this through openness and publicity so that everything was explicitly above board and not to be feared. The scientific foundations of the experiment were also important in underpinning credibility.

The trial also demonstrated the limitations of scientific knowledge at the time. Dr Harness could honestly conclude that the Lucett treatment had a positive effect; he simply couldn't explain how this came about. The early nineteenth century was a period when there was an increasing impetus to apply science in medicine and this extended to the understanding of mental illness. Some practitioners such as Dr Andrew Harper and Thomas Arnold MD were both frustrated that post mortem dissection had been inconclusive in identifying physical manifestations of insanity. The exactly contemporaneous development of phrenology was an attempt to satisfy the need for a more scientific basis for predicting mental function in individuals. The use of the shape and measured contours of the skull provided a method of recording individual differences using the available technology of the age. This was to prove a dead end but again demonstrated the limitations imposed by the technology of the age. Science couldn't deliver at this time because the mental processes of patients were undetectable and could not be applied to the king's delusions or any other patient diagnosed as insane.[16]

The Committee had been looking for what was essentially an illusion. To use the cliché they were looking for the 'magic bullet' which would cure insanity in all its forms. It was done in the name of science and the Committee used scientific methodology to assess the Lucett curative process. The failure of the Committee to fulfil its original aims led to a tacit admission that there was no single remedy for insanity. The trial of the Lucett process had provided no revelation in the basic understanding of insanity itself. It had provided a useful therapy but not a cure all. It had also endorsed the perspective that insanity was a more complex problem involving not a single illness but several and that some of the conditions which were included within the definition of insanity were misplaced. Sir Alexander Halliday's statement which opens this chapter looks entirely complacent at first sight yet he pinpoints the fact that the true nature of insanity was still a mystery but that practitioners were developing therapies as the result of experience which helped. Halliday's comments could almost be an alternative conclusion for the final Committee report.

This could be seen in hindsight as the moment when psychiatry began as a separate discipline even if this was not directly driven by the Committee experiment. Psychiatry was to prove to be an inexact science precisely because the mental processes which led to the king's delusions could not be tracked. The doctors treating George III had to deal with the difficult question of determining when their patient's behavioural symptoms had achieved normality. The subjectivity involved in defining 'normality' was a problem for those caring for the king and remains a problem for psychiatry today. Over time psychiatry has developed away from the standards which the Committee and some contemporary practitioners were looking for and had to accept that there was no hard evidence for a psychiatric diagnosis. Observing patients and categorising behaviour is the key to psychiatric diagnosis. For the 'mad doctors' of the late Georgian period the search was for an identifiable treatment which would cure 'insanity' in a predictable scientific way. This was unrealistic and would continue to be so. But Dr Harness essentially encapsulated a genuinely psychiatric approach to the outcome of the Committee experiment. The Lucett process safely worked to some extent and it did not matter that Harness and Lucett didn't know why it worked. The important thing was to use it anyway as it brought real relief – even if it was temporary. Much modern psychiatry is based on practice and experience. 'If a treatment works use it! It is not necessary to understand why it works.'[17]

The probable conclusion over what practitioners in the early nineteenth century could realistically aspire to in managing patients was to provide the conditions in which an individual who suffered from any of the range of complaints which were included within the definition of 'insanity' at the time could recover naturally and spontaneously. The outrages practised on the patients at the York asylum which prompted the creation of The Retreat were not that and nor was the enforced solitary confinement of George III. The king was a special case, but the enforced treatment which he underwent was a precursor of the special legal status which the insane have so often experienced. Legally such patients and their family and friends have had to accept imposed treatment. In that sense George III and the royal family were like everyone else when a diagnosis of insanity is made. Fear of forced treatment was real then as it is now and may have been a driver in the actions of the Duke of Kent and his associates. Lucett was formally a quack but so too were all practitioners at the time. The record from Lucett's practice in Surrey is that he provided, at a price, the conditions of calm and respect which gave as good a chance of the patient self-healing as any and was all that any insane patient at the time could hope for. Certainly it was better than the treatment found at many celebrated asylums including Brislington House where John Perceval, the son of one of Lucett's eminent 'sponsors' suffered extended periods of restraint in 1831.[18]

Lucett would have become quite well known in his own time through his association with the experiment of the Committee, his writing, and perhaps infamous through his conflict with the law. There would have also been reminders of his existence from time to time by his critics who claimed he was a charlatan and a quack. Yet there is some evidence that Lucett was taken seriously enough in his own time for his practice to be included in some contemporary medical text books. An example is Dr Robert Thomas' *Modern Practice of Physic*.[19] A mystery remains, however. What started James Lucett the banker down the avenue of treating the insane? The story of the foreign doctor saved by Lucett's father was the kind of necessary fiction required to explain the career change once it had happened but does not really explain what set him off in that direction. The answer may lie in some archive unregistered and may be discovered in due course. But Lucett and his career as a pioneer in the humane treatment of the insane should be more widely known now; even if it is definitely a case of 'warts and all'. This is particularly the case in the UK where Lucett's rejection of mechanical restraint for insane patients was subsequently to become a defining characteristic of the psychiatric system. It is also perhaps right to give him the last word by quoting again from his letter to the Ewell Vestry in which he set out his attitude to his patients and with crystal clarity defined what an asylum really should have been. 'I shall never consider my residence a mad house or a place of Confinement, as never having occasion to use these unhappy means resorted to in public and private receptacles for lunatics and if I should be so fortunate as not to be more annoyed by the inhabitants of Ewell than they will be by anyone in my house I shall be perfectly satisfied with the results.'[20]

The Diagnosis of George III's Insanity

The king's case, Dr Robert Willis remarked, has 'never borne the characteristic of insanity; it never gets beyond derangement'. Dr William Heberden also questioned the king's diagnosis stating 'nor is it a common case of insanity'. These comments were made by Drs Robert Willis and William Heberden on George III's case when questioned by the Privy Council on 28th and 29th November 1810.[1]

During his adult life George III was recorded losing his reason during four bouts of illness. The first occasion was during 1788/9 with further short episodes in 1801 and 1804. The onset of the behavioural manifestations of illness during the illness of 1788/9 provided a kind of coherence for the otherwise bewildering range of physical symptoms which the patient displayed and allowed the physicians of the time to conclude that George was actually suffering from insanity. At this point, as set out in chapter one, the specialist 'mad doctor' Dr Francis Willis was brought in to take charge of the case. The final illness which began in 1810 was of a wholly different order in its intensity and magnitude to the earlier episodes. By this time the king's loss of reason was simply assumed to reinforce the earlier diagnosis of insanity. Yet the professional perception of the king's case was a little more nuanced as the two comments above made by doctors who were treating the king during his last illness indicate. The simplicity of Dr Heberden's comment that it was no 'common case of insanity' encapsulates the unease which some contemporary doctors felt. The meaning of 'common' at the time and in context would have included the ideas of ordinary or regular. Dr Robert Willis, a specialist in treating the insane, went further and directly expressed doubt about the correctness of the king's diagnosis of insanity. In the absence of a viable alternative assessment of the symptoms of organic disease or a more refined definition of insanity, the limitations of Georgian medicine meant that it was inevitable that George would continue to be treated for insanity as it was understood at the time. It is worth bearing in mind that a range of illness and behavioural manifestations were included in the definition of 'insanity' during George III's lifetime which would not be included now. The king's case and his treatment have continued to exercise a fascination ever since and have led to refinements of the original diagnosis as well as complete reassessments of the king's illnesses made by later historians and physicians.

The record of George III's case made during his lifetime has, for the most part, continued to underpin subsequent attempts to refine the diagnosis of the king's illness in the light of advances in medical knowledge. This has been possible because the behavioural evidence is crucial to making any diagnosis of mental illness. The key contemporary assessment was made by Dr Francis Willis in evidence to a parliamentary committee at the end of 1788. 'That from the particular detail of His Majesty's mode and manner of life for 27 years, I do imagine, that weighty business, severe exercise, and too great abstemiousness, and little rest, has been too much for His Constitution'.[2] Willis' view therefore was that the king suffered a mental breakdown in response to the pressures imposed on him by his constitutional role and his family life. This view was perfectly reasonable within the parameters of his time. However while the behavioural manifestations of illness and their importance in diagnosing insanity have not significantly changed over the intervening time the capacity to determine underlying organic disease has changed fundamentally.

Dr Isaac Ray, an American doctor who specialised in the treatment of the insane, is credited with a more refined diagnosis in 1855. Ray took the view that the behavioural disturbances which George III suffered, rather than any physical symptoms, were the dominant manifestation of his illness. He concluded that the king had suffered from 'acute mania' and had therefore been insane.[3] It is perhaps an indication of how far treatment of the insane had developed that Ray commented on the use of restraint on the king that, 'There was nothing in his condition which would be considered at the present time a sufficient reason for its application'.[4] In view of the later assertions that George III suffered unbearable stress due variously to the pressures of business or his family life, Ray's comment 'Insanity had never appeared in his family and he was quite free from those eccentricities and peculiarities which indicate an ill-balanced mind' is important.[5]

Dr Arnold Chaplin, half a century later, would refine Ray's assessment of George III's illness. 'It was a case of delusional insanity attended by mania followed by periods of melancholia.'[6] The highlighting of melancholia is significant as the problem from the perspective of the physicians actually attending the king had been mania. Melancholia seems only to have been a significant behavioural manifestation of the extended period of seclusion during the king's final illness when George turned in on himself and had periods of withdrawal. Nevertheless this new emphasis fed through into later historical re-evaluations. The assessment also did nothing to question the basic diagnosis of insanity. The focus on mania had been consistent during George III's illnesses and had continued in commentaries thereafter.

The assessment of George's illness was taken to an extreme in 1941 in Manfred Guttmacher's *America's Last King*. Guttmacher concluded that George III had suffered from 'manic depressive psychosis'[7] or bipolar disorder as it is now called. In simple terms Guttmacher argued that George had not been up to the job of running country and growing empire and his mind had given way under the strain. The physical symptoms, which the king undoubtedly displayed, were dismissed as inventions of the court to cover the terrible truth of mental illness. The king himself was even implicated in the process by the claim that he 'was trying to delude himself into viewing his illness as primarily physical'.[8] There must be considerable doubt that the king was actually party to any supposed conspiracy as he admitted 'I prayed to God all night that I might die, or that He would spare my reason'.[9] George was in no doubt of the acute danger to his sanity which his illness implied and, despite Guttmacher's claims to the contrary, was prepared to say so. The problem with Guttmacher's dismissal of the physical symptoms which the king undoubtedly suffered from and which were consistent in each instance when he lost his reason is that it limits any assessment of a possible diagnosis of the king to a behavioural one which predisposes to the conclusion of some form of mental illness. In favour of Guttmacher's focus on bipolar disease is that sufferers often experience long periods with minimal symptoms as was the case with George III.

The impact of Freudian analysis in due course fed through into the assessment of George's illness with alleged sexual frustration becoming the claimed explanation for the king's mental breakdowns. Richard Pares was quoted in chapter one referring to George's 'resolute fidelity to a hideous Queen'.[10] This perspective gathered accretions over the years until it was summarised in 1999 as, 'Until a few years ago the general opinion was that it was a form of manic depressive psychosis brought on perhaps by the frustration felt by a man naturally highly sexed but married to a woman he had never wanted to marry and, despite their numerous offspring, never able to satisfy his sexual appetite.'[11] It seems odd that this perspective gained such currency given that the decision on who George should marry was made without external pressure on him.

This endorsement of the basic assumption that the king had suffered from periodic bouts of insanity continued until 1964 when Charles Chenevix

Trench published an account of the onset of the problem which concentrated on the illness of 1788/89 and the political implications of the Regency Crisis. Despite examining some previously overlooked primary source material in the diaries of Sir George Baker, who had been the king's principle physician in 1788, Chenevix Trench did not challenge the orthodoxy of George III's assumed insanity.[12]

The fundamental change in the assessment of George III's illness came in January 1966 with the publication in the British Medical Journal of *The 'Insanity' of King George III: A Classic Case of Porphyria* written by Drs Macalpine and Hunter.[13] Their paper, followed in 1969 by their book, *George III and the Mad-Business*, analysed and assessed both the physical symptoms recorded by the many doctors who had been responsible for the care of the king during his illnesses and the behavioural aberrations which they recorded. The conclusion of Macalpine and Hunter was that George III had suffered from a form of porphyria, a rare metabolic disease which while physical in its origins can have a severe psychological impact. Formally, they argued, the king had not been insane.

This revolutionary re-evaluation of George III's illness and the conclusion that he had not been insane went to the core of the assumptions about the king which had held sway for 150 years. The re-evaluation sparked a renewed interest in the king's reign as well as a renewed debate on the nature of the king's illness. Perhaps more significantly Macalpine and Hunter's re-assessment of the king's illness began to alter the popular perception of his illness. For the first time since George's own lifetime there was a move away from the simple perspective that he had been insane and that this defined his character and reign. Some writers have attempted to re-impose bipolar disease as the orthodoxy for explaining George's illness. An example is the recent focus on the change in the syntax and vocabulary of his writing when he was suffering serious illness. To this author however the impact of the deterioration in the king's eyesight is a more likely explanation for the radical change in his handwriting and the more abbreviated syntax.[14] Most of the debate has been serious and some has even been humorous, but some has not. Surprising heat has been generated and Macalpine and Hunter have come in for harsh criticism from some. One academic paper includes the comment about them, 'They also sought to remove "the taint of madness" from the House of Windsor for which they hoped to be appropriately rewarded'. There seems to be no evidence that they were rewarded - appropriately or otherwise![15]

Diagnosis of historical illness is extremely difficult and it is very often impossible to arrive at any categorical conclusion. At best historical diagnosis can arrive at some degree of hypothesis. The medical knowledge of even the best practitioners of George III's time was incredibly limited compared with practitioners to-day. The diagnostic tools available then were incomparably limited when set against what is available now. The stethoscope, for example, was only fitfully coming into use by physicians at the time of George's final illness. Indeed Sir Henry Halford, who was the king's principle physician and was later President of the Royal College of Physicians, did not use the stethoscope even when it became increasingly common to do so.[16]

While George's physicians were arguably the best available at the time their perspective was necessarily limited by the knowledge and the tools at their disposal and by the obvious diagnosis which they had to hand which was that the king was insane. They will have recorded what they regarded as significant within the limits of their knowledge and their diagnostic tools will have limited the range of symptoms which they could pick up on. Information which did not fit the diagnostic parameters of the day would almost certainly have been missed or discarded so that the record of the king's illness which the physicians did conscientiously put down may not represent a comprehensive picture of what would have been observable at the time. So although his illness must, without doubt, be one of the best documented cases of 'insanity' ever made, there can be no certainties in any historical diagnosis of George III's complex illnesses. There will always be an element of the subjective. The best hypothesis at the moment seems to this writer to be that he did suffer from a form of porphyria. Even so, account would still need to be taken of the probability that he also displayed some manifestations of the impact of his treatment during his extended last illness. After the relapse and the crisis of late 1810 the king was subjected to years of regular dosing with opiates and medicines containing heavy metals as was recorded in chapter eight. This would almost certainly have had a toxic impact on George. He was also kept in effective isolation for years; an isolation which was made more profound by his blindness. While it would be easy to argue that such treatment of the king would have had an impact on his behaviour there is no way in which the extent of such an impact could be judged now. He was also old by the standards of his time and may well have suffered from some form of dementia but again it is only possible to speculate on whether this was the case and if it was what degree of impact it might have had.

Ultimately it seems highly unlikely that a certain historical diagnosis of George III's illness can ever be made simply on the basis of the documentary record from the period of his reign and that a degree of hypothesis will always remain however well a protagonist for a particular diagnosis may argue. Indeed some commentators seeking an historical diagnosis may have been motivated in part by considerations beyond the immediate focus on the tribulations of George III. Even Macalpine and Hunter for example were concerned that the separation of psychiatry from the rest of medical practice meant that the consequent separation of diseases of the mind could overlook origins in physical illness.[17] The case of George III therefore had an additional importance for them as it seemed to exemplify the separation between purely behavioural and physiological illnesses. Their concern is hugely important. Modern psychiatry begins only when organic disease has been excluded as an explanation for behavioural change in patients. Behavioural manifestations of mental illness may be recognisably the same whether recorded in Georgian times or now, but the capacity to assess organic disease now is incomparably more sophisticated than it was when George III was on the throne. The problem with all the subsequent attempts to produce an historical diagnosis of George III's illnesses is that they are entirely reliant on the records from the eighteenth and early nineteenth centuries. What would be needed to make a definitive assessment of the king's case and to justify the dependence on the record of the behavioural manifestations on their own would be to deploy modern scientific capabilities to eliminate underlying organic disease as an explanation for behavioural change.

It is just possible that the question of George III's illness could be settled scientifically and a case which ironically has a direct familial connection provides a pointer. When the remains of the Russian royal family were rediscovered in Yekaterinburg some years ago DNA analysis not only demonstrated that the remains were indeed those of the murdered Russian royal family but also enabled individuals within the family group to be identified. It proved possible to clarify that Alexei carried the very rare B form of haemophilia and that he would have inherited it from his mother Tsarina Alexandra. The daughters of Alexandra would have had a 50/50 chance of being carriers of haemophilia like their mother.[18]

Some commentators have claimed that Alexandra displayed the symptoms of porphyria during her lifetime and that the linkage for both haemophilia and porphyria goes back to Queen Victoria and possibly to her father the Duke of Kent.[19] If it was possible to test the genetic material from Yekaterinburg for porphyria then a familial link to George III and his illness would potentially be established. A conclusive determination whether George suffered from a form of porphyria would depend on the technology being available to test material which it could be proved came from the king.[20] Such an investigation would potentially determine whether an underlying physiological illness, and in particular porphyria, could be eliminated so that George's illnesses could be judged with some justification by the behavioural evidence alone.

In chapter eight, evidence that George III probably suffered from chronic arsenic poisoning was presented, based on the analysis of a sample of the king's hair. That sample of hair could not be tested for porphyria however because it had been respectfully cut from the dying monarch. Had it been pulled out literally with the roots it would in principal have included the right tissue to test for porphyria and the nature of the king's illness could perhaps be finally laid to rest.

Appendix

The Committee Members

The list of the members of the Committee 'who have undertaken to make enquiry into, and the extent of the process practiced by Messrs Delahoyde and Lucett' were recorded on the first page of the first report of the Committee. WWM/F64 in the Sheffield Archives is the copy which came from the records of Earl Fitzwilliam. Other copies exist in the Lambeth Palace Library for example.

The fifteen Committee members comprised the core of the men who supported the trial of the Lucett curative process. There was a wider group of individuals who supported the therapeutic trial and they were referred to as 'Subscribers'. A list of the subscribers is in WWW/F64 and included such varied individuals as Henry John Temple, Viscount Palmerston who was later to become Prime Minister and Sir Thomas Bernard who was educated at Harvard and founded the 'Society for Bettering the Condition of the Poor' in 1796. He was also the treasurer of the Foundling Hospital in London and an active promoter of vaccination.

As might be expected the Committee and subscribers can loosely be described as members of the 'establishment', but that encompassing term would not do justice to the range of people involved. It was not, of course, a mass organisation, but within the total of 35 contributors at the beginning there were representatives of the old landed aristocracy but also the new aristocracy of manufacturing. The political spectrum was covered with Whigs as well as Tories represented. This was not simply a case of supporters of the king doing what they could for their leader and should not be compared with modern political donors. A more unifying thread of thinking was a belief that the world could be improved and that science could contribute to finding answers to problems. So the names of several of the participants appear in other contexts where they showed a willingness to support what can be termed 'good causes'. The age range of participants included contemporaries of the king, but also encompassed the younger generation.

Short biographical notes on the Committee members are set out below.

His Royal Highness Edward Duke of Kent.
Fourth son of George III and Queen Charlotte, he was not apparently very highly esteemed by his father. He lived abroad for much of his adult life including a relatively happy period in Canada. He was constantly in debt and this caused friction with his father. He lived with Madame de Saint-Laurent for 27 years, but ended the relationship so that he could marry. This followed the death of Princess Charlotte in 1817 who was the only legitimate heir to the throne. The union produced the future Queen Victoria and it is for this that the duke is principally remembered. He was a straight forward character who did not engage in the distractions of gambling and excess alcohol.

His Royal Highness Augustus Duke of Sussex.
The sixth son of George III and Queen Charlotte. His marriage to an older woman when he was 20 and in defiance of the Royal Marriages Act caused a breach in relations between father and son. The marriage was declared null and void by the Privy Council although ironically it produced a male child who would otherwise have been the legitimate heir following the death of Princess Charlotte in November 1817. Sussex, like many of his siblings, lacked a fulfilling role throughout his life. His involvement in the Committee trial was perhaps an indication of his better qualities.

Lord Dundas.
Lord Dundas had been a Whig member of parliament for most of his adult life before being elevated to the peerage in 1794. He was no aristocrat however, despite his wealth. His father had been a trader when he was young and had made a great deal of money supplying the needs of the British army. A Fellow of the Royal Society Dundas took a direct interest in the application of steam power to ships.

Earl Fitzwilliam.
William Wentworth, 4th Earl Fitzwilliam was one of the richest men in the UK who derived his fabulous income not just from the traditional resources of a great landowner but from the rapid expansion of coal mining on his estates in Yorkshire. A political liberal on some issues, Fitzwilliam had sided with the American colonists in their confrontation with the British Government and had been dismissed in 1795 from his position as Lord Lieutenant of Ireland when he tried to end the Protestant Ascendancy and to achieve Catholic Emancipation. In the bitter aftermath of his dismissal Fitzwilliam was on the point of engaging in a duel when a magistrate ran onto the field and arrested him. Ironically in view of Fitzwilliam's involvement in the Committee an

element in his removal from Ireland was George III's view that ending the Protestant Ascendency there would run counter to his coronation oath to uphold the Protestant faith. After the 'Peterloo Massacre' in 1817, Fitzwilliam called for an enquiry and opposed the use of military force in a civil process. Surprisingly perhaps Fitzwilliam opposed electoral reform proposed by Earl Grey, which brought him into disagreement with his son Lord Milton.

Lord Milton.
Son of Earl Fitzwilliam who succeeded him as the 5th Earl. He was a strong and active supporter of electoral reform in Britain and specifically the 1832 Reform Act which widened the franchise.

The Hon. Lawrence Dundas.
Son of Lord Dundas, the Hon Lawrence Dundas MP, whose election expenses at York had apparently been covered by Fitzwilliam. [WWM/ F48/115-189]

Sir Joseph Banks, Bart.
Sir Joseph Banks the explorer, naturalist and President of the Royal Society was an outstanding scientist of the day. George III consulted him on scientific subjects, while Queen Charlotte used him as an advisor on her active involvement with Kew Gardens which had been founded by her predecessor, Caroline of Ansbach, wife of George II. Queen Charlotte was also a friend of the Banks family.

John Harness, MD.
Dr John Harness was no society physician and was not a member of some august family who might expect an impressive inheritance which would have placed him amongst the ranks of the very wealthy. He was a former naval surgeon who had worked for a living and had worked to improve the professionalism and status of the physicians who worked for the navy. In 1813 he was the medical officer at the Transport Office of the Admiralty which was responsible for naval and marine sick and infirm. The presence of Lord Melville First Lord of the Admiralty on the Committee was important as he would play an important role in underwriting Harness' role in the Committee activities.

John Dent, Esq.
John Dent was head of the Worcester glove makers and future owner of Sudeley Castle. He was also a shareholder in Child & Co, bankers to the

Committee, and a highly respected institution at the time. Child & Co is the oldest bank in the UK although it is now part of the Natwest group.

Thomas Smith, Esq. Alderman.
Thomas Smith was a wine merchant who had risen in the ranks of the city of London's management to become the Lord Mayor of London in 1809 and was still an Alderman of the city in 1813. He became a public health reformer and went on to found the Health of Towns Association in 1839.

Viscount Melville.
He was briefly First Lord of the Admiralty in 1804, a position he returned to in 1812 – 27 and again in 1828 – 30. He sat in the House of Lords from 1811 when he succeeded his father and sat on various Royal Commissions. He had a long standing interest in science and became a Fellow of the Royal Society in 1817.

Duke of Bedford.
The 6th Duke of Bedford was perhaps a more conventional member of the aristocracy, but he was not entirely predictable in the sense that he was a Whig politician, who had been briefly Lord Lieutenant of Ireland like Fitzwilliam, but who opposed British involvement in the Peninsula War.

John Julius Angerstein, Esq.
With his Russian birth and unclear family background, he would have brought an element of the exotic with him to the Committee. But his wealth, derived in part as the driving force behind the development of Lloyds insurance market in London and his connoisseurship which meant that his collection of paintings would form the core in the foundation of the National Gallery collection, would have ensured that he was in his element with the other members of the Committee. In any case he lived close to Lord Dundas in Pall Mall so was a familiar figure in the St James' area.

Richard Clark, Esq. Chamberlain.
An attorney, he became wealthy through marriage to an heiress from the woollen trade. He was made Lord Mayor of London in 1785.

Earl Cork.
Edmund Boyle the 8th Earl of Cork was perhaps a more politically conservative example of the aristocracy. He was a career soldier who became an aide de camp of George III in 1798.

Number 19 Arlington Street, the venue for the first meeting of the Committee in 1813, was a great aristocratic townhouse in St James' which had been built in 1732. At the time of the Committee meeting it was the London residence of the Dundas family and remained in the family until its demolition in 1936. *Country Life* magazine, in its issue of 17th September 1921, ran an article on the house which included photographs of the exterior and the interior. The architectural drawings made by Robert Adam during the 1760s are the only record of how the interior would have been in 1813. [Sir John Soane Museum Online.]

Acknowledgements

This book would not have been written without the initial impetus given me by my younger son Nicholas. 'I think there are some loose ends which you might like to explore' was the gentle fly he cast over me and which soon had me hooked. He had done a Masters in the history of medicine between the pre-clinical and clinical parts of a medical degree and in the process had discovered James Lucett. How seriously he was concerned about my ability to cope with impending retirement is not clear, but a strong dose of George III and Lucett was what he prescribed.

The other early influence was the eminent psychiatrist Griffith Edwards with whom I had lunch and who had the grace to take me seriously when I said I wanted to research and write a book related to early psychiatry. 'Don't start with too many preconceptions' was his advice. 'Let the story take you where it will.' So I discovered the world of archives and original documents populated with knowledgeable enthusiasts who were never anything other than welcoming and helpful as I followed the story from Lambeth Palace library to Cumbria archives via Leicester and Rutland, Sheffield and many others. I looked for and found excuses to spend time in the incomparable British Library and treated the Wellcome Library almost as my club. So good are the records in the UK and so well are they kept that I was almost resentful when a line of enquiry seemed to come up against a blank. As a resource for creativity the system of libraries and archives in the UK deserves nurturing rather than salami slicing to meet immediate budgetary needs and I can only express my gratitude as a newcomer for being encouraged to use that resource when it was in good order.

The danger in following a story 'where it will' is to continue indefinitely in the vain hope of achieving something called 'completion'. My wife Jan was instrumental in shifting my focus from the rather indulgent pleasure of researching to the discipline of actually writing. As the drafting advanced I was lucky to have Nick Foster as a friend. He not only encouraged me in my endeavours but demonstrated a talent for editing and had a vital impact in recommending how the distinct stories of the treatment of George III's 'madness' and the imperfect career of James Lucett as a clinician or 'quack' could be integrated.

I owe a debt of gratitude to my daughter in law Helen and through her to Professor Michael Clarke who drew the attention of Lester Crook, as commissioning editor, to my completed manuscript. It was Lester who made the transition from manuscript to publication possible. I am very grateful to Lester, to Harriet Fielding and the Pen and Sword team for turning aspiration into reality.

Without the encouragement of my wife, family and friends this project would not have happened or reached publication. I am grateful to them all for putting up with my almost obsessive fascination for George III and the story I was developing over several years; even if for the most part I have not named them. I will make an exception of Caroline Ball who is both a writer and editor and whom I have quizzed mercilessly on the arcane mysteries of the world of publishing. My one regret is that there is no magic process which could turn my enthusiastic effusions into 'deathless prose'. So I shall have to stand by what I did write and to accept the responsibility which is ultimately and entirely mine.

Bibliography

Archival Sources

British Library

Willis Papers: MS 41733F, MS 41733G, MS 41734, MS 41735, MS 41736, MS 54202, MS 54203 to 6, MS 54204.

MS 41695 Dr Robert Willis to Queen Charlotte.

MS 58868 Dropmore Papers.

MS 38283 Vol XCIVff161 Lord Liverpool.

MS 88883/1/57A. Memorandum Giving an Account of the Death of the Duke of York in 1827. Written by Col Taylor.

Harcourt Papers. The edition available in the British Library is one of 50 printed in 1925. This was a six volume edition edited by Edmund William Harcourt. It is not therefore a comprehensive collection of the letters and for the most part the letters are in fact extracts only. The originals are in the Bodleian Library.

Lambeth Palace Library

MS 2107 to 2139 cover the involvement of the Archbishop of Canterbury in his capacity as chairman of the Queen's Council in the management of the illness of King George III.

Sheffield City Archives

Wentworth Woodhouse Muniments. Papers of William Wentworth-Fitzwilliam, 4th Earl Fitzwilliam [1748-1833] WWM/F64.

Leicester and Rutland Record Office

Halford MSS. Correspondence of Sir Henry Halford.

Surrey History Center

'Chertseyana' 1827.

'Visits of Magistrates to Lunatic Asylums'

'Vestry Minutes of Ewell Church.'

Goulburn Papers.

Cumbria Archives

The records in the Cumbria Archive of the correspondence between Dr John Willis and Lord Lonsdale are listed under DLONS/L1/2/33.13/6/13 as 'Collection of 60 unbound letters'.

Royal College of Physicians

'The Royal Sufferer - or letters on the malady of the Sovereign' held by the Royal College of Physicians under barcode 36959.

Committee Meeting dated 5/2/1830. RCP Register of Committee Meetings – page 176.

Bank of England
Bank of England House List dated 25th April 1797.
Directors' Minutes.

Bethlem Hospital Archives
Admissions Registers, Bethlem Incurable Patient Admission Registers and Case Books.
  ARA-15, ARB-01, ARA-07 and ARA-18.

London Metropolitan Archives
Metropolitan Commissioners in Lunacy records August 1830 to August 1831.
Sun Insurance Company records.

National Archives. Kew
C/13/860/32 Page V Lucett. Two Bills and Two Answers. 1825 and 1826.
HO 17/82/94 Criminal Petition in the case of Peter Fenn. 1828.
C 13/2945/6 Lucett V Lomax.
South Australia Maritime Museum. Passengers in History.
Wellcome Library. London.
Sir John Soane's Museum Collection Online.
1841 England, Wales and Scotland Census.

Primary Sources
Anon. *Quacks and Quackery. A remonstrance etc*. A Medical Practitioner. 1844. Wellcome
  Library.
Anon. *The Quackery of the Medical Profession*. 1846.
Adair, Dr James Makittrick. *Medical Cautions: Chiefly for the consideration of invalids etc*. 1787.
Aspinall, Arthur. *The Later Correspondence of King George III*. 1962.
Aspinall, Arthur. *The Correspondence of George Prince of Wales, 1770–1812*. 1963.
Aspinall, Arthur. *The Letters of King George IV. 1812–1830*. 1938.
Arnold MD, Thomas. *Observations on the nature, kinds, causes and prevention of insanity*. 1806.
Bakewell, Thomas. 'Letter to the Chairman of the House of Commons Select Committee on
  Madhouses.' Wellcome Library.
Balbirnie, John. Letter from *Water Cure and Hygiene Magazine* 1848.
Belcher, William. *Belcher's Address to Humanity*. 1796.
Buckingham and Chandos, Duke of *Memoirs of the Court of England during the Regency 1811
  to 1820*. London 1856.
Browne, Dr William. *What Asylums Were, Are and Ought to Be*. 1837.
Burrows, George Man. *An inquiry into certain errors relative to insanity etc*. 1820.
Burrows, George Man. *Commentaries on Insanity*. 1828.
Chambers, Neil. [Editor] *The Letters of Sir Joseph Banks. A Selection 1768–1820*.
Clarke, Sir Arthur. *An Essay on Warm Cold and Vapour Bathing*. 1827.
Connolly, John. *The Treatment of the Insane Without Mechanical Restraints*. London. 1856.
Courteney, Francis Burdett. *Revelations of Quacks and Quackery* a series of letters by "Detector".
  10th edition. 1885.
Cox, Joseph Mason. *Practical Observations on Insanity etc*. London 1813.
Croker, Margaret Sarah. *Monody on His Late Royal Highness the Duke of Kent*. 1820.
Dunne, Dr Charles. *Brand's Lunacy Case etc*. 1831.
Edinburgh Medical and Surgical Journal. Volume 10, page 251.
Ellis, William Charles. *Treatise on the nature, symptoms, causes and treatment of insanity*. 1838.
Este, Michael Lambton. "On Baths, Water, Swimming, Shampooing etc." London. 1812.

McKno Bladon, Frank. [Editor] *The Diaries of Colonel the Honorable Robert Fulke Greville.* 1930.

Granville, Countess [Editor] *Lord Granville Leveson Gower, Private Correspondence 1781-1821.* London 1917.

Hallaran, William. *An Enquiry into the Causes Producing the Extra-ordinary Addition to the Number of Insane.* 1810.

Halliday, Sir Alexander. *A General View of the Present State of Lunatics and Lunatic Asylums in Great Britain and Ireland.* London. 1827.

Haslam MD, John. *Observations on Insanity.* London 1798.

Haslam MD, John. *Considerations on the Moral Management of Insane Persons.* London 1817.

Harper, Dr Andrew. *A Treatise on the real cause and cure of Insanity, etc.* London 1789.

Healde, Thomas. *The New Phamacopoeia.* 1788.

Robert Gardiner Hill. *A Lecture on the management of Lunatic Asylums and the Treatment of the Insane.* Published 1839.

Robert Gardiner Hill. *A concise history of the entire abolition of mechanical restraint etc.* Published 1857.

Huish, Robert. *The public and private life of His late excellent and most gracious Majesty, George the Third, etc.* London. 1821.

Jesse, John Heneage. *Memoires of the Life and Reign of King George the Third.* London 1867.

Jerningham, Frances. *The Jerningham Letters 1780-1843.* London. 1896.

Kassler, Michael. [Editor] *Memoires of Charlotte Papendiek.*

Knight, Miss Cornelia. *Autobiography of Miss Cornelia Knight.* Third Edition. Edited by Sir J W Kaye.

Lady Knighton [Editor]*Memoirs of Sir William Knighton, Bart.* 1838.

Laing, William. *An account of the new cold and warm sea baths at Peterhead etc.* 1804.

Lucett, Edward. *Rovings in the Pacific, from 1837 to 1849; with a glance at California.* 1851.

Lucett, James. *Exposition of the Reasons which have prevented the process for relieving and curing idiocy and lunacy and every species of insanity from having been further extended.* London. 1815.

Lucett, James. *Address to a Candid and Impartial Public.* London. 1822.

Lucett, James. *A Statement of Facts Relevant to the Nature and Cure of Mental Diseases.* London. 1833.

Lucett, James. *La Folie.* Published in Paris 1838 by Duverger. Copy in the National Library of France.

Morison, Alexander. *Outlines of lectures on mental diseases.* Edinburgh 1825.

Neal, Erskine. *The Life of His Royal Highness, Edward, Duke of Kent etc.* 1850

Pargeter, William. *Observations on Maniacal Disorders.* 1792.

Childe-Pemberton, William Shakespeare. *The Romance of Princess Amelia Daughter of George III (1783-1810) Including Extracts From Private and Unpublished Papers.* 1911.

Poole, Dr Richard. *Memoranda regarding the Royal Lunatic Asylum, Infirmary and Dispensary of Montrose with observations on some other institutions of a like nature and an appendix of documents partly relating to Restraint in the treatment of insanity.* 1841.

Prichard, James Cowels. *A Treatise on Insanity and other Disorders Affecting the Mind.* 1837.

Ray, Dr Isaac. *Insanity of King George III.* Read before the Association of Superintendents of Insane Hospitals – 22nd May 1855.

Report from the Committee appointed to examine the physicians who have attended His Majesty during His illness etc. Ordered to be printed 13th January 1789. Note the report is reprinted in various formats and the pagination varies with each version.

Rose, George. *Diaries and Correspondence of the Right Hon George Rose.* Edited by L V Harcourt. London 1860.

Rowley, William. *Truth Vindicated; or, the specific differences of mental diseases ascertained.* 1790.

Rowley, William. *The Rational Practice of Physic.* 1793.

Sedgewick, Romney. [Editor.] *Letters from George III to Lord Bute. 1756 to 1766.* 1939.

Sharpe, James Birch. *Report together with the Minutes of Evidence, and an appendix of Papers, from the Committee appointed to consider provision being made for the better regulation of Madhouses in England and Ordered to be printed 11th July 1815. Each subject of evidence arranged under its distinct head by J B Sharpe.* London. 1815. Note. The House of Commons ordered the original publication of the results of their enquiries on 11th July 1815. However they did so in such small numbers and in a series of pamphlets that it is unlikely that they would have survived as a coherent whole if Sharpe had not gathered them at the time and made them available in a bound reprint. The background as well as Sharpe's compendium are available in the British Library.

Sharpe, James Birch. *Elements of Anatomy; designed for the use of Students in the Fine Arts.* 1818.

Shelford, Leonard. *A Practical Treatise on the Law Concerning Lunatics etc.*

Sutleffe, Dr Edward. *Essay on Insanity or mental Aberration.* 1827.

Thomas, Robert. *Modern Practice of Physic.* 1824.

Tuke, Samuel. *Description of the Retreat near York.* 1813.

Turton MD, William. *Treatise on Cold and Hot Baths with Directions for their Application in Various Diseases.* 1803 in a private edition. Wellcome Library.

Twiss, Horace. *The Public and private Life of Lord Chancellor Eldon.* London 1846.

Uwins, Dr David. *A treatise on those disorders of the brain which are usually considered and called mental.* 1833.

Ward, Robert Plumer. *Memoirs of Robert Plumer Ward.* Edited by Edmund Phipps. 1850.

Williams, John W. *Essay on Sea Bathing.* 1820.

Withers, Philip. *History of the royal malady, with variety of entertaining anecdotes etc.* 1789. British Library reprint.

Wheatley, Henry Benjamin. [Editor] *The Historical and Posthumous Memoirs of Sir Nathanial Wraxall.* London 1884.

Philip Yorke. [Editor.] *The Letters of Princess Elizabeth of England Daughter of King George III etc.* London 1898.

London Gazette.

London Medical Repository.

Journal of Mental Science Volume 14.

London Medical Gazette. Volume 7.

Medical and Physical Journal.

Monthly Magazine.

British Newspaper Archive at the British Library.

Victorian Review Volume 22 No1 Summer 1996.

Secondary Sources

British History Online. Survey of London.

Oxford Dictionary of National Biography.

Acres, W. Marston. *Bank of England from Within.* Vol. 2. 1931.

Arnold, Catharine. *Bedlam. London and Its Mad.* 2008.

Baker, Kenneth. *George III. A Life in Caricature.*

Bewley, Thomas. *Madness to Mental Illness. A History of the Royal College of Psychiatrists.* 2008.

Brooke, John. *King George III.*

Bryne, Paula. *Perdita. The life of Mary Robinson.* 2004.

Burns, Tom. *Psychiatry: a very short introduction.*

Carter, Harold Burnell. *Sir Joseph Banks*. 1988.

Chaplin, Arnold. *Medicine during the reign of George III*. 1927.

Crainz, Franco. *The life and Works of Matthew Baillie*. 1995.

Edwards, Griffith. *Matters of Substance. Drugs and Why Everyone's a User*. 2005.

Fraser, Flora. *Princesses. The Six Daughters of George III*. 2004.

Glover, Michael. *A Very Slippery Fellow. The Life of Sir Robert Wilson 1777-1849*. 1977.

Guttmacher, Manfred. *America's Last King. An Interpretation of the Madness of George III*. 1941.

Hadlow, Janice. *The Strangest Family. The Private Lives of George III, Queen Charlotte and the Hanoverians*. 2014.

Hibbert, Christopher. *George III. A Personal History*. 1998.

Hilton, Boyd. *A Mad, Bad, and Dangerous People? England 1783-1846*. 2006.

Hunter, Richard and Macalpine, Ida. *Three hundred years of psychiatry 1535 – 1860: a history presented in selected English texts*. 1963.

Macalpine, Ida and Hunter, Richard. *George III and the Mad-Business*. 1969. [Pimlico Edition of 1991 used for references.]

Macalpine, Ida and Hunter, Richard. *Some Effects of the Royal Malady on the development of Psychiatry*. History of Medicine Volume 1. 1968/9.

Munk, William. *The Life of Sir Henry Halford*. 1895.

Parry-Jones, Edward. *The trade in lunacy; a study of private madhouses in England in the eighteenth and nineteenth centuries*. 1972.

Porter, Roy. *Mind Forg'd Manacles*.

Porter, Roy. *Quacks Fakers and Charlatans in Medicine*.

Porter, Roy. *Flesh in the Age of Reason*.

Porter, Roy. *Bodies Politic. Disease, Death and Doctors in Britain, 1650-1900*.

Priestley, J B. *The Prince of Pleasure and His Regency*.

Ronson, Jon. *The Psychopath Test*. 2011.

Rohl, Warren and Hunt. *Purple Secret. Genes, "Madness" and the Royal Houses of Europe*. 1998.

Rushton, Alan. *Royal Maladies: Inherited Diseases in the Ruling Houses of Europe*. 2008.

Samuel, Ian. *An Astonishing Fellow*. 1985.

Sellar, W C and Yeatman, R J. *1066 and All That*. 1961.

Shelford, Leonard. *A Practical Treatise on the Law Concerning Lunatics etc*.

Smith, E A. *George IV*. 1999.

Watson, J Steven. *The Reign of George III 1760-1815*. 1960.

Wise, Sarah. *Inconvenient People. Lunacy, Liberty and the Mad-Doctors in Victorian England*. 2012.

Articles and Academic Papers

The Lancet. 1996. Page 1811. Wilfred Niels Arnold.

The Lancet. 2005 Issue 9482. July 23rd-29th. Vol. 366. Pages 332-335. *King George III and Porphyria: an elemental hypothesis and investigation.'* Author: Timothy M Cox et al.

Mad King George: The Impact of Personal and Political Stress on Mental and Physical Health. Dean, Keith Simonton. University of California, Davis. 1998.

In Search of Personality: Reflections on the Case of King George. Read and Nasby. *Journal of Personality* 66-3 June 1998.

Charles Palmer (1777-1851) Soldier, Politician, Vineyard Owner and Theatre Proprietor. Brenda J Buchanan. *Journal of the Society for Army Historical Research* Vol 90, No 361. Spring 2012.

Non-restraint and Robert Gardiner-Hill. Frank, J. Bulletin of the History of Medicine. Vol 41. [1967] page 144. Johns Hopkins.

Madness and Poor Wretches: Changing Perceptions of Madness in Early Nineteenth Century London. Sarah McCance. 2004.

King George III, bipolar disorder, porphyria and lessons for historians. Timothy Peters. Clinical Medicine 2011, Vol 11, No 3: page 262.

Porphyria – A Royal Malady. British Medical Journal. 1968. Macalpine, Hunter, Rimington, Brooke and Goldberg.

Infantile Convulsions in the early nineteenth century etc. Brigo, F. el al. July 2018.

Maddening business of King George III and Porphyria. Trends in Biochemical Sciences 21, Pages 229 to 34. [1996] Warren, Martin et al.

Diagnosing the dead: the retrospective analysis of genetic diseases. A R Rushton. In Journal of the Royal College of Physicians, Edinburg. 2013.

The Shorthand of Robert Willis, Physician-in-Extraordinary to King George III. Timothy Underhill and Timothy Peters. Electronic British Library Journal. Article of 2018.

Notes and References

The references to the newspaper articles in the main text include the title and date. These can all be accessed in the British Newspaper Archive at the British Library or many local libraries. Many of the genealogical sites on the internet, such as Find My Past, also include access to newspaper archives. For the most part the newspaper articles are not included in the references below. Exceptions are where the newspaper articles reprint official statements or documents. The style for titles of publications in the eighteenth and nineteenth centuries was for long descriptive pieces. In the references below sufficient to identify the titles is given, but where the titles were very long 'etc' is used to signify that the full title is longer. The complete title of such works is in the bibliography.

Introduction
1. Sir Alexander Halliday. *A General View of the Present State of Lunatics and Lunatic Asylums in Great Britain and Ireland.* London 1827.
2. *Memoires of Charlotte Papendiek. Late 1788.* Page 146.
3. *The Letters of Sir Joseph Banks. A Selection 1768–1820.* Edited by Neil Chambers.
4. Introduction to *An inquiry into certain errors relative to insanity* etc. George Mann Burrows. 1820.
5. Ibid.
6. *George III and the Mad-business.* Ida Macalpine and Richard Hunter. Pimlico edition – page 167.

Chapter One: Assuming His inheritance
1. *The First Four Georges.* J. H. Plumb. Page 97. 1956.
2. See *Letters of George III to Lord Bute. 1756 – 1766.* Edited by Romney Sedgwick.
3. Ibid. Letter 47 dated to winter 1759–60.
4. Ibid. Letter 47.
5. Ibid.
6. Ibid. Letter 48 dated to winter 1759–60.
7. *King George III and the Politicians.* Richard Pares. 1953. Page 65. It is perhaps worth quoting Pares perspective at greater length as it seems extraordinarily judgemental: 'Perhaps his madness can best be explained as the breakdown of a too costly struggle to maintain this official character – the reserve and equanimity imposed upon a hot temper and anxious nerves, to say nothing of his resolute fidelity to a hideous queen, and a regime of violent exercise and exaggerated abstinence designed to counteract strong passions and a tendency to fat.'
8. Quote from Horace Walpole – see *The Strangest Family* Janice Hadlow, page 149. Walpole was not a commentator who was noted for his generosity so his assessment of Charlotte was significant.
9. The period from mid-October to mid-November 1788 was apparently when George III first lost his reason. Both Chenevix Trench in *The Royal Malady* and Macalpine and

Hunter in *George III and the Mad Business* both had access to Sir George Baker's private diary for the period 17th October to 7th November which was then in the possession of Sir Randle Baker Wilbrahim.

10. *The Diaries of Colonel the Honorable Robert Fulke Greville.* Edited by Frank McKno Bladon. 1930.

11. Lady Harcourt and her husband were private friends of George and Charlotte and the people in whom the royal couple had the greatest confidence. Lady Harcourt was also a surrogate grandmother for many of the royal children.

12. *Practical Observations on Insanity.* Joseph Mason Cox pages 62/3.

13. *Observations on Maniacal Disorders.* William Pargeter. 1792.

14. *Practical Observations on Insanity.* Joseph Mason Cox.

15. See *Memoirs of the Years 1788 and 1789.* Harcourt. Also see Robert Fulke Greville – *Diaries* as above.

16. *The Diaries of Colonel the Honorable Robert Fulke Greville.* Edited by Frank McKno Bladon. See also *The Strangest Family* which has an excellent extended account of the king's treatment of his wife during his first illness.

17. See *George III and the Mad-Business.* Page 89. Also the Countess of Pembroke to George III, 8th April 1789 in *The Later Correspondence of George III.* 1962. Edited by A Aspinall.

Chapter Two: The Onset of the Crisis

1. *Memoires of the Life and Reign of King George the Third.* John Heneage Jesse. 1867.

2. *Diaries and Correspondence of the Right Hon George Rose.* Edited by L V Harcourt. London 1860.

3. Buckingham Papers Volume IV.

4. *Autobiography of Miss Cornelia Knight.* Third Edition. Edited by Sir J W Kaye Vol 1. Pages 174–5.

5. Princess Elizabeth to Lady Harcourt dated 9th November 1810. Harcourt Papers IV.

6. *George III. A Life in Caricature.* Kenneth Baker. The original quotation comes from the Harewood MSS and is longer than the one in *A Life in Caricature.*

7. *The public and private life of His late excellent and most gracious Majesty, George the Third, etc* Robert Huish. 1821 London.

8. Ibid.

9. DG24/822/3. Leicester and Rutland Records Office.

10. DG24/822/4+5.

11. DG24/822/5 Princess Mary to Sir Henry Halford.

12. John Heneage Jesse. *Memoires of the Life and Reign of King George the Third.* Also in a fuller version in *The Diaries and Correspondence of Charles Abbot, Lord Colchester.*

13. Ibid , quoting Lord Colchester.

14. Ibid.

15. W. H. Freeman to the Marquis of Buckingham 2nd November 1810 and W.H. Freeman to Earl Temple, 11 November 1810, quoted in *George III and the Mad-Business* pages 145 and 6.

16. *George III and the Mad-Business.* Page 144.

17. Jesse. Reference for 1 November 1810.

18. Jesse. Reference for 11 November 1810.

19. Ibid.

20. Ibid.

Chapter Three: Specialists or Generalists?

1. Add MS 54202 Willis Papers Vol I – stuck to the inside cover. British Library. However, this doggerel appears in several versions and is usually entitled, *King's Doctors*. It is a fine example of the popular view of the time that seeing a doctor was potentially more dangerous than not.

2. DG24/831/1. Leicester and Rutland Records Office.

3. *George III and the Mad-Business* pages 132–3.

4. Dr Robert Darling Willis quoted in *George III and the Mad Business* page 275.

5. *Report together with the Minutes of Evidence, and an appendix of Papers, from the Committee appointed to consider provision being made for the better regulation of Madhouses in England and Ordered to be printed 11th July 1815. Each subject of evidence arranged under its distinct head by J B Sharpe.* James Birch Sharpe. London. 1815.

6. MS 41734 Folio 18. Willis Papers. British Library.

7. MS 41734. Folio 18.

8. MS 41734 Folio 23.

9. MS 41734 Folio 25.

10. MS 41734 Folio 28.

11. *What Asylums Were, Are and Ought to Be.* Dr William Browne 1837.

12. MS 41734. Entry for 28th November 1810.

13. MS 41734. Entry for 28th November 1810. It is not clear whether Robert Willis took down his own and his colleagues' views during the meetings or whether he simply copied the official record. The latter seems the more likely.

14. *George III and the Mad-Business.* Page 150.

15. Ibid. Although the *Examination of the physicians attending His Majesty*, which was the official record of the questioning of the physicians by the Privy Council and is quoted from page 150 of *George III and the Mad-Business*, Dr Robert Willis kept his own record which is in MS 41734 in the British Library for the appropriate dates. Unfortunately he did not add his own gloss of the proceedings.

16. RCIN 1047014 Robert Fulke Greville MSS Volume II October 1788–4th March 1789. Royal Library Windsor. Copyright HM Queen.

17. *Journals and Letters of Fanny Burney* (Madame D'Arblay) for 2nd February 1789, but quoted in *The Insanity of King George III* by Dr Isaac Ray as part of his historical re-assessment of the king's illness. See the Afterword.

18. See page 508 of *The Strangest Family* which in turn quotes Princess Sophia's views from page 206 of *Princesses* by Flora Fraser. The original source of Sophia's conflicting views about the change in her father's personality brought on by illness – even during convalescence – is in her correspondence with Theresa Villiers in early December 1804 held in the Royal Archives at Windsor.

19. See A Aspinall. Volume V of *Correspondence of George Prince of Wales.* Also see *The Strangest Family* Janice Hadlow page 508.

20. MS 54202 for 27 January 1811 for example. Willis Papers. British Library.

21. MS 41695 Folios 93/6. Willis Papers. British Library.

22. MS 54202 for 8 and 9 February 1811.

23. See *An Astonishing Fellow* by Ian Samuel or *A Very Slippery Fellow* by Michael Glover for background of Wilson's attacks on Bonaparte as well as biographies of this colourful character.

24. See A Aspinall. Volume V of *Correspondence of George Prince of Wales,* memorandum 1958, for the account of Wilson's visit to Weymouth and his contacts with George III. The incident of 1st October recounted by Sir Robert Wilson was also used by Manfred Guttmacher in his book *America's Last King.* Although the general sense of both versions

is the same unaccountably his version is markedly different from that collected by Aspinall. Guttmacher's version is as follows, 'The King commenced the conversation whilst taking some Papers out of a green box by observing "Mrs Deas, you look very well, very well indeed, Dear lovely Mrs Deas, what a pretty ass you have got. How I should like to pat (this word is more decent than the one he actually used and which would not bear repetition) such a pretty ass"'. See *America's Last King*.

Chapter Four: Regency

1. *A treatise on those disorders of the brain which are usually considered and called mental.* Dr David Unwins. 1833. Page 234.
2. *Memoirs of Robert Plumer Ward* Edited by Edmund Phipps. 1850. Entry for 11th January 1811.
3. Ibid. Entry for 15 January 1811.
4. Ibid. Entry for 18 January 1811.
5. Ibid. Plumer Ward quoting Croker 21st January 1811.
6. Ibid. Plumer Ward quoting Perceval 27th January 1811.
7. Horace Twiss. *The Public and Private Life of Lord Chancellor Eldon.* Vol 2 p162.
8. MS 54202 for the appropriate dates. Willis Papers. British Library.
9. *Diaries and Correspondence of the Right Hon George Rose.* Edited by L V Harcourt Volume II page 477 and MS 54202.
10. *Memoires of Robert Plumer Ward.* Entries for 2nd and 3rd February 1811.
11. Ibid and *Morning Chronicle* of 1st February 1811.
12. Add MS 58868 Folio 43. Dropmore Papers. British Library.
13. MS 54204 for 5th February 1811. Willis Papers. British Library.
14. *Memoirs of the Life and Reign of King George the Third.* John Heneage Jesse. London 1867.
15. Walpole letters Vol iii p437 1857.
16. See A Aspinall (ed) *The Correspondence of George Prince of Wales, 1770–1812.* Volume V pages 6–7 of the introduction in which Aspinall quotes Lady Bessborough.
17. Lord Grenville to Earl Temple in *Memoirs of the Court of England, during the Regency 1811 to 1820.* Duke of Buckingham and Chandos 1856. Volume I page 50. Also replayed in Jesse for March 1811.
18. See MS 54202 for 3 April 1811.
19. MS 2107 Folio 21. Lambeth Palace Library.
20. MS 41734 Folio 77 of 9 March 1811. Willis Papers. British Library.
21. MS 41734 Folio 74
22. MS 2107 Folio 21.
23. *Mad King George: The Impact of Personal and Political Stress on Mental and Physical Health.* Dean Keith Simonton University of California, Davis 1998 and *In Search of Personality: Reflections on the Case of King George.* Read and Nasby. *Journal of Personality* 66–3 June 1998.
24. MS 54202 for 30 March 1811. Willis Papers. British Library.
25. MS 41736 Folios 17 and 18. Willis Papers. British Library.
26. MS 2107 Folio 84 of 20 April 1811.
27. MS 54202 for the relevant dates.

Chapter Five: Relapse

1. MS 2110 Folio 141. Lambeth Palace Library.
2. MS 41734 Folio 105 dated 27 April 1811. Willis Papers. British Library.
3. MS 41734 Folio 106 dated 11 May 1811.
4. MS 54202 entry for 5 May 1811. Willis Papers. British Library.
5. MS 2107 Folio 45. Lambeth Palace Library.

6. 304/A1/2/1/8 Surrey Archives/History Centre. The paper is filed with the GOULBURN family papers of Betchworth under the personal papers of Henry Goulburn [1784–1856].
7. MS 2107 Folio 41.
8. MS 2107 Folio 50.
9. MS 2107 Folio 64.
10. MS 2107 Folio 50.
11. MS 41734 Folio 136.
12. MS 41734 Folio 136.
13. *The Strangest Family* page 79.
14. MS 2110 Folio 141. Lambeth Palace Library.
15. There is a reference in MS 54202 for 30th May 1811 to Mr Penlington taking charge of the new attendants responsible for the king.
16. MS 2110 Folio 139.
17. *Correspondence of George Prince of Wales* Volume VIII, 3099. Edited by Arthur Aspinall.
18. *The Letters of Princess Elizabeth of England etc.* Yorke, P C. Editor.
19. *Correspondence of George Prince of Wales*, Vol VIII, 3113.
20. *Correspondence of George Prince of Wales*. Vol VIII, 3120.
21. *Princesses. The Six Daughters of George III*. Flora Fraser. Page 255.
22. DG 24/835/30. Leicester and Rutland Records Office.
23. DG 24/835/31 for all the quotes in this paragraph. Leicester and Rutland Records Office.
24. *The Life of Sir Henry Halford*. Dr William Munk. Page 147.
25. *The Public and Private Life of Lord Chancellor Eldon*. Horace Twiss.
26. *Correspondence of George Prince of Wales*. Vol VIII, 3128.
27. 152M/C1804/OR12 of 15 February 1804 in the Devon Archives is a copy of the decision to bring in one of the Willis brothers to take over responsibility for treating the king.
28. *Correspondence of George Prince of Wales*. Edited by Arthur Aspinall. Volume IV. Letter 1806 dated Monday Night 13 February 1804.
29. MS 2107 Folio 100.
30. *Correspondence of George Prince of Wales*. Vol VIII 3128.
31. The most explicit statement lies in *George III and the Politicians* Richard Pares 1953 page 65. However, the theme was replayed subsequently by other writers and in its origins reflects contemporary comments on Queen Charlotte's coldness.
32. MS 2107 Folio 102.
33. William Black. Letter to the editor of the *Morning Chronicle* dated 8 December 1788.

Chapter Six: Bringing in the Specialists

1. DG 24/835/31. Sir Henry Halford probably to the Prince Regent dated from June or July 1811. Leicester and Rutland Records Office.
2. The summary is in MS 2110 folio 153. Lambeth Palace Library.
3. See also MS 41735 folio 3 of 4 August 1811. Willis Papers. British Library.
4. MS 2107 Folio 104. Lambeth Palace Library.
5. MS 2107 Folio 106.
6. 'nervous debility' was increasingly seen during the first third of the nineteenth century as meaning a fear of impotence. It was classified as "mens' secret disease" and was associated with quack medicine. See *Nervous Debility: A Disorder Made To Order* Judith Knelman. *Victorian Review* Vol 22 No1 Summer 1996.
7. John Willis to Lord Lonsdale – Cumbria Archives. Note. The records in the Cumbria Archive are listed under DLONS/L1/2/33.13/6/13 as 'Collection of 60 unbound letters'.
8. John Willis to Lord Lonsdale of 5/8/1811.
9. John Willis to Lord Lonsdale of 23/9/1811.
10. MS 2107 Folio 123.

11. MS 3011 Folio 49 of 13 August 1811. Royal College of Physicians.
12. MS 2107 Folio 158.
13. MS 2107 Folio 168.
14. MS 2107 Folio 118.
15. DG 24/862/20. Leicester and Rutland Record Office.
16. DG 24/835/30.
17. MS 41733F Folio 10. Willis Papers. British Library.
18. MS 41733G. Willis Papers.
19. MS 41733G.
20. MS 41733G.
21. MS 2107 Folio 186.
22. MS 41733 G.
23. MS 2107 Folio 188.
24. MS 2108 Folio 244.
25. MS 2107 Folio 194.
26. MS 2107 Folio 196 of 18th September 1811.
27. MS 2110 Folio 153.
28. *Correspondence of George Prince of Wales* Vol VIII 3185.
29. *The Life of Sir Henry Halford etc.* Dr William Munk – page 146.
30. MS 41733G.
31. John Willis to Lord Lonsdale of 9/10/1811. See under DLONS/L1/2/33.13/6/13.
32. MS 2108. There is a series of folios dated in November 1811 which cover questions and answers between the Queen's Council and the Specialists. Lambeth Palace Library.
33. MS 2107 Folio 258.

Chapter Seven: Confinement
1. Dr Andrew Harper *A Treatise on the real cause and cure of Insanity, etc* London 1789.
2. MS 2108 Folio 5. Lambeth Palace Library.
3. MS 2108 Folio 15.
4. *Memoirs of the Court of England, during the Regency.* Volume 1. Page 145.
5. John Heneage Jesse. *Memoires of the Life and Reign of King George the Third.* Volume 3 entry for 25 October 1811.
6. *The Letters of Princess Elizabeth of England etc.* Yorke P C. Also see Princess Elizabeth to Lady Harcourt 24 October 1811 in the *Harcourt Papers.*
7. Lady Bessborough to Granville Leveson Gower dated 22 December 1811. The italics are Lady Bessborough's. *Lord Granville Leveson Gower, Private Correspondence 1781–1821.* Edited by Countess Granville.
8. MS 2110 Folios 182–205. Lambeth Palace Library.
9. MS 2110 Folio 206.
10. MS 2108 Folio 52 and DG24/835/33. Lambeth Palace for the first reference, Leicester and Rutland Records Office for the second.
11. Dr John Willis to Lord Lonsdale. 9 February 1812. See under DGLONS/L1/2/33.13/6/13. Cumbria Archives.
12. MS 2108 Folio 57 of 15 February 1812.
13. MS 2108 Folios 63–68.
14. DG 24/835/32. Leicester and Rutland Record Office.
15. DG 24/835/32 and postscript.
16. MS 41736 Folio 25.
17. MS 2108 Folio 82.
18. DG 24/835/34 Princess Mary to Sir Henry Halford. The letter is undated but from the context is from late Spring of 1812. Leicester and Rutland Record Office.

19. *The Life and Works of Matthew Baillie.* Page 142.
20. DG/24/834/15.
21. MS 2108 Folio 89.

Chapter Eight: What orthodox "medicine" meant for the King

1. George Mann Burrows, *An Inquiry into certain errors relative to insanity etc.* 1820.
2. MS 41735 folio 3 and MS 2110 folio 153 both dated 4 August 1811. British Library and Lambeth Palace Library respectively. The paragraph quoted is part of a longer original document contained in the two folios, but is conveys the essentials of the general practitioners account for the specialists.
3. See Dr Weir's testimony in *Report together with the Minutes of Evidence, and an appendix of Papers, from the Committee appointed to consider provision being made for the better regulation of Madhouses in England and Ordered to be printed 11th July 1815. Each subject of evidence arranged under its distinct head by J B Sharpe.* London 1815. See entry for J. B. Sharpe in the bibliography.
4. MS 41736. Willis Papers. British Library.
5. *Considerations on the Moral Management of Insane Persons.* John Haslam. London 1817. Page 31.
6. *Observations of the Physician and Apothecary of Bethlem Hospital upon the Evidence taken before the Committee of the Hon House of Commons for Regulating Madhouses.* London 1816. See entry for J B Sharpe in the bibliography.
7. Thomas Healde's *The New Phamacopoeia* of 1788 is an example. Royal College of Physicians.
8. William Pargeter, *Observations on Maniacal Disorders* 1792. Page 64.
9. Ibid. Page 63.
10. MS 41736 Folio 13.
11. *The Letters of George IV*, Volume I. Letters 310 and 312. Arthur Aspinall editor.
12. *The Lancet* 2005 Issue 9482. July 23–29. Vol. 366. Pages 332–335. *King George III and Porphyria: an elemental hypothesis and investigation.* Author: Timothy M. Cox et al. See MS 54203–54206 for daily doses. Willis Papers. British Library.
13. MS 41733G.
14. MS 2108 Folio 52 postscript. Lambeth Palace Library.
15. Andrew Harper. *A treatise on the real cause and cure of insanity, etc.* London 1789. Page 57.
16. MS 41733G. Willis Papers. British Library.
17. MS 41735 Folio 145.
18. Dr Edward Sutleffe. *Essay on Insanity or mental Aberration.* 1827.
19. *The Treatment of the Insane Without Mechanical Restrains.* John Connolly. London 1856 pages 205–6.
20. *Report together with the Minutes of Evidence, and an appendix of Papers, from the Committee appointed to consider provision being made for the better regulation of Madhouses in England and Ordered to be printed 11th July 1815. Each subject of evidence arranged under its distinct head by J B Sharpe. John Birch Sharpe.* London. 1815.
21. Andrew Harper. *A treatise on the real cause and cure of insanity, etc.* London 1789. Page 61.
22. *Brand's Lunacy Case etc.* Dr Charles Dunne. 1831. Pages 14–15.

Chapter Nine: A New Approach to Insanity

1. *The Letters of Princess Elizabeth of England etc.* Letter to Lady Harcourt dated 11th October 1811. Phillip Yorke. Editor. 1898.
2. Bank of England House List dated 25 April 1797. E20/6.
3. The painting is in the National Gallery, Washington DC. Painted in 1778 by John Singleton Copley it sets out the dramatic rescue of Brook Watson from a shark in Havana harbour.

4. 1841 Census records his birth as 'about 1771'.
5. Bank of England E41/8.
6. British History Online. Survey of London Volume 24, Chapter 12, Somers Town.
7. *The Letters of Princess Elizabeth of England etc.* 26 October 1811. Philip Yorke. Editor. 1898.
8. DG24/834/3. Leicester and Rutland Records Office.
9. Bethlem Admissions Registers, Bethlem Incurable Patient Admission Registers and Case Books. ARA-15, ARB-01 and ARA-07.
10. MS11936/413/689475. London Metropolitan Archives.
11. James Lucett, *Exposition of the Reasons which have prevented the process for relieving and curing idiocy and lunacy and every species of insanity from having been further extended.* London. 1815.
12. Ibid. Page 10.
13. Ibid. Page 15.
14. Ibid. Page 11.
15. Add. MS 38283 Vol XCIVff161. British Library.

Chapter Ten: Concern for the House of Hanover?

1. The last two lines of *Monody on His Late Royal Highness the Duke of Kent* by Margaret Sarah Croker. 1820.
2. DG 24/835/36 dated 11 June 1811. Leicester and Rutland Records Office.
3. *King George III.* John Brooke. Pages 314/5. This is one of the many similar accounts of the incident.
4. *The Letters from George III to Lord Bute. 1756–1766.* Edited by Romney Sedgwick.
5. *Harcourt Papers.* Volume IV. Lady Harcourts account of the king's views on insanity are in pages 12 to 16. And *King George III.* John Brooke. Also *Letters from George III to Lord Bute. 1756–1766,* Sedgwick. London 1939.
6. *An inquiry into certain errors relative to insanity and their consequences: physical, moral and civil.* George Mann Burrows. 1820 pages 9 and 10.
7. *Lord Granville Leveson Gower, Private Correspondence 1781–1821.* Editor Countess Granville, London 1917. Volume 2. Page 421.
8. *Practical Observations on Insanity etc.* Dr Joseph Mason Cox. 1813.
9. Quoted from *George III and the Mad Business* page 259 which was in turn translated from records in Niedersachsiche Staatsarchiv, Hanover.
10. *Later Correspondence of George III.* A. Aspinall editor, page 493.
11. *The Correspondence of the George Prince of Wales* Volume V in the letter series as 1958. Noted by Aspinall as 'A copy, in McMahon's hand.' McMahon was the Prince of Wales' private secretary. Sir Robert Wilson was a Whig sympathiser but also a monarchist. He would have been concerned at anything which undermined the prestige of the Crown. In his public statements Wilson always presented himself in the best possible light. He could also be indiscreet. His account from Weymouth was private and has clear internal indications of discretion being exercised.
12. Ibid. Letter 3285 of 14 December 1811.
13. *Memoirs of Sir William Knighton,* Bart. Vol I page 285.
14. *The Authentic Medical Statement of the Case of HRH the Late Princess Charlotte Of Wales with some Observations.* Dr Anthony Tod Thompson. Extracted from the 48th Number of *London Medical Repository* published on 1 December 1817.

Chapter Eleven: Psychiatry's First Therapeutic Trial

1. William Rowley in *Truth Vindicated etc.* 1790. 2. Sir John Soane's Museum Collection Online.

2. Sir John Soane's Museum Collection Online.
3. WWM/F64/193. Wentworth Woodhouse Muniments, Sheffield Archives.
4. WWM/F64/216.
5. *Monthly Magazine* of 1 June 1813.
6. *George III and the Mad Business*. Page 167.
7. WWM/F64/193. Page 2.
8. ADM 105/23. National Archives, Kew.
9. Testimony to the House of Commons Committee given by Dr Monro dated 19 May 1815.
10. Testimony to the House of Commons Committee given by Mr Haslam. Page 123.
11. Testimony to the House of Commons Committee given by Dr Harness on 6 June 1815.
12. Bethlem Admissions Register ARA-15.
13. Account in the *Monthly Magazine*. Volume 35 No 241, dated 1 June 1813.
14. MS 2109 Folio12. Lambeth Palace Library.
15. MS 2109 Folio 21.
16. *Edinburgh Medical and Surgical Journal*. Volume 10, page 251.
17. Royal College of Physicians, card index under 'Harness'.
18. MS 2109 Folio 95.
19. MS 2111Folio 37. Lambeth Palace Library.
20. MS 2111 Folios 41 and 42.
21. MS 2109 Folio 2 for the document actually shown to the physicians.
22. See MS 2111 folios 43 to 53 for the doctors' responses.
23. MS 2111 Folio 35.
24. MS 2109 Folio 33.
25. MS 2109Folio 33.
26. MS 2109 Folio 25.
27. WWM/F64/196.
28. MS 2109 Folio 33.
29. MS 2109 Folio 15.
30. MS 2109 Folio 41.
31. WWM/F64/199.
32. MS 2109 Folio 43.
33. *Medical and Physical Journal*. Volume 30 July/December 1813. Pages 124 to 128.

Chapter Twelve: The Trial Continues

1. *General View of the present state of Lunatics and Lunatic asylums in Great Britain and Ireland and some other kingdoms.* Sir Andrew Halliday, London 1828. Page 75.
2. WWM/F64/200. Sheffield Archives.
3. WWM/F64/201.
4. WWM/F64/202.
5. *Harcourt Papers*. Volume IV. See also *Sir Joseph Banks* by Harold Burnell Carter – page 448.
6. WWM/F64/203 dated 25 August 1813.
7. The vicar at the time was Charles Daubeny who was active in the area and had endowed an 'asylum' for four elderly men. In this instance, however, the word asylum indicated alms houses for the elderly rather than for the insane.
8. MS 2109 Folio 45 dated from the Transport Office on 30th August 1813. Lambeth Palace Library.
9. *Medical and Physical Journal*, No 177, pages 433–6.
10. *Infantile Convulsions in the early nineteenth century etc.* Brigo F. *et al* July 2018.
11. See *The Royal Sufferer – or letters on the malady of the Sovereign* held by the Royal College of Physicians under barcode 36959.

12. MS 2109 Folio 47.
13. MS 2109 Folio 49.
14. MS 2109 Folio 51.

Chapter Thirteen: Things Fall Apart

1. WWM/F64/189. Sheffield Archives.
2. MS 2109 Folio 2 and WWM/F64/189.
3. WWM/F64/216. Letter from John Dent to Earl Fitzwilliam dated 27 April 1815. Attached is a further letter from Alderman Thomas Smith to Dent in which he explains the circumstances of September 1813 when Lucett and Delahoyde admitted that a writ for debt had been issued against them and that Smith had advanced £200 to keep the pair from jail in order to keep the therapeutic trial going. In 1815 he had still not been reimbursed.
4. QS 2/6/1813/MIC/33. Surrey History Centre.
5. WWM/F64/205.
6. WWM/F64/206.
7. WWM/F64/207.
8. WWM/F64/208 folios 1 to 3.
9. WWM/F64/209.
10. Testimony given to the House of Commons Committee on 5 May 1815 by Dr John Weir.
11. MS 11936/413/689475. London Metropolitan Archives.
12. ADM 105/28. National Archives, Kew.
13. WWM/F64/211.
14. WWM/F64/212.
15. WWM/F64/191.
16. WWM/F64/212.
17. ADM 102/23.
18. ADM 105/22 Transport Board Medical Committee. In letter book – Dr Weir.
19. ADM 105/28 of 13th November 1812. National Archives, Kew.
20. *King George III*. John Brooke. Page 385.

Chapter Fourteen: Lucett. A New Career

1. W. H. O. Sankey MD. Presidential Address, *Journal of Mental Science* Vol 14, page 297. 1868.
2. WWM/F64/214. Sheffield Archives.
3. Bank of England. Directors' minutes. See Court of Directors Minutes 1814–15 pages 63 and 101.
4. WWM/F64/215.
5. James Lucett. *An Exposition of the reasons which have prevented the process for relieving and curing idiocy and lunacy and every species of insanity from having been further extended.* 1815. Radcliffe Science Library, Oxford. [Part of the Bodelian Library.]
6. *Exposition* page 3.
7. Ibid page 4. The capitals and italics are Lucett's.
8. Ibid pages 5 and 6.
9. Ibid page 10.
10. Ibid page 13.
11. Ibid page 15.
12. Ibid page 16.
13. Lucett's italics. *Exposition* page 16.
14. Ibid page 17.

15. Ibid page 18.
16. WWM/F/64/216.
17. *Exposition* page 26.
18. Ibid page 63.

Chapter Fifteen: 'Insanity Cured Without Confinement.'
1. *A concise history of the entire abolition of mechanical restraint etc.* Robert Gardiner Hill. 1857.
2. See *Chertseyana* 1827 a contemporary scrapbook of Chertsey held by the Surrey History Centre which includes a line drawing of Weston House.
3. *Morning Post.* 2nd December 1817.
4. See Joseph Mason Cox' *Observations on Insanity etc* of 1813 for an exactly contemporary perspective of excess blood in the brain producing mania.
5. QS 5/5/4 *Visits of Magistrates to Lunatic Asylums* for 21 March 1815. Surrey History Centre.
6. Ibid. 11 July 1815.
7. Ibid. 9 February 1816.
8. *Outlines of Lectures on mental diseases.* Published in Edinburgh 1825 by Sir Alexander Morison.
9. *George III and the Mad-Business.* Page 308.
10. QS5/5/4 *Visits of Magistrates to Lunatic Asylums.*
11. Epiphany 1819 III Folio 90. QS/2/6. Surrey History Centre.
12. See *Treatment of the Insane without mechanical restraint.* John Connolly. London. 1856.
13. LMA-P90/Pan1/79. London Metropolitan Archives.
14. Minutes of Vestry of Ewell Church. 3831/1/1 1770 to 1830. Surrey History Centre.
15. Ibid.
16. QS5/5/4 *Visits of Magistrates to Lunatic Asylums.* Surrey History Centre.
17. QS5/5/4.
18. *Mind Forg'd Manacles.* Page 225. Roy Porter.
19. Add MS 38283 Vol XCIV folio 161. British Library.
20. Add MS 38283 Vol XCIV folio 213.
21. Hume Tracts. Held by University College London Library.
22. QS 5/5/4.
23. *Jackson's Oxford Journal.* 2 August 1823.
24. See Financial Accounts for the Magistrates Visits to Lunatic Asylums for December 1824. These are bound in to the end of QS 5/5/4. Surrey History Centre.
25. QS 5/5/4 for 14 October 1825.
26. Hume Tracts. Held by University College London Library.
27. *Morning Post* for 22 August 1823.

Chapter Sixteen: Ruin and Recovery
1. Andrew Duncan MD Senior quoted in *Some Effects of the Royal Malady on the development of Psychiatry* – Ida McAlpine and Richard Hunter. *The History of Medicine.* Volume 1 – 1968/9.
2. *George III and the Mad-Business.* Pages 295/6.
3. Surrey Burials 1813–1861. Page 32. 2374/1/10. Surrey History Centre.
4. *London Gazette* for 1824. Page 901.
5. QS/5/5/4 for 14 October 1825. Surrey History Centre.
6. Affadavit of W A Rocher. Dated 18 December 1828. The dispute between Lucett and others in the case of the asylum in Mitcham is filed under C13/860/32. National Archives Kew.

7. C13/860/32. Dated 22 December 1825.

8. C13/860/32. Dated 22 December 1825.

9. C13/860/32. Dated 11 January 1826.

10. *Morning Post* for 9 February 1826. Kirke's Nursery was a well-established nursery which seems to have specialised in fruit trees with a purple plum named after the proprietor. Its heyday was in the eighteenth century but it was still a successful business when Lucett began his association with the place.

11. Attachment to HO17/82/94 in the National Archives Kew.

12. *Morning Post* for 23 February 1828.

13. The *Examiner* 14 September 1828.

14. Ibid.

15. HO 17/82/94. Letter from James Chapman dated 28th November 1828. National Archives, Kew.

16. HO 17/82/94.

17. The papers covering the petitions for clemency are un-numbered within 'Criminal Petition – Peter Fenn'. HO 17/82/94. National Archives, Kew.

18. *London Gazette*. 1828 Page 2436.

Chapter Seventeen: Taking on the Medical Establishment

1. *Treatise on Insanity and other Disorders of the Mind*. James Cowles Prichard. 1837.

2. MS 88883/1/57A. "Memorandum Giving an Account of the Death of the Duke of York in 1827." Written by Col Taylor. British Library.

3. *George III and the Mad-Business*. Page 259.

4. *London Medical Gazette*. Volume 7. 25 December 1830.

5. Royal College of Physicians Committee Meeting dated 5/2/1830. RCP Register of Committee Meetings – page 176.

6. *Mind-Forg'd Manacles*. Roy Porter. Page 153.

7. Metropolitan Commissioners in Lunacy records August 1830 to August 1831. London Metropolitan Archives.

8. *A Practical Treatise on the Law Concerning Lunatics etc*. Leonard Shelford. Page 482.

9. Survey of London Volume 42, Chapter X – Hereford Square Area: The Day Estate.

10. *Treatise on the nature, symptoms, causes and treatment of insanity*. William Charles Ellis. 1838.

11. A picture of the house is in the Orleans House Gallery, Twickenham.

12. Introduction to *Rovings in the Pacific etc*. Edward Lucett. 1851.

13. C 13/2945/6. National Archives, Kew.

14. The *Sun*. 31 January 1834 and other newspapers.

15. *A Statement of Facts Relevant to the Nature and Cure of Mental Diseases*. James Lucett. 1833. Hume Tracts. Held by University College London.

16. *Belcher's Address to Humanity*. William Belcher 1796. Page 8.

17. *The Lancet*. 3 May 2014.

18. See *Inconvenient People* by Sarah Wise for an account of John Perceval's plight. Chapter Two.

Chapter Eighteen: Back on the Campaign Trail

1. Letter to the governors of Bethlem Hospital from General Palmer dated 9th October 1835 from Clarges Street. Reprinted in full on 14 October 1835 by the *Sun* newspaper and other 'papers.

2. *Charles Palmer (1777–1851) Soldier, Politician, Vineyard Owner and Theatre Proprietor*. Brenda J Buchanan. Journal of the Society for Army Historical Research Vol 90, No 361. Spring 2012.

3. Letter to the governors of Bethlem Hospital from General Palmer dated 9th October 1835. Reprinted in the *Sun* newspaper on 14 October.

4. Bethlem Admissions and case notes for Ellen Mack. ARA-18 for 22nd May 1835. Bethlem Royal Hospital, Archives and Museum Department.

5. *Evening Mail* of 11th September 1835 and other papers.

6. Recorded in the Sub-Committee meeting of Bethlem Hospital reported in the *Morning Post* of 24 September 1835 and *London Evening Standard*. 26 September 1835.

7. See the *Sun*, London, Wednesday October 14th 1835 and other newspapers which reprint Palmer's letter in full.

8. Admissions and patient casebooks register Bethlem. ARA-18.

9. The Sun. 14 October 1835.

Chapter Nineteen: A Sorry End

1. Page 513 of the 8th American edition of *The modern practice of physic etc.* by Robert Thomas, 1825, quoting the impact of the Lucett treatment of mania as related by Mr Tardy.

2. *La Folie*. Published in Paris 1838 by Duverger. Copy in the National Library of France. NUMM-5463124.

3. Ibid.

4. Ibid.

5. FO 687/8. National Archives, Kew.

6. 1841 census H107/1050/9.

7. *Camberwell*. Volume 4 page 43.

8. *Rovings in the Pacific, from 1837 to 1849; with a glance at California*. Edward Lucett. 1851.

9. Passengers in History. South Australia Maritime Museum.

10. Church of England Marriages, St Mary Newington. 1820–25. Page 131 certificate 392 of 17 July 1824.

11. Register of Deaths for the Parish of St Giles, Camberwell. 19th March 1851.

Chapter Twenty: George III the Last Years

1. *The Royal Sufferer – or letters on the malady of the Sovereign*. Charles Dunne. Royal College of Physicians. Barcode 36959.

2. MS 2108 Folio 52. Lambeth Palace Library.

3. MS 2132 Folio 143. Lambeth Palace Library.

4. *The Letters of Princess Elizabeth of England etc.* Yorke ed. P.88.

5. Ibid.

6. *Journals and Letters of Fanny Burney* (Madame D'Arblay) Volume VII. Letters 632–834. Edited by Edward and Lillian Bloom. 1978. Letter 694 dated 14 May 1813.

7. *The Letters of Princess Elizabeth of England etc.* Yorke P. C. Letter dated 20th October 1814.

8. Ibid.

9. Quotations from page 385 of *King George III* by John Brooke. References are to letters written to the Prince Regent by Queen Charlotte and Princess Mary in the Royal Archives series.

10. *The Gentleman's Magazine*. December 1818, page 559.

11. References in this paragraph are from MS 2139 for the dates. Lambeth Palace Library.

12. *The Life of Sir Henry Halford*. Dr William Munk. Page 146.

13. *King George III*. John Brooke. Page 385. The same figures are recorded in *The Life and Works of Matthew Baillie*. Franco Crainz. PelitiAssociati.

14. MS 41736/10. Willis Papers. British Library.

15. References are to John Willis' letters are in uncatalogued papers held in date order by Cumbria Archives under DLONS/L1/2/33.13/6/13.

Chapter Twenty-One: They never met

1. *Medical Cautions: Chiefly for the consideration of invalids.* Dr James Makittrick Adair. 1789. and Sir Alexander Halliday. *A General View of the Present State of Lunatics and Lunatic Asylums in GB and Ireland.* London 1827.
2. *Quacks and Quackery* by a medical practitioner. Wellcome Library.
3. *Quacks, Fakers and Charlatans in Medicine.* Roy Porter. Page 102.
4. *The Journal and Correspondence of William, Lord Auckland.* R J Eden 1861. Quoted in *George III and the Mad-Business* on page 52.
5. Presidential Address. Journal of Mental Science, Volume 14, 1868.
6. See the introductory note of *Remarks On Baths, Water, Swimming, Shampooing etc* by M L Este.
7. *Treatise on Cold and Hot Baths with Directions for their Application in Various Diseases.* W. Turton MD. Published in 1803 in a private edition. British Library.
8. John W. Williams, *Essay on Sea Bathing* 1820 and William Laing writing about Peterhead Spa in 1804.
9. *An Essay on Warm Cold and Vapour Bathing.* Sir Arthur Clarke. 1827. Page 86.
10. *Description of the Retreat near York.* Samuel Tuke. 1813.
11. Thomas Bakewell. *Letter to the Chairman of the House of Commons Select Committee on Madhouses.* Wellcome Library.
12. *Non-restraint and Robert Gardiner-Hill.* Frank. *Bulletin of the History Medicine.* Vol 41. [1967] page 144. Johns Hopkins.
13. *Memoranda regarding the Royal Lunatic Asylum, Infirmary and Dispensary of Montrose with observations on some other institutions of a like nature and an appendix of documents partly relating to Restraint in the treatment of insanity.* Dr Richard Poole 1841. Page 48.
14. *A Lecture on the management of Lunatic Asylums and the Treatment of the Insane.* Robert Gardiner Hill. Published 1839.
15. *A concise history of the entire abolition of mechanical restraint.* Page 59. Robert Gardiner Hill. The italics are Hill's.
16. References for Harper and Arnold are: *A Treatise on the real cause and cure of Insanity, etc* London 1789 and *Observations on the nature, kinds, causes and prevention of insanity.* Thomas Arnold MD. 1806.
17. See *Psychiatry: a very short history.* Tom Burns.
18. See *Inconvenient People* by Sarah Wise. Chapter two.
19. *Modern Practice of Physic.* Dr Robert Thomas. 1824 edition for example – page 189.
20. Minutes of Vestry of Ewell Church. 3831/1/1 1770 to 1830. Surrey History Centre.

Afterword: The diagnosis of George III's Insanity

1. See page 150 of *George III and the Mad-Business*.
2. *Report from the Committee appointed to examine the physicians who have attended His Majesty during His illness etc. Ordered to be printed 13th January 1789.* Page 105. Note the report is reprinted in various formats and the pagination varies. Available in the British Library.
3. *The Insanity of King George III.* Dr Isaac Ray. This paper was read before the Association of Superintendents of Insane Hospitals in the United States on 22 May 1855. It was based on accounts written in the UK by commentators such as Sir Nathanial William Wraxall.
4. Ibid.
5. Ibid. Page 4.
6. *Medicine in England during the reign of George III.* Arnold Chaplin.
7. *America's Last King.* Manfred Guttmacher.
8. Ibid. Page 190. The full comment by Guttmacher was, 'The probability is that, abetted by false interpretations of those about him, he was trying to delude himself into viewing

his illness as primarily physical'. It would be helpful if Guttmacher had said more about the 'false impressions' apparently being fed to the king. It is not obvious who might have been the source of such 'impressions'. See also page 10 *Porphyria – a Royal Malady*. This is a reprint of Macalpine and Hunter's *The Insanity of King George III: A Classic Case of Porphyria*.

9. *George III*. John Brooke. Quoted on page 370.
10. *King George III and the Politicians*. Richard Pares.
11. *The Royal Malady Again*. Chapter 9 in *George IV*. E. A. Smith. 1999.
12. *The Royal Malady*. Charles Chenevix Trench. 1964.
13. *The insanity of George III: A Classic Case of Porphyria*. British Medical Journal, 8 January 1966. Pages 66–71.
14. Pages 140 and 141 of *George III and the Mad Business* have representative examples of George III's writing from 1789 and 1809.
15. *King George III, bipolar disorder, porphyria and lessons for historians*. Timothy Peters. *Clinical Medicine* 2011, Vol 11, No 3: page 262.
16. *Medicine during the reign of George III*. Arnold Chaplin 1927.
17. See *George III's illness and its Impact on Psychiatry* page 1025. *Proc. Roy. Soc. Med.* Volume 61, October 1968.
18. The events in Yekaterinburg and examination of the remains were widely covered in the general media and the specialist press. Accounts are available on the internet and in print.
19. An example of the view that Edward, Duke of Kent was the source for porphyria passing into the royal houses of Europe can be found in *Royal Maladies: Inherited Diseases in the Ruling Houses of Europe* by Alan Rushton.
20. *The Lancet*. 2005 Issue 9482. July 23–29. Vol. 366. Pages 332–335.

Index